Dementia Nursi

A *Guide to Practic*

Dementia Nursing
A Guide to Practice

Edited by Rosalie Hudson

Foreword by Pauline Ford

Radcliffe Medical Press

Radcliffe Medical Press Ltd
18 Marcham Road
Abingdon
Oxon OX14 1AA
United Kingdom

www.radcliffe-oxford.com
The Radcliffe Medical Press electronic catalogue and online ordering facility.
Direct sales to anywhere in the world

This book was originally published in Melbourne, Australia by Ausmed Publications Pty Ltd

British Library Cataloguing in Publication Data

A catalogue record for this book is available from the British Library

ISBN 1 85775 899 4

Typeset by Egan-Reid Ltd, Auckland, New Zealand
Printed and bound by T J International Ltd, Padstow, Cornwall, UK

Contents

Acknowledgements

Radcliffe Medical Press would like to acknowledge the advice and help of several individuals in the preparation of this edition of the book. These include Professor Mary Marshall and her colleagues at Stirling University, who wrote several chapters, and Pauline Ford, Gerontological Nursing Adviser at the Royal College of Nursing, who wrote the Foreword for this edition. Our special thanks are extended to Barry Aveyard, School of Nursing and Midwifery, University of Sheffield, who reviewed the entire text and made some amendments to reflect the NHS and UK practice.

Foreword

This book is a tribute to expert nursing. It should be seen as a celebration of all that is good in nursing. It also sets out the path for nursing that is centred on relationships—the essence of person-centred nursing is based on the quality of relationships both between the nurse, the client and their significant others, and also between nurses and their colleagues and peers. I believe that to practise nursing in a person-centred way is only possible if the nurse holds a value system that demonstrates a level of relating which truly values the 'other' in that relationship. This requires an approach that focuses on the human aspects of nursing. This book achieves that and as such is a cause for celebration.

Increasingly, it is a challenge for nurses to hold on to humanistic care when we practice in a world of healthcare which is performance and fiscally driven.

Nursing deals with the here and now of personal experience and demands exceptional intuitive skills and compassion. Rather than focusing on the cost benefits (although these are considerable) nursing a person with dementia is a moral endeavour where everyone is considered to be of equal worth.

The concept of partnership and reciprocity runs through the book like a golden thread, gleaming in a rich tapestry of person-centred practice expressed via the perspectives of the contributors. Expert practitioners working with people who have dementia, have led the way in the development of person-centred practice.

As a student nurse in the 1970s, one of the few placements that I really enjoyed was the mental health placement. Here I experienced first hand the needs of people with dementia. My placement was positive because I was allowed to be me, and so were all the patients. I didn't realise at the time that I was working in a very forward thinking unit which strove to deliver what I now understand as person-centred nursing. As a student nurse I found myself valued as an individual for the first time in my training, I experienced person-centred care from the qualified members of staff, and as a consequence felt valued for what I could contribute. This memory of a tremendous sense of well being has stayed with me, as has my admiration for those nurses who provided me with my very first experience of truly expert person-centred nursing..

The challenge of course is how to teach such an approach. Nurses who work with older people who have dementia, have had to fight for recognition of their skills and what they can offer to the lives and health of their patients. These nurses have had to be open to the realities and challenges of practice, flexible and responsive to needs and creative in finding new ways of working to develop practice and services within which they work. Nurses working with older people, particularly those older people who have dementia, have consistently challenged the prevailing value system. As a result there is a strong nursing contribution to the greater understanding of the needs of older people.

Pauline Ford
Advisor in Gerontological Nursing
Royal College of Nursing
October 2003

Preface

Dementia Nursing: A Guide to Practice is written primarily for nurses who have twenty-four hour responsibility for the care of people with dementia in the context of residential aged care. The book will also be valuable for doctors, allied health professionals, personal-care workers, volunteers, families, and carers of people with dementia in a variety of settings. It will empower them all with practical strategies for clinical management and will encourage reflective care in which they enter into the experience of the person with dementia. Dementia nursing depends on partnerships with a variety of people. The book therefore provides knowledge and encouragement for all members of a team of care who support and accompany the person with dementia.

Drawing on current research and international expertise, this book challenges nurses throughout the world to respond with the latest knowledge and the best clinical practice in dementia care. Everyday clinical issues are described, and guidance is provided on practical management issues that are so important to the total well-being of the person with dementia—especially when dementia is compounded by physical frailty and other problems. Nurses are encouraged to go beyond the technical aspects of nursing practice to hear the deeply human needs of the people in their care. The purpose of the book is not only to identify physical problems and clinical needs, but also to capture the lived experience of those with dementia, and to encourage all carers to respond with creativity and imagination.

Throughout the book the reader is invited to enter the whole story of dementia, to trace its history, and to identify current trends in research and management. Personal accounts are interwoven with practical guidelines for nursing care. The importance of environmental ambience is highlighted, together with the value of skilled nursing interventions. Matters of wholeness and relationships that emphasise the *person* with dementia are fundamental to excellence in dementia nursing. When the person is treated as whole, matters of clinical importance are *integrated* with matters of leisure and lifestyle. Throughout this book nurses are called upon to engage creatively with residents during all aspects of care.

Dementia nursing is a highly skilled and important speciality. In facing the challenges of dementia nursing, nurses will find in this book the necessary practical guidance for excellent care, as well as renewed impetus towards those deeply personal elements that profoundly influence each episode of care. Nurses are encouraged to put these guidelines into practice and to experience the rich rewards that come from dementia nursing.

Rosalie Hudson

About the Authors

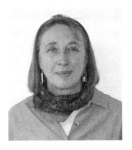

Carole Archibald
Chapter 10

Dr Carole Archibald has had a wide range of nursing experience in general hospitals including gynaecology, theatre, care of the elderly, and orthopaedics. Carole has worked in the field of dementia since the late 1980s, and is a senior fieldworker at the Dementia Services Development Centre at Stirling University (Scotland) where she is involved in consultancy, training, and research. Her consultancy work has included work in the acute sector facilitating multi-disciplinary focus groups and interviewing key members of staff in acute hospitals in Edinburgh (Scotland). Carole has also interviewed family carers and has held day workshops for staff on issues affecting people with dementia in acute settings. Carole's other areas of interest include activities and respite care for people with dementia, specialist dementia units, and sexuality in people with dementia. She has published widely in many of these subject areas.

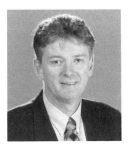

David Arthur
Chapters 7 and 15

Before moving to Hong Kong, David Arthur worked in Australia for 17 years in the fields of mental-health nursing and nursing education. He is now professor in the Department of Nursing and Health Sciences at Hong Kong Polytechnic University and a visiting professor in the School of Nursing at the Peking Union Medical College, Beijing. David serves on the editorial boards of a number of international nursing journals and is convenor of the East Asian Forum of Nursing Scholars. He has co-authored a text on mental-health nursing and has published numerous journal papers on different aspects of nursing theory and research. David's research interests include nurse-initiated early intervention in alcohol problems, expressed emotion in the families of Chinese people with schizophrenia, postnatal depression in Chinese women, the professional self-concept of nurses, and the cultural aspects of caring and communication in nursing. David is currently a member of a research team that is examining the caring attributes of nurses involved in the care of the elderly in Hong Kong, Scotland, and the United Kingdom.

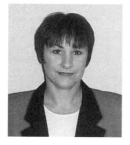

Jill Beattie
Chapter 11

Jill Beattie is a registered nurse and midwife with postgraduate qualifications in nursing and education whose doctoral research at La Trobe University (Melbourne, Australia) has been on the subject of medication management in residential aged care. Jill represents the Royal College of Nursing, Australia on a number of committees concerned with the role of nurses in medication management. She has presented at several conferences and has conducted continuing education in a number of organisations on issues related to the quality use of medicines. Jill also works as a consultant in her own business focusing on enhancing performance with individuals and within organisations. She has an interest in enhancing people's ability to work harmoniously together in pursuit of common goals.

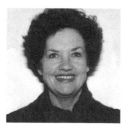

Sally Bowen
Chapters 21 and 22

Sally Bowen comes from a teaching background and holds a degree in social sciences and postgraduate qualifications in aged care. She began working in aged care in 1994 as an activity director, and has become committed to the implementation of various activities and programs as part of her holistic understanding of dementia care. Sally has developed a particular interest in validation therapy, and this has enhanced her communication with people with dementia and her skills in providing leisure opportunities for older people in general. Sally is committed to a team-oriented approach in which the skills of nurses are combined with the skills of teachers and other activity leaders in many areas, including massage, outings, music, story-telling (and listening), floral arranging, and so on.

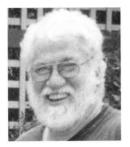

Graeme Cameron
Chapter 22

Graeme Cameron is a sculptor, but before his retirement from active professional life he was an architect, health-care design consultant, and project manager. During his professional career Graeme was responsible for the detailed functional briefing and planning of many health-care facilities, including the relocation and amalgamation of major teaching hospitals, community housing for the intellectually disabled, community health centres, facilities for the aged, and psychiatric care accommodation. Graeme's interest in working with his hands began at an early age, and he created his first piece of sculpture at around the age of fourteen. After his retirement, Graeme met the sculptor Kevin Free who taught him the essentials of his craft, working mostly with limestone. Graeme's works range in size from 100 mm to 2 metres high, with most of his work coming from commissions and limited exhibitions. The work varies from the abstract and angular to more rounded and recognisable forms based on the human figure. Working with dementia sufferers is a relatively new and rewarding experience which began when Graeme started working with Sally Bowen at the Lynden Aged Care Centre (Melbourne, Australia). In a sense he has gone full circle from building health facilities to now working in them.

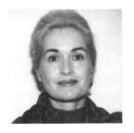

Lynn Chenoweth
Chapter 14

Dr Lynn Chenoweth began working as a clinical nurse in 1966 and has worked as a nurse manager, educator, and researcher. In her doctoral studies Lynn evaluated outcome standards in aged care and the effect of these standards on the lives of older residents in nursing homes. Since then she has taught and conducted research in the areas of dementia management, improving care practices, and health outcomes for older people in a range of care settings. Lynn is currently the director of the Health and Ageing Research Unit, South-Eastern Sydney Area Health Service, and is professor of Aged and Extended Care Nursing at the University of Technology, Sydney (Australia).

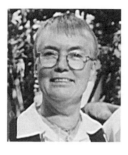

Jane Crisp
Chapter 9

Jane Crisp retired recently as a senior lecturer in the School of Film, Media and Cultural Studies at Griffith University, Brisbane (Australia), where she now holds an honorary adjunct position. Jane's doctorate in English literature was obtained from the Australian National University, and she has taught and published in the fields of nineteenth-century fiction, film and media, cultural studies, and communication studies. More recently, Jane has applied ideas from her professional work to communicating with people who have dementia—inspired by her experiences with her mother. She has spent time in New Zealand, Australia, Britain, and France meeting fellow researchers and professional carers and visiting specialised care units. Jane has presented papers at international conferences and talked to many carer groups. She has published extensively in both English and French. Jane's book, *Keeping in Touch with Someone Who Has Alzheimer's* was published by Ausmed Publications (see page 336).

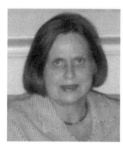

Barbara Davison
Chapter 22

Barbara Davison is an occupational therapist who has worked extensively in community and residential settings with older people, including those with dementia. After teaching at the School of Occupational Therapy at the Lincoln Institute of Health Sciences (Melbourne, Australia) from 1980 to 1987, Barbara returned to clinical work with the Extended Care Unit at Caulfield Hospital (Melbourne, Australia) from 1987 to 1988. From 1989 she worked as a research fellow at the Lincoln Gerontology Centre at La Trobe University (Melbourne, Australia) where she conducted qualitative research that included a study examining best-practice issues for people with dementia in adult day care. Barbara contributed to *Better Care for People with Alzheimer's: A Practice Manual for Day Centres*. From 1996 to 1997 she was project officer for the Ministerial Task Force on Services for People with Dementia in Victoria (Australia) and contributed to the major reports published by the task force. Since her retirement, Barbara has cared for aged relatives and indulged her long-term interest in painting. Her involvement with people with dementia in the Sefton Day Club Art Project has brought together her two major interests.

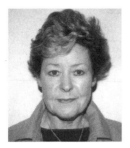

Sandy Forster
Chapter 22

Sandy Forster is a former secondary schoolteacher who, in 1992, was appointed as reminiscence historian at the Kingston Centre—a large aged-care facility centre in suburban Melbourne (Australia). In this role, Sandy coordinated a reminiscence program with assistance from care staff, pastoral-care volunteers, local secondary school students, and family members and friends of residents at the centre. In 1997 Sandy presented a paper of her work at the 'Widening Horizons in Dementia Care Conference' in London. Age Exchange Theatre Trust published her paper the following year in a book entitled *Reminiscence in Dementia Care*. When funding for her program ceased in 1998, Sandy set up 'Memories Revisited', a consultancy service that promotes the use of reminiscence and life-review therapies. Sandy continues to record the life stories of older people—either as a therapy or as a legacy for future generations. She has a special interest in working with people with dementia.

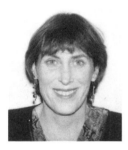

Julia Fountain
Chapter 2

Julia Fountain is the regional program manager for Asia for Australian Volunteers International. Julia's interest in dementia care was triggered by her mother's need for care in the last twelve months of her life, and Julia made it her business to learn as much as she could about dementia nursing from the perspective of an intelligent, concerned, and committed relative. During this difficult time, Julia studied the legislation governing nursing homes and acquainted herself with all the 'ins and outs' of dementia and the care of aged people. Julia acted as her mother's advocate and closely observed the care that her mother received. She was prepared to praise what she perceived to be 'good' care, but she also observed much that concerned her. Written by a concerned and informed relative, this chapter will help nurses to be aware of how their dementia care affects family members, both negatively and positively. Nurses and relatives alike will learn much from the observations contained in this chapter.

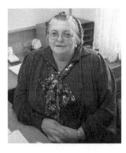

Sally Garratt
Chapter 1
Professor Sally Garratt has has been involved in aged care for more than thirty years, and has held senior positions in the field as both an academic and a practitioner. Sally has co-written three previous books and has published numerous papers on various aspects of aged-care nursing. Her research has concentrated on dementia nursing, with special emphasis on the effect of the environment on nursing practice, including the ethics of restraint. Sally has conducted numerous workshops and seminars on many aspects of aged care, and has been widely sought for consultant advice in Australia and internationally. Sally manages the clinical nursing school at the Caulfield General Medical Centre in conjunction with La Trobe University (both Melbourne, Australia). Her work involves responsibility for graduate and undergraduate educational programs for nursing staff, and the undertaking of clinical care projects and research.

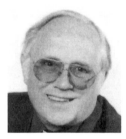

Malcolm Goldsmith
Chapter 19
Malcolm Goldsmith was, until his retirement through ill-health, the rector of St Cuthbert's Episcopal Church in Colinton, Edinburgh (Scotland). During the past ten years or so Malcolm has developed a particular interest in dementia. This has involved his spending two years as a research fellow within the Dementia Services Development Centre at the University of Stirling (Scotland), writing *Hearing the Voice of People with Dementia*, and preparing various training aids on the subject. Malcolm has also contributed to various books and journals on matters relating to dementia and communication, ethics, and spirituality. In his day-to-day work as a parish priest, Malcolm ministered to people with dementia and their families in their homes and in specialised settings. He is engaged in further writing on the subject in retirement.

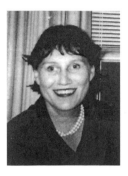

Julie Goyder
Chapter 20
Julie Goyder has worked as an enrolled nurse in several nursing homes, a hostel for the multi-handicapped, and a respite centre for people with disabilities. Her PhD thesis, later published in book form in 2001 under the title *We'll be Married in Fremantle* focused on the people she was still nursing while undertaking work on her doctorate. Julie holds degrees in English and Aboriginal and intercultural studies, and a graduate diploma in creative writing. She is currently a lecturer in creative writing at Edith Cowan University (Bunbury, Western Australia).

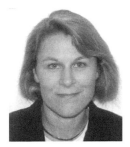

Jane Hecker
Chapter 5

Dr Jane Hecker is a senior consultant physician in geriatrics and general internal medicine at Repatriation General Hospital and Flinders Medical Centre, Adelaide (South Australia) where she has established a memory disorders studies unit. Jane is a lecturer at Flinders University with involvement in teaching at both the undergraduate and postgraduate levels, and has clinical and research interests in the assessment and management of memory disorders, Alzheimer's disease, and other dementias, with more specialised interests in dementia and driving, and dementia and the role of the caregiver. Jane has been the principal investigator in several clinical trials of treatment in Alzheimer's disease, and has published extensively in the academic medical literature and in textbooks. She is on the board of the Rosemary Foundation of the South Australian Alzheimer's Association, the executive committee of the Australasian Consortium of Centres for Clinical Cognitive Research, and the Federal Council of the Australian Society for Geriatric Medicine.

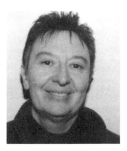

Heather Hill
Chapter 22

Heather Hill has worked as a dance therapist with people with dementia since the mid 1980s. A holder of degrees in arts and education, and postgraduate qualifications in dance and movement, Heather has also pursued doctoral studies on person-centred care at La Trobe University (Melbourne, Australia). She was commissioned by the University of Stirling to write a book on dance and dementia, and this book, *Invitation to the Dance*, was published in 2001. By engaging people through dance and the whole domain of the non-verbal, she works to affirm the individual and offer opportunities for expression, communication, and positive interaction with others.

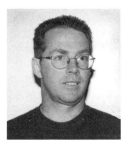

Keith Hill
Chapter 13

Keith Hill is a physiotherapist with more than 20 years of experience in rehabilitation and aged care. Keith's PhD thesis was entitled 'Balance studies in older people', and he has published numerous papers in this area. Keith is a senior research fellow at the National Ageing Research Institute and co-director of the falls and balance clinic at the Melbourne Extended Care and Rehabilitation Service (Victoria, Australia). He was recently project manager for a falls-prevention project in seven residential aged-care facilities, as a result of which falls were reduced by half.

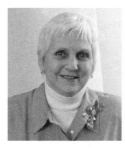

Rosalie Hudson
Chapters 18 and 22

Dr Rosalie Hudson's varied nursing and theological career is now focused on aged care and palliative care. As an aged-care consultant she explores end-of-life issues for people in residential aged care, and as an author, teacher, and associate professor with the University of Melbourne (Australia) she seeks to raise the profile of gerontic nursing. Rosalie has presented and published numerous papers and articles internationally on the subjects of spirituality, palliative care, dementia, pastoral care, and ethics at the end of life. She has co-authored two books on death and dying, and has contributed chapters to several other Ausmed publications. Rosalie has had 12 years' experience as a director of nursing of a 50-bed nursing home and, more recently, has served as the Victorian project officer for the Australian Palliative Aged Care Project. She enjoys family life with her husband, adult children, and grandchildren.

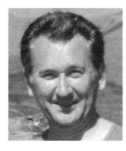

Graham A. Jackson
Chapter 16

Dr Graham A. Jackson is a consultant psychiatrist in Glasgow (Scotland). He is also an honorary lecturer at the Dementia Services Development Centre at Stirling University and is co-author, with Dr Alan Jacques of the book *Understanding Dementia*. Graham has been involved in research into behaviour problems in dementia and has published numerous papers on the subject. Before training in psychiatry, Graham was a general medical practitioner.

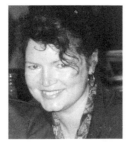

Kirsten James
Chapter 22

Kirsten James is a registered and practising nurse manager with tertiary qualifications in massage and relaxation techniques, health and healing in other cultures, and adult education. In 1995 she established her consultancy 'Complementary Care Resources' to facilitate the safe and professional introduction of complementary therapies into a variety of health-care settings. Kirsten frequently presents to various organisations and community support groups and has contributed to Australian and American nursing textbooks and journals on a range of topics on the subject of complementary therapies. Kirsten has also been a lecturer in complementary therapies at RMIT University and Victoria University of Technology (both Melbourne, Australia). Kirsten is now unit manager of the residential aged-care dementia unit at Mt Alexander Hospital, Castlemaine (Victoria, Australia), where a variety of complementary therapies are incorporated into daily care.

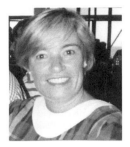

Susie Kerr
Chapter 14

Susie Kerr is a registered nurse with experience in general nursing, paediatric intensive care, and operating theatres, and more recently as a clinical nurse consultant in pain management. She completed a postgraduate diploma in pain management at the University of Sydney (Australia) in 1998. Susie teaches and and conducts research within a multidisciplinary team in her role as clinical nurse manager in the Department of Pain Management, Prince of Wales Hospital, Sydney (Australia). She is a member of the International Association for the Study of Pain, the Australian Pain Society, the Pain Interest Group of New South Wales, the Special Interest Group Pain in Childhood, the Australian Pain Relief Association and the Australian Clinical Nurse Consultant Association.

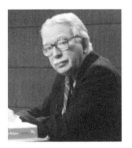

Melvin A. Kimble
Chapter 3

Melvin A. Kimble PhD has been professor of pastoral care at Luther Seminary, Minnesota (USA), since 1965. In 1993, he established the Center for Aging, Religion and Spirituality and has served as director since its inception. In 1999, he was elected professor emeritus of pastoral care and remains on the faculty as distinguished senior lecturer. Melvin was a contributing author to *Handbook on Humanities in Aging* (1999) and *Aging and the Meaning of Time* (2001), editor of *Viktor Frankl's Contribution to Spirituality and Aging* (2001), and senior editor of *Aging, Spirituality, and Religion: A Handbook* (1995, 2003). He has been the recipient of a number of prestigious awards from the American Society on Aging and National Council on Aging (USA). Melvin also received the American College and Health Care Administrators Research Award in 1986.

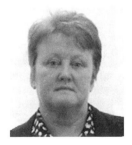

Mary King
Chapter 12

Mary King has been involved with continence management in nursing since 1987. In 1988 she was awarded a nursing fellowship from Royal Perth Hospital (Western Australia) to investigate continence facilities in Australia. Mary completed a course in continence with the Royal District Nursing and later established a nursing continence service at the Royal Perth Hospital. In 1992 Mary established a community-based family continence service with Silver Chain Nursing Service. Her current position is clinical nurse consultant in continence and urology at Royal Perth Hospital—a position that involves a multidisciplinary partnership in the aged-care and urology departments.

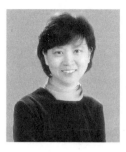

Claudia Lai
Chapters 7 and 15

Claudia Lai is an assistant professor in the School of Nursing at Hong Kong Polytechnic University. She is a clinical specialist in gerontological nursing and has a special interest in dementia care. Claudia's research interests include issues in long-term care including restraint reduction, wandering behaviour of people with dementia, interventions in improving the psychosocial well-being of people with dementia, and the use of information technology in care. In addition to teaching nurses and caring for older people, Claudia volunteers her time with the Hong Kong Alzheimer's Disease and Brain Failure Association.

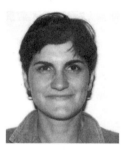

Dina LoGiudice
Chapter 13

Dr Dina LoGiudice is a consultant physician in geriatric medicine, a senior associate at the National Ageing Research Institute (Melbourne, Australia), and coordinator of the Cognitive Dementia and Memory Service at the Melbourne Extended Care and Rehabilitation Service. Her PhD thesis was entitled 'The Assessment of Services for Elderly People with Dementia'. Dina's main interests lie in assessment and management of older people with dementia and their carers, in particular those of non English-speaking background.

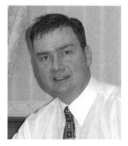

Colin MacDonald
Chapter 16

Colin MacDonald is a registered general and mental-health nurse. He is the charge nurse of a 30-bed long-stay hospital ward for people with dementia who have challenging behaviour. The ward is situated in Bonnybridge Hospital (Scotland)—a small community hospital for older people. Colin also works on a part-time basis with the Dementia Services Development Centre (DSDC) at Stirling University (Scotland) as an associate trainer in delivering training sessions on dementia and challenging behaviour. In 1997 Colin completed a research pilot study questioning the use of antipsychotic drugs in the care and treatment of people with dementia, and this led to the publication of 'Who's in Control?' (MacDonald & Teven 1997, DSDC, Stirling University).

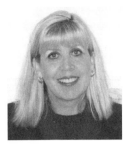

Dawn MacKenzie
Chapter 23

Dawn MacKenzie is a registered nurse and midwife with qualifications in occupational health and safety and dementia care and services. Dawn is a company director of Aged Care Service Group Pty Ltd, a private organisation which she started 15 years ago with her husband, Peter. The organisation now has responsibility for the care of more than 350 aged-care residents. Dawn has served as a consultant to Box Hill Institute of TAFE (Victoria, Australia) in curriculum development of personal-care courses, and has a long involvement with government and non-government bodies responsible for standards of care in nursing homes and private hospitals. Dawn is an Eden Alternative associate and is enthusiastic about the Eden Alternative described in this chapter.

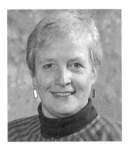

Mary Marshall
Chapter 6

Professor Mary Marshall is the director of the Dementia Services Development Centre at the University of Stirling (Scotland). The centre, which began in 1989, extends and improves services for people with dementia by providing information, consultancy, training, research, conferences, and publications for staff and volunteers in all aspects of dementia care. Mary has worked with older people as a social worker, researcher, teacher, and manager for more than thirty years. She is the author of several books on working with older people and people with dementia. In the field of dementia care, Mary's special interests are design, technology, and food.

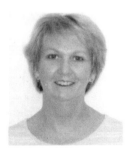

Virginia Moore
Chapter 2

Virginia Moore is an occupational therapist who has worked for more than twelve years with the Brightwater Care Group (Western Australia) which provides services to people with disabilities in residential-care facilities and in their homes. Virginia is the dementia services consultant and manager of specialist support services. In this role she provides expert consulting and support to a range of people, including those providing dementia care. Virginia has had extensive experience in the aged-care area including acute care, rehabilitation, and long-term care. She also spent several years as clinical coordinator and lecturer with Curtin University School of Occupational Therapy (Western Australia). In 1998 Virginia was the recipient of a Churchill Fellowship to travel to the UK and Scandinavia. Her area of special interest was an evaluation tool known as 'Dementia Care Mapping', the subject of this chapter.

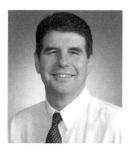

Richard Osborn
Chapter 8

Richard Osborn is an audiologist and educator working in private practice. Over the past thirteen years, his clinical practice has focused on addressing the hearing and general communication needs of older people. In this time he has been especially involved in the development of a range of rehabilitation services for people who experience dual sensory (vision and hearing) loss. The designing and delivery of specialised training programs for service providers working in the aged-care field has been an important component of this role. Richard is a frequent presenter at conferences and seminars, and has published more than twenty articles in professional journals.

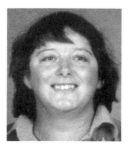

Sue Piccoli
Chapter 22

Sue Piccoli is a diversional therapist who holds a diploma in community services (aged care). Sue has worked in dementia care since the mid 1980s—initially at Carunya, a dementia day-care centre in Warilla, and then with the Illawarra Dementia Support Team (both New South Wales, Australia). She has been interested in social-management strategies to manage challenging behaviours in nursing homes, hostels, and the community. In recent years Sue has become especially interested in using dolls as therapy to settle agitation in people with a moderate to severe dementia. She is currently employed as dementia respite coordinator with Shellharbour City Council (New South Wales, Australia).

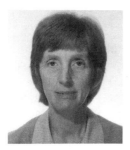

Carole Quinn
Chapter 22

Carole Quinn is an occupational therapist who holds a degree in applied science (occupational therapy) and postgraduate qualifications in dementia care and service. She is an aged-care quality assessor and has worked in residential aged care since the mid 1980s. Carole currently works as therapy recreation coordinator and quality manager of Andrina Private Nursing Home—a 60-bed dementia high-care facility in Brighton (Victoria, Australia).

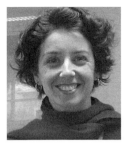

Wendy-Mae Rapson
Chapter 8

Wendy-Mae Rapson is a speech pathologist and educator who works in private practice in aged care. She has been employed as an ageing and sensory loss specialist by Baptist Community Care and the Royal Freemasons' Homes of Victoria (Australia), and has wide experience working and consulting in dementia units—with special emphasis on assessing residents' sensory needs, staff practices, and environmental modifications to improve communicative competence. Wendy-Mae has presented numerous conference papers on ageing and sensory loss, and is involved in communication training programs for staff and caregivers in Australia and internationally.

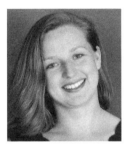

Tanya Ryszczak
Chapter 22

Tanya Ryszczak is a registered music therapist with a degree in music and postgraduate qualifications in psychology. She is currently working as a consultant music therapist in Melbourne (Australia) where she provides group music therapy for people with depression and dementia. She also works as a sessional lecturer in music therapy, educating students on topics of music therapy in aged care. Tanya's work with people with dementia has focused on music therapy interventions in conjunction with multidisciplinary teams. Her particular interest is in reducing depresion through specific music therapy programs that focus on communication. Tanya lectures and frequently presents conference papers on these topics.

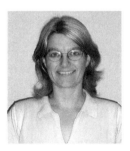

Robyn Smith
Chapter 13

Robyn Smith is an occupational therapist specialising in aged care and rehabilitation, and is a researcher with an interest in health services and health promotion. She is director of the public health division of of the National Ageing Research Institute (Melbourne, Australia) and has had a lead role in many research projects, with a focus on fostering sustainable change in community and residential aged-care environments. Robyn has a particular interest in falls prevention, and in strengthening staff capacity to apply current research evidence in everyday practice.

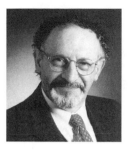

Geoff Sussman
Chapter 17

Geoff Sussman is a senior lecturer and director of wound education and research in the Department of Pharmacy Practice, Monash University (Victoria, Australia), an associate of the National Ageing Research Institute, and director of the Wound Foundation of Australia. Geoff has been involved in wound management for more than 25 years, has undertaken clinical research, product evaluation, and clinical practice, and has written many articles on the topic. He has trained in several major centres for wound management including the wound-healing research unit in Cardiff and the Nordic wound school in Copenhagen. Geoff is the co-author of a textbook on wound care published in the USA and has written several other book chapters. Geoff is a member of the editorial board of the *Australian Wound Management Journal*.

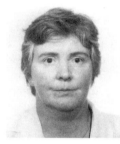

Margaret Winbolt
Chapter 13

Margaret Winbolt is a nurse with 20 years of experience in the care of older people and is currently a clinical nurse consultant in gerontic nursing at Bundoora Extended Care Centre (Melbourne, Australia). In this role, Margaret has been involved in the development and implementation of a falls-prevention and injury-minimisation program at the centre. Margaret has a keen interest and expertise in the care of older people with dementia and was previously a nurse unit manager of a dementia unit specialising in the management of challenging behaviours.

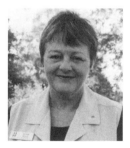

Kim Wylie
Chapter 4

Dr Kim Wylie is a general and mental health nurse with extensive experience in the care of older people. Kim holds a bachelor's degree in health sciences and a master's degree in nursing, the latter involving a phenomenological study of the lived experience of busy-ness for aged-care nurses. Kim also holds diplomas in community health and gerontology. In 1993, she was awarded a Churchill Fellowship and spent three months studying innovative practice in dementia care internationally. In 1997 and 1998, she returned to the United Kingdom to undertake training in dementia care mapping with the Bradford Dementia Group, and in 2001 she presented the keynote address at the Alzheimer Society Conference of Washington (USA). Kim's PhD involved a critical evaluation of the outcomes of enriched sensory environments for people with dementia, and the material presented in this chapter is largely taken from that thesis (Wylie 2000). Kim is currently employed as the senior nurse educator at Calvary Retirement Community, Cessnock (New South Wales, Australia).

Introduction

Rosalie Hudson

Dementia has been described as 'the disease of our time'—one of the greatest challenges for medicine, nursing, and society in the twenty-first century. It is estimated that about 5% of people over the age of 65 and 20% of people over 80 have some form of dementia. Nearly half of the people with moderate to severe dementia in Australia live in residential care and require 24-hour attention. No definite cause of dementia has yet been identified; nor is there a cure.

In the face of these demographic factors, dementia nursing has important roles to play in addressing urgent present-day issues and in planning for the future. It is also evident that more research is needed to guide nurses—if dementia care is to be based on the best available evidence.

Dementia nursing goes to the heart of what it means to care for a person holistically. Because there is no direct access to the inner subjective world of a person with dementia, and because such people are often unable to articulate their needs, nurses are challenged to use their intuitive skills in addition to their clinical skills and knowledge. In the spirit of true advocacy, nurses are often called upon to be the 'voice' of residents. By developing a relationship and 'tuning in' to a person, a sensitive and well-informed nurse might well be able to 'hear' what that person is experiencing and feeling. Entering the unique story of a person with dementia in the context of his or her family, the nurse creates a trusting environment for the continuation of that story. This does not mean the choosing of esoteric 'soft' options of care to the exclusion of soundly based therapeutic treatments; the whole repertoire of holistic care is needed. Far from being remote and idealistic, relational care actually grounds dementia nursing—for it deals with the here and now of personal experience.

Dementia nursing is thus founded on well-practised assessment skills and the choice of skilled interventions for all of a person's physical needs—based on the best available evidence and an ability to evaluate the outcome.

Nurses are also challenged to evaluate their interventions in the spiritual, psychological, social, and emotional realms, and to observe and describe the effect that their care has on the total well-being of a person with dementia. The aim of dementia nursing is not to cure or change a person, nor to modify or manage particular behaviour merely to suit other peoples' expectations. The aim of dementia nursing is to acknowledge the significant challenges, fears, and insecurities that surround this mysterious malady, and to move beyond the dilemmas to a true meeting of persons in relation.

There is no 'one size fits all' remedy in dementia care. Nurses are encouraged to try various options, to try again when a genuine effort does not bring the desired response, to support one another, to acknowledge the place of humour, and to be prepared for surprises. As many carers testify, an unexpected response from a person with dementia can dispel myths and shatter illusions—thus calling into question some of the misperceptions of that person's cognitive abilities. A skilled dementia nurse is alert for the cues that indicate the capacities that have been retained, rather than those that appear to have been 'lost'. In this two-way process, a person with dementia might well become the nurse's teacher.

Dementia nursing is always aware of the role of the family. Throughout this book, the importance of family involvement is emphasised in formulating plans of care that are addressed to the specific needs of each person with dementia. Many family members have cared for their relatives for months or years, with all the joys and frustrations that accompany such a 24-hour role. When a person with dementia is transferred to residential care it is essential that opportunities be provided for family involvement in all aspects of the resident's ongoing needs. Careful assessment of the family's needs is integral to the care of a person with dementia, especially when family circumstances change (for example, the death or increasing frailty of a spouse or other significant carer). Dementia nursing is a dynamic partnership involving many relationships, and these relationships provide nurses with numerous opportunities to achieve the highest quality of care for each resident, in the context of his or her unique social environment. The role of the family is thus crucial to good dementia nursing, and is to be encouraged and nurtured at all times.

In the ordering of chapters in this book, no hierarchy is intended in terms of priorities for care. However, the book does have a logical progression—beginning with an outline of the history of dementia care. This first chapter raises significant issues for contemporary nursing practice, and thus informs the discussion in the chapters that follow. The second chapter is written from a relative's perspective—relating one person's experience of the rocky road that leads to residential care and the various responses that follow. As noted above, an important aspect of understanding the effects of dementia nursing is to hear from relatives. The book thus reflects the importance of the relatives' perspective by emphasising, in an early chapter, how such insights offer a significant guide for all aspects of dementia nursing practice as detailed in subsequent chapters. The third chapter follows with an emphasis on the importance of the 'whole person'—again providing an overview that has applications in all subsequent chapters.

In these subsequent chapters, important clinical issues such as memory loss, nutrition, wandering, sensory loss, restraint, the quality use of medicines, incontinence, falls prevention, pain management, depression, aggression, wound care, and many others are covered. Communication skills are explored, together with matters of intimacy and the kind of physical ambience best suited to the person with dementia. Palliative care is also explored—not merely as symptom management at the end of life, but as a skilled sensitive approach that nurtures hope throughout the final chapter in a person's life. The final chapter describes a well-researched method of evaluating the outcome of care from the perspective of a person with dementia, paving the way for dementia nursing that responds directly to a person's identified needs.

Many chapters focus on the dangers of treating a person with dementia as merely a combination of disparate, fragmented parts. Rather, the emphasis is on caring for a whole person who is more than the sum of various defining characteristics or the accumulation of various deficits. In this context, dementia nursing integrates matters of clinical importance with leisure activities, and the book encourages nurses to engage creatively with residents at any time of the day or night, rather than at designated 'program times'. This is not intended to imply that busy nurses should somehow find additional time for these pursuits. Rather, specific guidance is offered for incorporating creative care into other areas of daily nursing practice.

The concepts of partnership and mutuality are highlighted throughout the book. This focus is not new, and it applies to all nursing practice. Various contributors, however, rekindle this framework of person-centred care. In so doing, they are following in a long and noble tradition of theological, philosophical, and anthropological insights into the meaning of personhood and relationships. Contemporary dementia nursing will be enhanced by further building on this foundation.

In a textbook such as this there will, inevitably, be gaps. Although the book is primarily intended for nurses in the residential aged-care setting, nurses caring for people with dementia in other settings will also gain valuable insights for their caring practice. However, it is acknowledged that dementia nursing in other contexts (such as home care, community care, and acute hospital care) requires different responses in certain situations—matters that are beyond the scope of this book. There are no separate chapters on documentation, cultural issues, or ethical issues; it is the intention of the book that these important factors permeate all the chapters. The debate surrounding physical design of facilities for 'dementia-specific' care is not directly addressed. However, descriptions are offered to show ways in which the physical ambience can facilitate a calm, gentle approach to dementia care. Staff support is not addressed specifically; however, it is acknowledged that dementia nursing can be frustrating and personally taxing, while also being professionally fulfilling. Dementia nursing flourishes in an atmosphere of collegiality and good humour in which relationships of trust and professional fulfilment are fostered by management and permeate the entire care environment. When dementia nurses care for one another, their care for people with dementia is enhanced.

In dementia nursing, typical nurse–patient relationships are challenged because a person with dementia might not even recognise his or her own name or status, or the reason for dependence on nursing care. Indeed, a person with dementia might not even recognise the nurse as nurse—leaving nurse and resident to rely on their shared humanity. In the face of such communication difficulties, and in the context of stringent constraints on resources, nurses are to be commended for their continued commitment to dementia nursing. It is hoped that this book will empower nurses to take up this guide to practice in such a way that dementia nursing, because it is goes to the heart of humanity's deepest needs, becomes a model for all nursing.

Chapter 1

History and Issues

Sally Garratt

> We need to remind ourselves constantly that the purpose of gerontic nursing is to prevent untimely death and needless suffering, always with the focus of doing *with* as well as doing *for*, and in every instance to attempt to preserve personhood as long as life continues.
>
> DORIS SCHWARTZ (EBERSOLE & HESS 1998, P. 24)

Nursing knowledge about caring for older people with dementia develops through three interrelated streams—(i) the personal beliefs, attitudes, and values of nurses; (ii) the educational preparation of those nurses; and (iii) their personal experience of dealing with older people. For those beginning a career in nursing, learning about ageing is thus coloured by previously accepted value systems and social understandings of ageing, their educational preparation for their nursing role, and their personal experiences with respect to ageing and older people—experiences that might have been limited to exposure to ageing relatives or perhaps to some time spent working with older people in the community.

Nursing as a profession does not have a good record in promoting a positive value system with respect to gerontic nursing. Many studies have been conducted of nurses' attitudes to old people, working with old people, and studying aged care (for example, Stevens 1996). In general, nurses do not *choose* to work in aged care, and they often feel that gerontic nursing is the least exciting aspect of nursing work. This is partly due to the development of the specialty from a chequered past, and partly due to a current lack of recognition of the skills needed to provide what is, in reality, a complex and demanding nursing role.

This chapter sets the scene for better practice in dementia nursing care, and this requires a brief review of the past, the implications for the present, and a glimpse of what the future might hold.

A brief history of aged care
Earlier paradigms of care

A review of the past is necessary as a reminder of how current practice has been shaped. Such a review draws attention to the positive and negative aspects of change, and helps to ensure that past failures are not repeated. The experience in Australia is typical of that of many Western countries.

In Australia, formal care of older people began with the select committee established in New South Wales in 1861 to review the 'adequacy of provision made for the destitute' at the Sydney Benevolent Asylum. By today's standards, conditions of care at the asylum were horrendous, with overcrowding, poor food, no beds, no blankets, inadequate clothing, and substandard care. The committee recommended the development of a separate institution for the aged and infirm (Schultz 1991). From these humble beginnings of asylums for the insane, and poor houses for the destitute, large government geriatric institutions later developed. Older people who exhibited dementia were considered senile and were confined to asylums. The need for more sophisticated specific aged-care programs grew from government concern regarding the number of older people who required care, and from the steadily increasing costs of providing it. Benevolent groups throughout Australia gave attention to the plight of the aged and infirm, and charitable homes were also established.

In the twentieth century, governments and benevolent societies gradually increased their involvement, but formal nursing care was not provided as part of the care of the aged. Committees of ladies managed most services, and the inmates themselves did the daily work (Schultz 1991).

In the United States, the *American Journal of Nursing* published the first article on care of the aged in 1904, and aged care as a specialist field of nursing became recognised by this journal by 1925 (Ebersole & Hess 1998). By 1950, geriatrics had become a recognised specialisation in nursing in America, and there has been a steady increase in the dissemination of knowledge about aged care in nursing ever since.

As awareness of aged-care nursing developed, nurses were gradually employed in benevolent aged-care institutions and in government agencies responsible for the alleviation of destitution. However, the prevailing attitude to older persons was still essentially founded on sympathy, paternalism, and dependency. The emphasis was on 'doing things for' people, and the desired outcomes were cleanliness, food provision, and good housekeeping practice. Older people were expected to be grateful for the care they received. Extra events, such as outings or celebrations, were considered to be 'luxury treats' that were made available through the 'goodness' of auxiliaries or committees who supported aged-care institutions. Fundraising by these groups provided equipment and activities, and the professional role of nurses was limited to advising on the latest mattress for pressure relief, or to accompanying residents on an outing.

> 'The prevailing attitude to older persons was still essentially founded on sympathy, paternalism, and dependency.'

Good clinical care involved use of medications to improve illnesses associated with ageing, together with adjunct therapies adapted from the hospital model (including physiotherapy, occupational therapy, and podiatry). Care was considered 'good' if wounds healed, if new pressure sores were prevented, and if nutrition was maintained. 'Activity' formed the major part of the usual daily routine, and aged persons were encouraged to take part in occasional craft activities and domestic chores. The push towards 'activity' as a means to prevent physiological deterioration became mandatory, and a philosophy of 'use it or lose it' prevailed. Every aged person was expected to be up and dressed before breakfast, and all meals had to be taken in a communal dining room. Showering became a daily event and activities of daily living were considered to be a major means of keeping active. This mindset was derived from a 'rehabilitation model' of aged care, and good care was understood to involve the fostering of independence at all costs. Dementia was considered to be a psychiatric problem, and older people who could not be managed in aged persons' facilities (or 'homes') were swiftly relocated to mental health institutions.

The reforms of the 1980s and 1990s

In the 1980s and 1990s there was a rapid process of reform in Australia and other Western countries. This shifted the delivery of residential aged-care services from a medical model of health and disease to a socially constructed model of ageing. Philosophically, the arguments in support of the ideological shift could not be effectively challenged. Home-like environments, expression and maintenance of human rights, and ageing-in-place were ideals that most people supported.

These philosophical changes were associated with a move towards greater accountability among service providers. Steps were taken to impose accreditation and the provision of quality care outcomes through standards monitoring.

The reform process of the 1980s and 1990s thus shifted the focus from the older model of benevolent care with a medical and rehabilitation approach to one of social justice, equity, and rights. Residential care became less institutional and more like a personal 'home'. Nurses were confronted by regulations and standards that upheld the freedom of choice of residents, their involvement in decision-making, and personal control over their lifestyles. This was a huge philosophical swing that most nurses came to embrace as being positive. Nursing homes became focused on the activities of daily living, family and community involvement, and management systems to guide every facet of care. These changes, and the pressure to meet accreditation standards and provide evidence of quality outcomes, altered the focus of gerontic nursing away from matters of a purely clinical nature.

> 'The reform process shifted the focus to a model of social justice, equity, and rights.'

Implications for current nursing practice
Problems and benefits in the new paradigm

There were problems with the new aged-care paradigm. It soon became apparent that it was not easy to meet the personal preferences and rights of residents and their families in a setting of communal living. As a consequence, nurses began to leave aged care work as the demands of individual care in an institutional setting became too difficult to meet. The changes in work practices meant that 'routines' were no longer acceptable practice, that supervising and delegating work to minimally skilled workers meant much more accountability, and that resources were not always available to promote good care.

On a more positive note, the advent of accreditation standards meant that a shift back to good clinical care took place (see Figure 1.1. page 5). Such issues as infection control, pain management, wound care, continence management, and hydration maintenance all required contemporary clinical nursing skills.

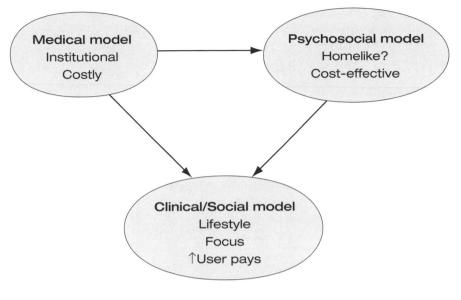

Figure 1.1
Changing models of aged-care services
Author's presentation

Before the advent of rigorous accreditation standards, nurses had become so intent on providing a 'home-like' environment that they almost lost sight of the need for specialist nursing practice in aged care.

There is now a recognition that older people in residential care are very frail and highly dependent, and that they have a range of co-morbidities that require skilled staff and good clinical leadership. This is a positive change. However, the nursing workforce in aged care has been so devalued and so deskilled that practitioners are not developing the necessary expertise at a pace required to meet the demands of the task at hand.

The advent of the paradigm of the 1980s and 1990s assumed that every registered nurse was automatically an expert in aged care. It was expected that any nurse could deal with the emotional, psychological, spiritual, cultural, and physical needs of older persons and their families. It was also assumed that nurse managers, as a matter of course, could adopt new quality systems and the documentation associated with such systems. The reality is that aged-care nursing requires a degree of clinical expertise comparable to any other area of nursing. Indeed, it could be argued that nurses working with older people require more skills, or at least distinctive skills. Older people in residential services are more likely to require dementia care and palliative care, and these call for distinctive specialist knowledge and skills.

Most nurses are responsive to human needs and adapt their nursing practice to care for such needs, but they require work structures that allow their expertise to be recognised and valued. Aged care work is under-valued, and this is reflected in poor funding, an undeveloped workforce, and a lack of proper recognition of the necessary skills in the workplace.

Containing costs is always a factor in the delivery of human services. It is not possible to meet the needs of all involved, but it is possible to recognise the worth of people. Nurses have attempted to adapt to the constant changes that surround them and are imposed on them. However, they have not engineered changes themselves. They alone can re-examine their practice and ensure a return to the traditional nursing values—values that are easily forgotten or misplaced in modern approaches to care.

Nursing values in the new paradigm

Nursing work is human work. The very nature of nursing means that nurses become involved in personal, close, and powerful relationships with others. People are most vulnerable when they are unwell, uncertain of their future, or in the process of dying. Nurses are privileged to share these journeys in ways often denied to other care providers. Their educational preparation and practical experience gives nurses the skills to enter the life of another person and to be of service.

To be of service is not merely the provision of 'customer satisfaction' and other indicators of 'service quality'. Service means giving and receiving personal 'entry'. It means *involvement* in the lives of others. A true service framework values others, despite not always sharing the same beliefs, and it enables a *caring* transaction to take place. It involves searching for the differences in people. People should not all be treated in the same way; nor should they be treated as special groups. Rather, each person should be treated with *individual understanding*. When a nurse understands another person there is enlightenment in which new knowledge is shared and new bonds are formed. Watson (1985) has referred to this as a 'caring event', and has stated that this is the true foundation of nursing practice.

> 'A "caring event" is the true foundation of nursing practice.'

Because of current dissatisfaction in the nursing workforce, a large percentage of nurses choose to undertake casual or agency work, and there is consequently a lack of continuity in residential care. Only a small fraction of staff on a shift are full-time. The impact on aged care is severe. A lack of stable staffing is not conducive to nurses getting to get to know the residents, or getting to know each other, and this situation compounds the dissatisfaction they feel from a lack of recognition of the value of their work. Continuity of care for older persons is essential for the development of mutual personal knowledge and understanding.

Students of aged-care nursing often say that they admire nurses who 'know the residents', 'know aged care', and 'put people before routine'. If routines and 'efficiency' dictate the work environment there is a lack of flexibility, and people become frustrated as tasks are not accomplished. Frustration leads to anxiety and intolerance. These feelings are manifested in relationships with others, and this creates the antithesis of a caring person-centred environment.

Unless nurses take a stand and change their work environment, the treadmill of 'surviving the shift' can take precedence over getting to know the residents. Blaming management, governments, or each other for changes that have been forced upon nursing is futile. Nurses themselves govern the manner in which nursing work is undertaken. Nurses themselves determine their nursing values and how they view people. Care is best provided by a team approach that takes account of all those involved—including residents, families, and co-workers. Such a team approach should include (rather than exclude), consult (rather than dictate), and facilitate personal growth (rather than accept defeat).

> 'Nurses themselves govern the manner in which nursing work is undertaken. Nurses themselves determine their nursing values and how they view people.'

Improving dementia care

The approach of this chapter (and this book) is to promote excellence in dementia care, with special attention to the following three factors.

- ▶ Nurses who work in aged care must have current clinical knowledge and skills, especially in the areas of dementia and palliation.
- ▶ Nurses who work in aged care must revisit and apply the fundamental precepts of good nursing practice—knowing the other; sharing the values of person-centred practice; putting people before tasks; and taking responsibility and accountability for care.
- ▶ Nurses must establish an understanding within their profession that working with older people, especially those who have dementia, is a complex, dynamic, and rewarding field of practice.

Each of these is discussed below.

Current knowledge and skills

Nurses who work in aged care must have current clinical knowledge and skills, especially in the areas of dementia and palliation. This knowledge is acquired through:

‣ personal responsibility for undertaking further education;
‣ reading current information;
‣ asking questions; and
‣ seeking answers.

Nurses must carefully re-examine any assumptions they might hold with respect to aged care, rather than routinely adopting these without thought. Good practice demands current knowledge, and should never be based on habit and guesswork.

The diagnosis of dementia is made by astute observation, history-taking, and special tests (such as scans and blood tests). To make the diagnosis, it is often necessary to eliminate other possible causes of the presenting signs and symptoms. Different types of dementia present in various ways, and the nurse is often in the best position to observe behaviour and personality change, and thus make valuable observations to aid in differential diagnosis.

Some forms of dementia (for example, cerebrovascular dementia) can be treated, and even if it is not possible to offer a cure, symptoms can often be ameliorated. Nurses should be able to contribute to the diagnostic process by being knowledgeable and astute in recognising the different presentations of conditions affecting behaviour. As research has uncovered the various pathological processes involved in the many forms of brain malfunction, the days have long gone when all presentations of dementia were considered untreatable.

Nurses also need to know the pharmacokinetics and dynamics of modern medication used in treating older people. Nurses are responsible for the administration of many powerful mind-altering substances, and should be aware of the synergistic or antagonistic interactions among medications.

Nurses also require practical skills in the application of alternative ways of delivering care. Restraint is not a desirable option—even if the objective is the safety of older people. There are many alternative strategies that can be tried. But the use of these alternatives depends upon the willingness of carers to try different techniques and to take responsibility for minimising the use of restraint. Practical knowledge is also required to maintain adequate nutrition and hydration for older persons who do not want to eat or drink, or who cannot sit down long enough to do so.

Fundamental precepts of good nursing practice

Nurses who work in aged care must revisit and apply the fundamental precepts of good nursing practice:

▶ knowing the other;
▶ sharing the values of person-centred practice;
▶ putting people before tasks; and
▶ taking responsibility and accountability for care.

Good nursing is not only 'doing for' people. It also involves 'doing with' people. Such a philosophy requires an ability to understand others with tolerance and mutual acceptance.

All too often, carers have a desire to control the behaviour of others to make 'management' easy. 'Management', in this sense, usually implies controlling the actions of people in a way that suits the prevailing practices of the institution. Keeping people 'safe' thus becomes an excuse for keeping them in a chair so that they cannot wander, fall, and cause themselves physical damage. Good practice becomes a matter of 'risk manage-

> 'Good nursing . . . requires an ability to understand others with tolerance and mutual acceptance.'

ment'—in which the possibility of personal injury is assessed against the values of personal freedom and self-determination. Such risk management often becomes overshadowed by the need of staff to maintain order and control over the environment, thus decreasing creativity and innovation in trying other means of providing safety.

Family involvement can also affect risk-management strategies. Well-meaning family members often have difficulty in accepting the need for some degree of risk-taking in older people. There is often a lack of understanding of the competence of people with dementia. The overwhelming presentation of cognitive loss can lead family members to assume that people with dementia cannot do anything on their own. However, older people themselves often prefer to take a risk—rather than be confined to a boring and frustrating existence in an environment that is not of their choosing.

In their professional roles as caregivers, nurses should be aware of these issues. Indeed, they have a professional responsibility to educate families and the wider community regarding good dementia care. Communication can promote informed understanding of the care delivered, and can enhance mutual cooperation among all the parties involved.

Recognition of professional role

Nurses must establish an understanding within their profession that working with older people, especially those who have dementia, is a complex, dynamic, and rewarding field of practice. Nursing older people:

- is special;
- requires sophisticated knowledge;
- is very rewarding;
- is an essential service to the community;
- is a growing field;
- is conducted within a research-based, well-recognised practice framework; and
- is a challenging area in terms of ethical practice.

Recognition by the nursing profession that gerontic nursing is a positive career option is essential if advanced clinical practice is to be developed and if the community is to accept that aged care is important. Attitudes to this work will change if nurses themselves see value in gerontic nursing work, and if they promote the clinical knowledge necessary to promote good practice.

> 'Recognition by the nursing profession that gerontic nursing is a positive career option is essential.'

Nursing research in gerontic nursing will help to establish the clinical outcomes that guide good practice. The adaptation of research from other disciplines should also be utilised to facilitate the assessment skills and knowledge that are required for good clinical decision-making (Koch & Garratt 2001).

Knowledge of ethical developments assists in dealing with end-of-life decisions, and an understanding of the legal and ethical responsibilities of aged-care nursing is essential to good practice (Nay & Garratt 1999).

Conclusion

The approach of nurses to dementia nursing is driven by their knowledge, values, and experience. A stimulating intellectual environment is required to promote the nature and work of gerontic nursing as a worthwhile career choice for nurses. The chapters in this book provide the stimulus for a recognition of the complexity and challenge offered by gerontic nursing. Through the knowledge available in these pages, nurses will be able to take responsibility for the development of gerontic nursing in general, and for the excellence of their own clinical practice in particular.

Chapter 2

The Relatives' Perspective

Julia Fountain

Introduction

The family and friends of people with dementia have much to learn when confronted with the question of how best to care for their relatives. Family members want to provide their relatives with the best quality of life possible. At the same time, there is much to be learnt about the illness, the health-care system, and various types of residential accommodation. In undertaking this difficult journey, relatives and friends also learn much about themselves.

Nurses can share in this journey, and can benefit professionally by having a sensitive awareness of the trials and tribulations faced by relatives. An essential aspect of the best nursing is a sensitive empathy with those in their care. Extending this empathic awareness to the relatives and friends of those in care is an essential part of best nursing practice.

'Extending empathic awareness to the relatives and friends of those in care is an essential part of best nursing practice.'

In most legislative jurisdictions there is a requirement for a plan of care for every aged-care resident. In most cases, this individualised plan of care is formulated in consultation with the resident and/or the resident's family. The family is thus considered part of the unit of care. In dementia care, family members become the spokespersons for the residents—particularly if residents are unable to speak effectively on their own behalf. In addition, relatives and close friends know and understand residents much better than do the nurses. In many cases family members have been caring for the person for months or years before admission to full-time care. For these reasons, input from families and close friends is vitally important to good nursing care.

It is hoped that nurses who understand the importance of reflective practice will gain important insights from this chapter, written by a concerned and committed relative on the basis of personal experience. The chapter explores some of the issues faced by loving relatives who strive to do their best in what can be a strange and disconcerting new world.

Finding new accommodation

Being moved from one's own home into residential care, perhaps involving transfer from one part of the country to another, is a significant life event for the person involved. Some people are intensely private persons and can resent being institutionalised and 'handled' by others, even when it is apparently in that person's own best interests. Family members observe the distress of their relative, and are inevitably affected by it.

If standards of care are poor, family members might see their realtives sedated and physically restrained. They might see sedatives used as 'management' tools, and watch a relative who was previously able to walk unaided now become chairbound, confused, and dishevelled. Security might be unsatisfactory, and elderly folk who have always loved walking outdoors in the fresh air might be found wandering outside the nursing home, much to the distress of relatives.

Family members might be forced to search for alternative accommodation for their relative—perhaps in a town far distant from where the family members live and work themselves. Alternatively, they might be faced with moving their relative away from his or her home town to be closer to the family. In searching for new accommodation, the family might be forced to visit dozens of establishments before finding a suitable and available placement. It can be a daunting challenge to tackle the logistics of commuting between cities, gathering information, arranging appointments, visiting places, inspecting the facilities, talking to staff formally and informally, calculating costs, and then weighing up the advantages and disadvantages. Family members might even meet others in the same situation on group tours of various establishments, and find themselves sharing information with others in a car park after a tour. They might find themselves wishing that there was a better way of making an informed decision about such an important matter—an acceptable practical solution to providing their relative with comfort and security in the last years of his or her life.

Understanding the medical condition and learning how to respond to a person with dementia is not easy. Family members often wish to let their elderly relatives make decisions for themselves for as long as possible and to retain a sense of independence. It can be difficult to judge when the time has come to step in and take more responsibility. In making such judgments, family members ask themselves many questions. How much do I need to know about dementia? How much can I allow my relative to participate in decision-making? Who can I rely on for sound judgment and advice? To what extent should I question and challenge professional advice? When should I seek a second or third opinion?

Relatives can find themselves relying on their own intuition in making assessments of residential establishments, their residents, and their staff. They observe people, noting their dress, behaviour, and body language, listening to how they speak to each other, the words they use, and their tone of voice. They learn to note the design of the rooms, the lighting, the smells, the furniture, and how much space is available for people to sit or move around comfortably. They find themselves asking whether they would accept these living conditions for themselves.

All in all, arranging suitable care for relatives who can no longer care for themselves can be a difficult experience. It can involve family members in having to make assessments of unfamiliar people, places, and procedures, and the whole experience can be disconcerting, confusing, and daunting.

And after the exhaustive assessments have been made, and the difficult decisions have been taken, the real practical problems begin. Arriving and moving into new accommodation is no simple task.

A new world and new people

Most of us have several worlds that we inhabit during our lives—some more intense and demanding than others. The world of a nursing home or other aged-care accommodation is a thriving community of people into which new arrivals and their relatives have to work to be accepted and accepting.

The director of nursing (DON) is obviously an important person in this new world. The DON provides leadership to the whole staff, and a good DON can

The arrival

The move took place on the day that would have been my parent's 57th wedding anniversary. I don't think Mum really knew where we were going but she graciously accepted everything I organised—the flight, the wheelchairs provided by the airline, the taxi to the nursing home. The director of nursing and the staff were prepared for Mum's arrival and were very welcoming. Someone had put fresh flowers on her bedside table—a gesture that meant far more to me than it did to Mum, who could not see them.

Despite the warm welcome, we felt strange and out of place. We gradually became used to Mum's new environment, but during the months that followed, I watched other people having the same experience when they first arrived. When new people came I watched them going through the same motions of settling into this strange new place that was to be their home.

From the beginning I tried to get to know everyone who worked in Mum's new home. I tried to establish good communication and a comfortable working relationship with the director of nursing, other nurses, therapists, office staff, kitchen staff, laundry staff, and cleaning staff, as well as with other residents and visitors. I kept asking questions in an attempt to understand how the aged-care system works, and I tried to provide as much information as possible for Mum's care plan, including Mum's personal likes and dislikes. The resident-classification scale gave me an indication of how Mum fitted in. I also needed reassurance that her nursing-care plan would be frequently reviewed and adjusted to meet her changing needs.

I made a point of putting time aside for private conversations with Mum and others, and tried to include Mum in discussions with staff whenever possible and appropriate. The formality of some of these meetings gave Mum a sense of someone being in charge and taking responsibility.

Although I had moved Mum to another state, away from family and familiar places, there happened to be a staff member who came from the same small country town where my parents had lived for thirty years. This person became an important link with the past, and it made such a difference to Mum's day to be able to talk about people and places that she could recall more readily than events from recent times.

Finding a nursing home close to where I lived and worked made it possible for me to visit frequently and to come immediately if there was an urgent problem. Although Mum did not know where she was, she had a sense that I was not far away, and staff could reassure her when she fretted or became agitated.

inspire confidence and trust in staff and residents alike through sound professional judgment and warm personal support. Relatives of residents soon become aware that managing a nursing home is a complex and responsible task, and should try to establish a good working relationship with the DON and other key people who will be caring for the person with dementia.

Relatives need to become familiar with the various roles and responsibilities of the many people involved in running residential accommodation. Sometimes it is appropriate to consult with the DON. At other times it is more appropriate to discuss matters with the deputy DON, or the person responsible for a particular shift. At other times again it is appropriate to discuss an issue with administrative staff. It is often difficult for relatives to judge whether a problem is really a significant matter of health policy, or whether they have allowed a relatively minor matter to assume an importance out of proportion to its real significance. Understanding the roles of staff, and establishing good working relations with them, can be very helpful in sorting out these matters to everyone's satisfaction. Nurses can assist by helping relatives to understand who does what, and who is the best person to provide guidance in certain situations.

'Nurses can assist by helping relatives to understand who does what, and who is the best person to provide guidance in certain situations.'

If the new accommodation is a different locality, it will be necessary to find a new doctor. Family members often have the responsibility of finding the right doctor—someone who visits the establishment, someone who will provide appropriate and sympathetic treatment, and someone who will be accepted by their relative. The new doctor must also be someone with whom the family members feel comfortable, and whose judgment they trust.

Getting to know other residents is a time-consuming task, but it is important that family members do so—especially if their own relative finds it difficult to communicate with others and make new friends. This involves relatives in getting to know other residents, their families, and various other visitors. It also involves time in getting to know staff members, agency nurses, therapists, and various other people with a range of roles and responsibilities in care. Understandably, family members are essentially interested in the care of their own relative, but it is worthwhile to take the time and trouble to show interest in others, to remember their names and something about them, and to be as bright and friendly as possible. Nurses can be very helpful in facilitating these important relationships and interactions.

Older people can have fixed ideas about the roles of men and women, and can have difficulty in accepting some aspects of institutional life. It is inevitable that privacy will be invaded to some degree in institutional life, and arrangements such as male nurses showering and dressing female residents can be disconcerting for older ladies. Nurses need to be sensitively aware of these sorts of issues, and can play an important role in helping relatives to smooth the transition from the privacy of home. Various other gender and cultural issues can arise, but with the increasingly diverse cultural mix in Australia, greater

A new home

I tried to lessen the division between my world and Mum's world by treating the nursing home as if it were Mum's own home—dropping in at any time just to say hello and have a chat, or to share a cup of tea, or to tidy clothes and possessions. I tried to create as normal a life as possible for Mum's sake and for my own sake. In some ways it was a game that had to be played out—otherwise it would have been overwhelmingly sad.

I presumed, and was given, access at any time of the day or night. I was pleased to meet the night staff who were otherwise the silent partners—rarely seen or heard by daylight visitors. When I discovered this group of dedicated people I felt a great sense of relief that Mum was in good hands throughout the night.

Mum shared a room with others. The advantage of a shared room was that other more able residents could keep an eye on Mum, and she could keep an eye on them. Although I hoped that Mum might make new friends, this turned out to be an unrealistic expectation. Even though these people never became 'real friends' of my mother, I was unprepared for my own grief when some of them died. Even though I tried to make it all seem like 'home', there were problems. Of the several communal rooms that could be used by all the residents, some were unavailable at certain times, and there was often no suitable place for a private conversation or just a quiet cup of tea together. Because she was so thin, Mum found that most of the chairs were very hard, and although there was usually a supply of sheepskins to sit on, Mum could not find these by herself or remember where she had left hers.

I arranged to have fresh flowers delivered every week. Mum could not see the flowers but I believe that she still liked receiving them. They provided another talking point and other people enjoyed them.

Sometimes essential oils were used in oil burners, but these were too costly for the nursing home to supply for long. It really made a difference when they were used. I have heard of places with sensory rooms with fishtanks and lava lamps for colour and movement. This would have been nice if they had such a thing in Mum's place. I sometimes brought lavender and rosemary creams to give Mum a hand and foot massage. She appreciated this, and might have reminded her of treatments in her days as a beautician.

Moving from a warm climate to a much cooler one that meant she had to spend most of her time indoors was quite hard for Mum. She was used to the heat and being able to sit outside and enjoy the sun and fresh air. She did not have enough warm clothes, and it was quite difficult to find new clothes for her that fitted, that she liked, and that could be easily looked after.

cross-cultural awareness among both staff and residents promises to make for a more harmonious environment.

New daily routines

Despite the security provided to residents by a nursing home or other residential accommodation, adult children often feel a strong need to protect their aged parents. This forms part of a role reversal between parent and child that can be disconcerting for both. Nursing home staff are invariably caught up in the dynamics of these changing family roles, and they should respect advocacy on behalf of an aged parent if those representations are put fairly and reasonably.

As residents experience increasingly limited ability to do the things they like, family members need to think more creatively about providing simple pleasures and enjoyment for their relatives. Simple things such as movement in a rocking chair, going for a drive in a car, hydrotherapy, and talking books can all bring significant pleasure, especially if they reflect past experiences and habits.

However, even with the best efforts from relatives in terms of advocacy and small entertainments, residents can still become frustrated and angry. The sheer frustration of not being able to do things for themselves, or being ordered to do something at a certain time or in a certain way, can be very difficult to accept. The transition from independent living to assisted accommodation is hard for everyone involved—residents and loving relatives alike.

Because they spend so much time indoors, and because they are sometimes unable to see to tell the time (or remember the time if they can see it), residents often do not know know whether it is day-time or night-time. Meals are often the only regular activity because it is not always possible for everyone to be bathed or showered at a set time each day. Having a shower every day has been an important lifelong routine for many residents, and it can be distressing if this is not possible because staff are too busy. Many elderly people have also become accustomed to a nap in the afternoon, even though this might mean that they might not sleep through the night. Such personal routines are sometimes difficult to continue in a new environment, and life can seem chaotic and miserable without them.

> 'The transition from independent living to assisted accommodation is hard for everyone involved— residents and loving relatives alike.'

Food can still be one of the simple pleasures of life, and many residents maintain a good appetite and a desire to manage for themselves. However, increasing debility can mean that every meal requires patient and sympathetic assistance to get food from plate to mouth, and approriate supplements might be needed to maintain good nutrition.

Failing health

Family members can find themselves trying to understand what is going on in the head of their aged relative, and can find themselves always watching for signs of improvement or deterioration. The state of mind of residents can vary enormously—being affected by general ill-health, infections, medication, or agitation as a result of an unfortunate interaction with a staff member or other resident.

It can be hard to change residents' attitudes if they take a dislike to particular members of staff. Some staff members have a friendly manner with everyone, but others can have a particular style that endears them to only some of the residents. Such staff members are borne with resignation by residents who, after all, cannot leave at the end of the shift.

Activities

People who have been creative and busy all their lives find it frustrating to have their sight, dexterity, and memory desert them. But many never give up trying, and long to have something to do with their hands. Any little job can help. But it can be hard for relatives to watch the frustration that comes with increasing disability. Many residents are aware of their increasing disability, and some can become obsessed with wanting to regain old skills—such as learning to write again. Family members can experience the anguish of encouraging their relatives in their efforts, while knowing that it is all a desperately futile exercise.

'Family members can experience the anguish of encouraging their relatives in their efforts, while knowing that it is all a desperately futile exercise.'

Residents who have been keen walkers can get some exercise by wandering up and down passageways. If there are people available, a walk outdoors in pleasant weather can be most enjoyable, but fatigue is always a potential problem.

Deteriorating health

Sadly Mum's sense of time and place became increasingly confused. On many occasions I did not know which decade she was talking about, and so I just played along and encouraged her to talk. I tried to find distant relatives and people who might be able to help Mum make connections, but it was not easy to bring them together.

It took me a while to work out that her belief that there was a dead baby in a box in her room might have been about the baby she lost more than fifty years ago, and I alternated between contradicting her and comforting her. These times left me sad and confused, because the death of this child had been mentioned only once or twice before. Mum also talked about other things that I did not know whether to believe or not.

Sometimes she would get into other people's beds. I thought that this was rather strange until I worked out that the bed was in the same place as hers, but in a different room. Because of her confusion, her being in a new place, and her poor vision, it was understandable that she would make these sorts of genuine mistakes.

Mum was always losing something and often believed that people were stealing things. To minimise the problem I left her with very few possessions in her little bedside cabinet, which had one small drawer. Because I was aware of how she used to treasure and enjoy all her things, her sparse possessions in a little drawer looked terribly bare and depressing, but I knew that this was in her interests. I put her favourite painting on the wall above her bed and that brightened things up a bit. I also put a photo frame on the wall with old family photos. Although she could not see them, others might have initiated conversation about the people in the photos.

Failing sight seemed to be the main cause of Mum's frustration and depression. Like everyone, Mum was dependent on visual cues for recognition and communication to help maintain her independence and dignity. It takes a long time to learn to compensate for loss of sight, especially with poor hearing. In addition, she suffered from bad circulation which increased her isolation as she suffered increasing loss of sensitivity in her fingertips.

Hydrotherapy is an alternative form of useful exercise, and a new experience for many residents. Relatives can go along with the group to see how it is managed. Many elderly folk love being in the water, and the freedom of movement this can give. Even experienced staff members can be surprised at the confidence and swimming ability of many older residents.

Talking books can provide much enjoyment, and relatives can ensure a steady supply of these from appropriate agencies. However, many residents will require help in choosing a cassette, and diminished sensation in the fingers and a lack of manual dexterity can also cause difficulties in using play and stop tabs. Radios can provide companionship and entertainment, but some older folk also have difficulties in using these, especially if they involve earphones and headphones. Unfortunately assistance is not always readily available.

Hearing impairment can be a great burden, and many staff members and visitors fail to realise that residents cannot hear, or cannot understand an unfamiliar accent. Hearing aids can be a constant problem because they are easily misplaced or lost. Relatives are often surprised to discover that many staff members seem unable or unwilling to put hearing aids in position, install batteries, or adjust the volume.

Many residents will want to use the telephone, but be unable to do so without special arrangements or supervision. A mobile phone is not usually a good idea because elderly people often need help to find the numbers and use

Personal care

Mum worked as a beautician in the 1930s, and all her life she had paid special attention to her grooming and appearance. She used to make all her own clothes and hats, and she dressed beautifully. She wore lipstick and simple jewellery every day, and continued to try to do this, even when she lost her sight. Fortunately there was a beautician who came to the nursing home and Mum enjoyed these sessions. She was always so pleased when I found and applied missing lipstick, or tweezed stray hairs on her chin—small things but they mattered a great deal to her.

Providing suitable clothes that could survive industrial washing and drying was a challenge. Once we had found something suitable, I often took Mum's dresses home to wash and iron them myself, rather than risk losing them.

Buying shoes for someone who is not able to visit a shoe shop was an unexpected problem. A solution was found—by cutting out cardboard outlines of each foot to take to the shop, and by purchasing shoes only if they could be returned.

Mum really liked the feeling of freshness in her mouth after cleaning her teeth. I often helped her do this. It was such a simple thing to do, but it made her feel so much better. She could still hold the toothbrush and scrub her teeth vigorously. Because this was something that she could still manage to do for herself, it gave her great satisfaction. It gave her gums a good massage too. I would clean her dentures when they were left dirty in an empty cup beside her bed.

When Mum wanted to get out of bed in the night it was often because she simply wanted to go to the toilet. She was not incontinent, but I often found her with pads in her pants which she did not want or need. I think she probably just gave in to nurses whose work would be easier if residents wore a pad just in case, and would not need to be washed and changed again.

At the end I slept on a mattress on the floor beside Mum's bed to prevent her from falling out of bed if she tried to get up to go to the toilet during the night. I also wanted to be there when she died.

Good things . . . and not so good

Things that worked well

- A DON who provided leadership, authority, compassion, and understanding.
- Access all hours for carers and relatives.
- A monthly activities program that was varied and thoughtfully designed.
- A large frequently updated noticeboard at the reception desk.
- Office technology that allowed me to stay in contact by email with the nursing home, especially when travelling overseas for my work, often in countries where communications were difficult.
- Regular sessions for residents—such as music therapy, bus trips, visits from the animal farm.
- A trusted doctor who would come when needed.
- Use of name tags—Mum was not the only one with a poor memory.
- Palliative-care volunteers.
- People who did little things—such as taking a photograph of Mum and me together, and giving me a copy; or giving Mum a shoebox of audiotapes to use in her talking book machine.
- Staff members who understood that appearances mattered and took the time to help Mum dress.
- Physical activities such as physiotherapy and hydrotherapy.
- Treats such as a glass of green ginger wine or a box of chocolates.

Things that were difficult

- As a single woman, trying to manage a full-time job, maintain relationships, and stay healthy, while still giving Mum the time and attention that she needed and deserved.
- Learning to pace myself, not knowing whether this condition would last for months or years.
- Trying to be responsible, constant, and creative in problem-solving.
- Learning to trust the nursing home staff to look after Mum in all sorts of situations—on an outing, in the shower, at mealtimes.
- Phone calls from the nursing home in the middle of the night to let me know that Mum was not too well, and I might like to come over.
- Mum's lifelong worry that something bad would happen to me.
- My fear about who would look after Mum if I predeceased her.
- Sensitivity to family expectations of the standard of care in this nursing home.
- Seeing a bereavement counsellor—a dreadful experience that only served to deepen my sadness about my impending loss.
- Aggressive residents—although I respected the policy of having a mix of residents with varying needs.

(Continued)

(*Continued*)

- Staff members who did not pay attention to residents' needs or did not care about details.
- Staff members who did not understand how to communicate with people whose sight and hearing are impaired.
- Mum pretending not to understand, being uncooperative, and behaving badly towards other residents (all of which were uncharacteristic of her).
- Mum thinking that people were stealing her things.
- My battle in resolving the dilemma between having realistic expectations but not accepting anything sub-standard.

the phone, and there is a likelihood of loss or misuse. Some relatives try innovative systems, such as ringing twice—the first time to give staff members an opportunity to find the resident, bring him or her to the nurses' station, and allow time for the person to settle comfortably; and the second time to make the actual call. However, staff routines sometimes do not allow this. Leaving a tape of familiar family voices is another good idea to provide companionship.

The desire for companionship and conversation should never be overlooked. Some establishments allow residents to sit up at night with the nurses at the nurses' station. It can be a bother for the staff, but residents often just want company. Relatives can help in satisfying this desire for companionship by organising others to drop in for a visit. Friends, acquaintances, and various other people are often willing to 'just drop in' for an occasional visit, and this can be useful not only for the resident, but also for the visitor who might otherwise never see the inside of an aged persons' establishment.

Conclusion

Family members learn a lot as they care for their aged relatives, but often these things are learnt too late to put them into practice. This chapter has explored some of the common issues faced by relatives, and provides useful food for thought for nurses who wish to provide professional empathic care for relatives faced with this responsibility.

Relatives need to know that they can always ask other people for help. Relatives are faced with the responsibility of finding out as much as they can about unfamiliar situations so they can make an informed decision about what is best. Nurses can provide invaluable information and assistance in this daunting responsibility.

Death

How do you discuss the death of other residents? How are people told? What words are used? Did Mum hear or understand them? How would you like to find out that the person living in the bed next to you had died overnight? When the curtains are pulled around a bed in an institution it signals something is happening. It signals that this is private. They might be washing or dressing. Or the doctor might be there. Or the person might be dead.

Looking back on photos taken throughout the year, Mum's deterioration was quite evident. There were a few good moments towards the end—such as the time we escaped to a nearby park with the wheelchair—but Mum's last coherent words were not the words of someone demented, just someone in pain wanting to end her life.

Palliative care requires a lot of explanation, and it is difficult to understand the implications of the use of morphine. The choice of words as death approaches is important. The wrong words, even if well meant, can be unhelpful. A well-meaning staff member told me: 'You will want to say goodbye, tell her you love her'. To me, those words implied that the relationship was over—which was not particularly helpful.

The night staff moved Mum's bed to another room and allowed me to sleep on the floor. They behaved as though this was quite normal, for which I am eternally grateful. Some people are so compassionate, even when they have so many to look after. So many people died that Christmas.

The funeral service was held in the chapel adjoining the nursing home, and the DON kindly allowed us to use one of the large rooms for afternoon tea. The minister was available, as was the organist. Lots of people came, including staff and residents. I felt overwhelmed by people's generosity of heart, many of whom had other commitments.

It was a huge relief to have made the decisions about the service and the cremation. We spread Mum's ashes with Dad's on Sydney Harbour, and installed a memorial seat for them both in the Botanic Gardens. This is a place that they both enjoyed. Now anyone can visit at any time to pay their respects.

The grief finally lessens with time. New routines replace the old. I have finally stopped looking at the shelf of chocolates in the supermarket, and wondering which ones Mum might like today.

Insightful relatives soon become aware it is not the facilities, fittings, and furnishings that make for good accommodation. Rather, the *people* make all the difference. Nurses can make all the difference between an 'ordinary' establishment and one that offers professional empathic care of the highest standards.

Relatives are often prepared to volunteer their time generously, but they soon discover that their lives can become a 'roller-coaster' of commitments—with one day being hectic and stimulating, and another being little more than a dull routine. The helpful guidance of experienced nurses can be invaluable in assisting relatives to develop a flexible routine to manage the potential chaos of their new lives as carers. Nurses can provide helpful professional advice in a whole range of areas. From their own experience of reflective practice, nurses might recommend to relatives that they keep a diary to record everything—dates, names, places, medications, and how they feel. This can be of great assistance in organising time and plans.

Relatives soon come to know that being a carer takes a lot of time, patience, empathy, and awareness. Nurses can help them in this journey of discovery, and should encourage relatives to laugh and cry as often as they feel the need.

Finally, nurses should always remember that their professional role involves more than the care of the resident in their midst. In a very real sense, they take on the care of the whole family.

Chapter 3

The Whole Person

Melvin A. Kimble

It is much more important to know what sort of patient has a disease than what sort of disease a patient has.

SIR WILLIAM OSLER

The meaning of life is in the relationship of the whole person to God, not in the relationship of the cerebellum.

EDNA HONG

Introduction

The dramatic increase in the longevity of older adults in our global society has brought an expansion in their numbers and in their potential for trauma and dementing illnesses, the most common of which is Alzheimer's disease. Dementia is one of the major health problems of our ageing society. It is the nightmare the elderly pray to avoid.

As their disease progresses, persons with advanced dementia are robbed of their cognitive capacity, bodily functions, dignity, and identity. Weeks blend into months as Alzheimer's steals its victims' memories, their personalities, and their relationships. Dementia of the Alzheimer's type has been called 'the disease of the century' for which there is no proven cure at this time. When it strikes, persons who were once resourceful and competent begin to suffer personality changes, memory loss, and confusion, and these changes create painful frustrations for spouses and others caring for them.

Persons suffering from dementia outlive the progressive destruction of their brains. Persons with Alzheimer's disease live an average of seven years after diagnosis, and some as many as twenty years or more. Of all persons over the age of 65 years, 10% are estimated to have Alzheimer's disease and, by the age of 85, this increases to an estimated 50%.

> 'A new perspective is emerging . . . a holistic understanding of dementia.'

A new perspective is emerging that sets forth a holistic understanding of dementia, moving beyond the standard biomedical paradigm. This chapter sets forth a holistic model for exploring the horrific complexities of dementia.

Beyond the biomedical paradigm

The orientation of the new paradigm of dementia involves a primary commitment to understanding the dementia patient as a whole person rather than understanding this person through a model that is limited to a medical and psychological diagnosis. When the medical community set forth a rigid biomedical approach to dementia, it created a limited view of a person with dementing illness. The new paradigm is opposed to reductionistic anthropology and emphasises the importance of a multidimensional conception of the whole person. This involves approaching a person with dementia as a whole person— not only in body and mind, but also in spirit. An inclusive anthropology is crucial in the medical and nursing care of persons regardless of their diagnoses.

What has been set forth at this point is nothing new. An increasing number of medical schools has introduced seminars and courses that include such a holistic model that incorporates the spiritual dimension in their operational definitions of health and medical care. There is a growing recognition that a wider frame of reference is required to explore the multifaceted and complex questions about dementia in particular, and about older adulthood and its meaning in general.

If an effective response is to be made to the profound multidimensional issues of ageing and dementia, the new paradigm insists that insights from medical and biosocial scientists must be brought into dynamic dialogue with religion and spirituality. There is a need to recognise that Alzheimer's patients, despite the accumulating neuritic plaques and tangle of their brains, have not lost their humanity.

All over the world, medical schools are recognising that the spiritual dimension is an important component in health care and healing, and are introducing courses in spirituality and health care. Medical research literature has increasingly confirmed the positive relationship between spirituality and holistic medicine. Dementia patients need to be seen as more than simply the results of scans and various clinical tests.

'Dementia patients need to be seen as more than simply the results of scans and various clinical tests.'

The inclusion of spirituality in medical care is more than simply adding another biomedical tool to the medical kit. It is a revolutionary expansion of the holistic understanding of a person suffering from a dementing illness. The ultimate context of medical care and health is spiritual. As Gunderson (1997, p. 9) has observed:

> . . . faith needs the language of health in order to understand how it applies to life. Health needs the language of faith in order to find its larger context, its meaning.

Frankl's dimensional ontology

A whole new interpretation of dementia is introduced once the validity of the spiritual dimension is acknowledged. It is at this point that Frankl's concept of 'dimensional ontology' is helpful in understanding Alzheimer's disease and other dementing illnesses. Frankl (1967) contended that an examination of dementia should reflect an understanding of the whole person as a dynamic blend of spiritual, physical, mental, emotional, and social dimensions. Each dimension needs to be acknowledged and valued in any evaluation of the person. A segmented approach to a person with dementia results in a reductionistic, one-dimensional caricature.

Frankl (1967, pp 136–42) set forth a 'dimensional ontology' to avoid a Cartesian body–mind dualism. In addition to the somatic and psychic dimensions of the person, Frankl's theory added an emphasis on the spiritual dimension—or, as Frankl, labelled it, the 'noetic dimension'. In contradistinction to the biological and psychological dimensions, this dimension is that in which uniquely human phenomena are located.

Frankl set forth a geometrical concept of dimensional ontology that reflects the rich multi-dimensionality of persons while still preserving their anthropological unity. Frankl (1967, p. 138) demonstrated this concept as follows:

> A glass on the table, if projected out of three-dimensional space into a two-dimensional plane, would appear as a circle. The same glass projected into its side view and seen in profile would appear as a rectangle. But nobody would claim that the glass is composed of a circle and a rectangle. Neither can we claim that man is composed of parts, such as a body and a soul. It is a violation of man to project him out of the realm of the genuinely human in the plane of either soma or psyche.

Dimensional ontology widens the lens through which Alzheimer's disease and other dementias are perceived. It permits the introduction of a fully developed anthropology that avoids reductionistic conceptions of the human person.

Alzheimer's patients as our teachers

Hermeneutics, broadly speaking, is the art and science of interpretation. Throughout life, at every stage, the developing self is confronted with the need to make interpretations of, and assign meanings to, what is experienced. A hermeneutical perspective is not concerned about predicting or controlling human behaviour. In this sense, it is radically different from the methodology of empirical science. Its aim is to describe what is observed and thereby to understand it. Phenomenology focuses on the importance of the individual as one who is actively and intentionally seeking meaning in his or her lived world. It examines the individual person and views that person as being embedded in a social, cultural, and historical context.

By examining the lived worlds of persons with dementia, expressions of meaning can be found in their feelings, actions, and values. Researchers and practitioners (such as chaplains and nurses) have documented examples of words and actions of persons with dementia that, when carefully observed, reveal personhood and meaning (McFadden, Ingram & Baldauf 2000). By the method of hermeneutical phenomenology, persons with Alzheimer's disease and other

'. . . the importance of the individual as one who is actively and intentionally seeking meaning in his or her lived world.'

dementias become our teachers. Phenomenological hermeneutics represents an attempt to challenge and replace the system of meanings set forth by tests and measurements. It attempts to balance an understanding of reality by recognising the role of the *subject* in perception. It cuts through the conflict between idealism and empiricism by stressing the *relationship* between the subject and the world. It is concerned with subjective reality.

> 'By examining the lived worlds of persons with dementia, expressions of meaning can be found in their feelings, actions, and values.'

A hermeneutical phenomenology views individuals as conscious and active, and as capable of symbol manipulation. Langer (1942, p. 29) has described symbol-making as:

> . . . one of man's primary activities, like eating, looking, or moving about . . . the fundamental process of the mind . . . essential to thought and prior to it.

In a similar vein, Frankl (1984, p. 153) has stressed that:

> . . . man is the being who is capable of creating symbols, and being in need of symbols.

Through symbolisation, people are able to represent their environments and thereby exercise existential choices that include alternative constructions, revisions, and replacements. This ability to symbolise allows people to transcend time and interpret all of life's events as they construct an individual 'reality'.

Spiritual intelligence

Spirituality can be difficult to recognise among persons with significant dementia, but spirituality is present even when severe intellectual disability makes consciousness limited or absent. As McFadden (2000, p. 71) has suggested:

> Perhaps because the symptoms of Alzheimer's disease are so frightening, there has been an insufficient effort to try to understand the inner, subjective world of persons with the diagnosis. In research articles, they are counted and the various behavioral outcomes of their cognitive declines are scored. The unique characteristics that form a whole person may become discrete variables entered into regression equations, but rarely do researchers actually converse with the person with dementia in order

to try to comprehend the subjectivity of dementia. This kind of careful listening is most often done by family members, nurses' aides, and chaplains or clergy.

Human beings are more than physical bodies and mental functions. Heuristic research on multiple intelligences suggests that there are separate human capacities (Gardner 1993). A concept of spiritual intelligence has been developed (Emmons 1999), and it has been suggested that persons with Alzheimer's disease can retain core components of this spiritual intelligence—even in the most advanced states of dementia. McFadden (2000, pp 72–3) has put it this way:

> Even when persons cannot comprehend language nor think in any way usually conceptualized as cognitive activity, still they retain personhood. This image of personhood as transcending reason, language, and thought itself stands in stark contrast to the secular 'hypercognitive' bias of our postmodern culture.

Spirituality is shared between persons with dementia and their caregivers. However, caregivers must first acknowledge their own spirituality if they are to recognise the spiritual essence of another person. In doing so, they gain insight into that which all persons have in common. Spirituality is an intensely personal unique quality that is not discovered through reason alone.

'Caregivers must first acknowledge their own spirituality if they are to recognise the spiritual essence of another person.'

This spiritual dimension does not require any specific religious connotation. The spiritual dimension is the energy within a person that strives for meaning and purpose. It is the unifying and integrating dimension of being that includes the experience of transcendence and the mystery. It is at once overwhelming and fascinating, and it renders existence significant and meaningful in the here and now.

The spiritual dimension is a mystery that is difficult to measure and lacks universal definition. It is easier to describe than define because it is the essence of the subjective self and thus resists objectification through definition. It cannot be partitioned or measured in relative terms. As Coulter (2001, p. 2) has observed:

> Spirituality is not lessened because conscious expression is lessened (as for example following severe brain injury). Consciousness may be the property

of the brain but spirituality is the property of the whole person (the subjective of essence of being). This suggests that consciousness may not be required for spiritual personhood and spiritual essence or being could be present in a person who no longer conscious . . . Perhaps spiritual consciousness can be considered a mediation between finitude of this world and on infinite aspect of being that transcend this world.

Such a spiritual definition of personhood starts with a fundamental affirmation that all human beings have within them a spark of divinity—or, as the Judaeo-Christian tradition expresses it, all human beings are 'created in the image of God'. This spiritual understanding of persons with dementia poses fundamental questions of meaning and purpose: What does it mean to be human?

As a result of a stroke or dementia, persons are often described as having lost their 'self'. The very core of who they were seems to have evaporated. But the self is relational. It is created through relationships with people in families, faith communities, institutions, and so on. Even when a person's memory fails, that person's social identity remains. This social identity can be strengthened to improve the person's quality of life and to retain his or her personhood. For Kitwood (1997, p. 8), personhood is ' . . . a standing or status bestowed upon one human being by others in the context of relationship and social being. It implies recognition, respect, and trust.'

Persons are more than their ability to link past, present, and future. However, a person is in jeopardy of losing personhood if he or she is unable to do this. For example, standard mini-mental examinations are used to assess Alzheimer's patients and to evaluate them on their ability to name the date and the year. Some mini-mental tasks require people to draw numbers and hands on the face of a blank clock. If they 'fail' such tests, dementia patients are perceived as objects without personhood.

'Even when a person's memory fails, that person's social identity remains.'

Is it possible for people with Alzheimer's disease to be spiritually alive and responsive? Persons with dementia do continue to respond to faith rituals that connect them not only with the present but also, in some mystical sense, with the transcendent. Worship services in nursing homes often foster this connectedness. Religious systems often provide a richness of metaphors that ushers the personal life story of the dementia person into a larger transcendent story. Religion can also serve as an identity maintenance system for persons in a faith community. Familiar hymns, prayers, and symbols have certain evocative powers. As Post (2000, p. 138) has observed: 'as the capacity for technical rationality fades, more contemplative and spiritual capacity may be elevated'.

In Alzheimer's disease, there is an inner spiritual core that remains intact in spite of the loss of instrumental and expressive faculties. The spiritual core of a person transcends all boundaries of ability and disability. People with Alzheimer's disease might lose the capacity to talk and to use language, but the spiritual core remains. Sometimes this is revealed by the warmth of a handshake, or a smile, or a tear. For this reason, the skilful use of familiar music, or a symbol, or a simple touch can evoke evidence of the innate spiritual core.

Conclusion

Spirituality is a dimension of authentic holistic personhood that enlarges and expands the definition of persons with Alzheimer's disease. This is a dimension that needs to be examined for its medical and nursing implications of treating and caring of persons who suffer from this disease. Being absent in mind or lacking a measurable IQ is not synonymous with being absent in spirit. The exploration of this holistic model has the potential to move the care and treatment of persons with Alzheimer's disease beyond plaques and tangles.

Chapter 4

Enriching the Environment

Kim Wylie

Introduction

Unfortunately, a significant number of aged-care facilities still fit Brooker's (1997) description of a 'kippers and curtains culture'. Such a culture exists when people pretend to be well-to-do by having expensive curtains on the windows, but exist on a diet of inexpensive fish—that is, the outward appearance is not matched by the internal reality. Using the same metaphor, a 'kippers and curtains culture' can be said to exist in certain dementia-care units that are housed in attractive buildings, publicise 'politically correct' mission statements, and speak in a language of proficient and caring practices—but which have a custodial atmosphere, a focus on performance of tasks, and a failure to value residents and staff as sentient and worthwhile people.

This chapter begins with an exposé of the everyday environments of care units as experienced by many people with dementia, and follows with a discussion of how and why such inappropriate and inadequate environments continue to exist. The chapter then discusses how practice can be transformed, how environments can be enriched, and how meaning can be restored to the lives of people with dementia.

The everyday lived world

Imagine yourself sitting for hour after hour, day after day, and perhaps even for year after year, in the same chair in the same room looking at the same wall (or ceiling if you happen to be seated in a 'tub' chair). Day in and day out, you smell the same unwelcome odours and listen to the same harsh sounds—trolleys clattering, doors slamming, people calling loudly to one another, and, occasionally, the person sitting next to you crying out that she wants to go 'home'. At meal times, strangers talk over the top of you and refer to you as a 'feed' or a 'purée'. They stand over you with a spoon, scooping food from a bowl that contains something that looks like porridge, smells like stew, but curiously tastes like potatoes and peas.

> 'Imagine yourself sitting for hour after hour, day after day, and perhaps even for year after year, in the same chair in the same room looking at the same wall . . .'

Every day these strangers insist that you cooperate with the same rituals (some very embarrassing) to ensure you are 'clean' and 'dry'. In the process, your naked body is exposed to the scrutiny of different men and women who wash and dress you, replacing your familiar and comfortable underwear with a plastic device that they call a 'pad'. You notice that these strangers approach you only when they want to do something to you (Armstrong-Esther, Browne & McAfee 1994; Hallberg, Norberg & Johnsson 1993).

You ache for the loving touch of another, a recognisable voice or sound, a significant fragrance or taste, and a comfortable and certain world. You long for something meaningful to do, rather than an existence filled with long periods of silence and boredom. But these vaguely recalled longings are rarely fulfilled.

In search of a more familiar and safe place, you try to find a way out (Zingmark, Norberg & Sandman 1993). But there is none. Your anger and frustration intensifies, and you are overwhelmed with a desire to protect yourself against some unknown and potentially threatening menace. Frequently, you notice strangers rushing by, and you ask whether they have seen your mother—because you know that when you find her she will rescue you from this barren hostile place (Häggström & Norberg 1996). The strangers tell you to sit down, and promise to return—but they never do. In desperation, you walk the corridors trying to find a safe haven, wherever and whatever that might be.

Although this is not necessarily a description of the lifestyle or environment experienced by all people with dementia, such an existence is not uncommon for a significant number of them.

The nurses' perspective

Many nurses and caregivers hold a quite different perception of the experience described above. Because many believe that people with dementia cannot remember, reason, or relate, it is easy for carers to consider that these people are no longer sentient human beings. In these circumstances, 'caring' becomes nothing more than attending to physical and 'hygiene' requirements, observing safety precautions, and managing so-called 'challenging behaviours'.

The reasons for this view of care practice are complex, and several factors are involved.

First, a significant amount of practice has been framed by the 'stage-theory of decline'. Although it provides some indications of the disease process, and although these can act as useful markers (Marshall 1996), such a theory constructs a view of dementia as a predictable syndrome with a stepwise process of degeneration. Nash (2000, p. 49) has described this view of dementia in the following terms:

> . . . your house [is] filled with lights. Now imagine someone turning off the lights one by one . . . there is no way to stop the lights from turning off, no way to switch them back on once they grow dim.

This view portrays persons with dementia as being terminally ill. Accordingly, their environments and social worlds are of minimal importance. But these people are living and vital people, most of whom remain sentient human beings for some time, and most of whom retain an ability to smile, laugh, and make others feel aware of the joy of life. Dementia care is not about the care of the dying; it is about meaningful life for the living.

'Dementia care is not about the care of the dying; it is about meaningful life for the living.'

A second factor in forming inappropriate views of dementia care practice is the sociotherapeutic model of 'normalisation'—which originated in the 1960s from Wolfensberger's work with intellectually disabled people (ACCS 1996). Care practice underpinned by such principles of 'normalisation' can be problematic. Garratt and Hamilton-Smith (1995) have explained that, from a normalisation perspective, integrating a person with dementia into a 'normal' lifestyle is crucial to care practice. The problem is that the notion of 'normal' is one imposed by those without dementia. As these authors explained, the pathology of dementia involves impairment of cognitive and physical abilities that can make it difficult, if not impossible, for a person with dementia to identify with role models or assume socially acceptable roles. The outcome is that when people with dementia do not behave 'normally', they are accused of exhibiting 'difficult', 'problem', or 'challenging' behaviours.

A third factor that has negatively influenced care practice is the implementation of a policy of highly regulated aged-care legislation, much of which confronts and consumes the commitment of nurses, and much of which serves to reinforce the perception that people with dementia are all similar—thus denying their individual distinctiveness and complexity. Funding arrangements in such highly regulated environments can monopolise care planning and have

> 'When people with dementia do not behave "normally", they are accused of exhibiting "difficult", "problem", or "challenging" behaviours.'

subtle influences on nursing discourse and practice. Under pressure to attract and maintain funding, many nurses write residents' care plans that focus on physical, social, and emotional deficits and that emphasise the need for physical and behavioural 'management' of such deficits. Nurses have little choice in this, because funding arrangements often reward such nursing interventions with greater financial incentives. In contrast, the provision of social, emotional, recreational, and healing care within an enriched sensory environment is accorded the lowest priority and the lowest rate of payment. Residents' care plans thus tend to be written with a view to gaining funding, rather than with a view to the promotion of well-being.

In addition to having a subtle effect on nursing practice, such a legislative and funding environment affects how people with dementia are perceived. The language of bureaucracy places an emphasis on residents' physical and verbal aggression, their abnormal behaviour, and their hygiene needs. Such language conjures up images of older people as deviant and decrepit, and in need of management and containment. The language is devoid of a recognition of the embodied experience, personhood, and humanness of people who are in need of aged-care facilities. As Lawler (1997, p. 45) has pointed out, this kind of language 'is not an authentic nursing discourse but an economically derived dialect that reflects the influence of economic games of truth on nursing'.

Transforming practice
Returning to traditional values

Enriching the sensory environment might seem somewhat removed from current approaches to care, but it actually represents a radical return to the very roots of nursing. For Florence Nightingale (published 1859, reprinted 1970), one of the most important principles of healing was a need to value patients as embodied, unique, and sensate beings. As Light (1997, p. 33) has observed with respect to Nightingale:

> [She] urged nurses to add a variety of colour and beautiful objects to the sickroom, especially with flowers and artwork . . . suggested methods for selecting soothing music . . . gave instructions for selecting and preparing healing foods, and discussed the value of pets in promoting health.

Embracing traditional values in this way helps nurses to rediscover the things that really matter in nursing—to find the inspiration to nurture the essential connection between the sensory world and the mind, body, and spirit of those with dementia. In doing so, nurses shape their own practice and ethics, rather than having such vital nursing issues determined by inappropriate theories or government policy. An alternative framework for shaping clinical practice is in keeping with a return to the traditional nursing values of healing and caring.

An alternative framework for nursing practice
Person-centred care

In their quest to improve the care of people with dementia, Kitwood (1993) and others developed what is commonly referred to as a 'person-centred approach'. Such an approach rejects the notion that dementia can be understood purely in terms of neuropathology or of established stepwise stages of physical and mental decline (Kitwood 1988).

The person-centred perspective challenges the commonly held notion that people with dementia require less social interaction as they deteriorate, and that they do not benefit from enhanced sensory experience and care. Rather, the person-centred approach argues that people with dementia require progressively *more* sensory stimulation, interaction, and human care, and that this helps to preserve their personhood until the moment of death

(Bradford Dementia Group 1997). This view asserts that an interplay of social, cognitive, historical, health, and environmental factors determines how individual persons experience dementia, and rejects the view that dementia is simply a matter of brain pathology of a certain severity and location (Kitwood 1993, 1997).

Person-centred care refers to an acceptance and regard for others in terms of their presence as fellow human beings. From this perspective, improving life for people with dementia ultimately depends on the human bond that develops between residents and staff. It does not depend on building designs or specific furnishings. Nor does it depend on the special effects produced by fancy equipment, as is so often used in sensory-enrichment approaches. However, it has been suggested that to look only at the person without recognising the importance of the environment they exist in and the relationships that support them, may be a limiting perspective (Nolan et al 2001).

> 'Improving life for people with dementia ultimately depends on the human bond that develops between residents and staff.'

Sensation as a source of healing and pleasure

As previously noted, Nightingale (1859/1970) believed that the senses are potential sources of healing and pleasure. Indeed, examples abound of how the healing value and hedonistic pleasure of sensory enrichment have been advocated and practised since antiquity. People have long appreciated good wine and food. The ancient Romans lounged in hot scented baths. Medieval physicians wore perfumed nosebags to shield themselves from the plague. Ancient cave paintings indicate that, even as far back as Palaeolithic civilisation, people enjoyed music and dance (Storr 1992). The Aztecs worshipped chocolate and considered it a gift from the gods (Ackerman 1990). Massage was used as a form of therapeutic touch as far back as 3000 BC (Hanson 1992). Pure essential oils have been used in prayer, rituals, celebrations, and meditation for more than 10 000 years (Newnham 1998).

Against that background, it is heartening to note that many nurses today are showing an increased interest in using sensory and complementary therapies. However, many of these approaches to care are yet to be properly acknowledged and valued.

Mary and Kathleen

Mary was walking with me in the garden one day when she suddenly stopped and commented: 'They grow rosemary here, not roses'. The rose was Mary's favourite flower, and she said that she missed the smell and feel of rose petals. Although she was confused and frequently agitated, Mary knew what flowers and shrubs grew in the unit's garden, and she also knew which ones she liked and which ones she did not.

Another resident, Kathleen, was with her daughter on a windy day. Suddenly, Kathleen stopped, turned her face into the wind and yelled: 'Naughty wind, go away!'. Kathleen then reminded her daughter that, when she was a young girl, she used to shout these words at the wind. For Kathleen, the sensation of the wind on her face transported her back to her childhood and her treasured memories of that time.

For both Mary and Kathleen, their senses provided memories and emotions—some joyous and some sorrowful, but theirs and theirs alone. For these two women, their sensory memories constituted a way of remembering, knowing about, and being in and of this world.

Valuing sensation for people with dementia

Although people with dementia might not sense in the same way that they did before the onset of their illness, they still perceive the world around them from the information gathered via their senses. Like all people, people with dementia perceive the current world through their senses, and are connected to their past world through the same senses. Although the memories evoked by sensory experience might not be as precise as they once were, they remain authentic and meaningful to the person involved, as illustrated by the stories in the Box above.

Implementing enriched environments
Simple strategies

Enriching the sensory experience of people with dementia does not necessarily require the purchase of expensive equipment (Willcocks 1994) or the preparation of special areas or rooms (Ellis & Thorn 2000). On the contrary, the following sorts of everyday simple events can enrich the sensory experience:

▸ the aroma of coffee percolating, fresh bread baking, or toast cooking;
▸ the sight of an interesting wall mural or pleasant garden area;
▸ enjoying favourite music or food;
▸ taking part in creative movement and dancing; walking in the park;
▸ singing, painting, creative writing, and poetry;
▸ enjoying pets and dolls; building bird feeders and feeding the birds;

- aromatherapy; a gentle hand massage;
- playfulness, humour, and storytelling;
- sitting around and chatting over a cup of tea; enjoying dining seated in the company of staff;
- meaningful work and leisure activities (such as washing a car; polishing furniture, shoes or silverware; and folding fresh washing still warm from hanging in the sunshine).

All of these simple activities are potential sources of pleasurable sensations. However, if they are to be truly effective in promoting residents' well-being, it is essential that nurses are committed to the value of these simple activities, and that they hold a genuine respect for the uniqueness of the person with dementia who shares in them.

More complex strategies

The Dutch word Snoezelen refers to an approach and practice that involves enriching the senses within a specially designed room. For readers who are

---

Snoezelen in action

The first room, a small activity area, was converted by dimming overhead lighting and covering windows to decrease external stimuli. The equipment purchased for the room included 200 fibre-optic strands that glowed in the dark and changed colour rhythmically, a vertical 'bubble-tube', and a suspended mirror ball that turned slowly and projected small colourful images across the ceilings and walls. A colour wheel that projected changing abstract patterns across one wall was added, and a music player, an aromatherapy burner, and various tactile and interactive aids were placed strategically around the room.

A similar approach was extended to a bathroom in the unit in which students of the local high school volunteered to create a special mural across one wall. The ceiling was draped with a large commercial fishing-net and decorated with fish and seashell mobiles. Like the activity room, the bathroom was filled with sensory equipment and aids—including aromatic shampoos, bath toys, massage sponges, and thick, soft bathrobes and towels.

Audiocassette tapes to be used in sensory sessions were recorded in accordance with the musical preferences of each resident. Staff assisted by finding out which favourite foods, beverages, photographs, soft toys, and precious possessions would be most enjoyed by each resident.

More than eighty sessions were undertaken in the sensory rooms. Several were group sessions that included two or three residents. In some cases, family members of residents joined in.

interested in a fuller explanation, this subject is explored in greater detail in Chapter 22, page 278. For the present, the Box below provides an indication of how it works.

Nurses who consider providing environments of this kind need to be sensitive to cues from residents indicating pleasure, boredom, discomfort, frustration, and so on. Enriching the sensory environment is not a panacea, and a certain set of interventions will not necessarily evoke the same responses from everyone, or even the same responses from any given person on different occasions. Careful and sensitive monitoring of responses is essential to appropriate care.

Being of their world
Story-telling

Story-telling is an important part of sensory enrichment. Stories are 'a way we try and make sense of our world' (Sutton & Cheston 1997, p. 159) and, for people with dementia, stories provide a means of reconstructing their identity (Crisp 1995). One resident's story might be of herself as the concerned daughter who nursed her parents. Another resident's story might be of himself as a son much loved by his mother. Another resident might speak in terms of herself as a mother and protector of young children. All of these residents are telling stories about themselves from their past worlds, and their significance in those worlds.

Walton and Madjar (1999, p. 6) have proposed that 'nurses learn from their own stories and from others' experiences, and [that] they remember important lessons through the stories they tell and hear others tell'. However, apart from the sort of opportunity afforded them in sensory rooms, residents are usually denied an opportunity to tell their stories, and thus to reconstruct their identities. After sensory sessions, nurses and caregivers often express a sense of surprise when, after having tended to people for some time, those same people are suddenly revealed to them for the first time.

A playful attitude

The development of a playful attitude and humour can become evident in many sensory sessions. People can be encouraged to seize the magic of the moment and delight in the uninhibited experience of playing with soft toys, hand puppets, bath ducks, ocean drums, and whatever else takes their fancy—free of the usual constraints about what others might think of such behaviour. In sensory sessions with the residents, staff members can allow their own childlike spirits to come to the fore, and can engage residents in playful activities.

Conversely, residents can show staff how to enjoy playful moments in their lives. Staff members often comment on how playful sessions make them 'feel great' for the rest of the day. In the same way, residents often communicate their pleasure and enjoyment of playful encounters.

Dolls, music and massage are technologically simple and readily available aids in such sessions. These and other sensory tools encourage playfulness and provide pleasure for residents, both within and outside the sensory rooms. Family members who recognise the significance of these simple items can purchase dolls for their relatives so that they can enjoy carrying them or cuddling them outside the sensory rooms.

In aged and dementia care, the focus is often on streamlining and programming 'care' such that more tasks can be accomplished with fewer human resources. Technical and mechanical interventions that reduce opportunities for human contact play a large part in such 'care'. It is little wonder that, in such an atmosphere, few see a need to encourage a playful attitude within an enriched sensory and social environment. But play, and having a playful attitude, are crucial to wholeness and humanness (Adams & Mylander 1993), As such, they are central to nursing.

Sounds and aromatic massage

In contrast to becoming distressed by the often harsh sounds of institutional life, a resident is likely to talk about special sensory music 'touching my heart'. Such sounds help people to remember particular places, events, and people. In the sensory rooms, people sit, close their eyes, and drift into a state of repose as they listen to their favourite music.

In a similar way, aromatic massage produces therapeutic effects. This can be of particular significance for residents who are restless and in need of constant motion. Such people can succumb to deep muscle relaxation and drift off to sleep with only a few minutes of massage. Some residents prefer to caress the hands and faces of staff. All of this can occur with residents who have never previously indicated any need to touch or be touched in such a manner.

Respect and affection

The need for residents to love and be loved is often expressed in spoken and unspoken ways during such sessions. Precious memories, respect, and affection often emerge as being essential to well-being. The personal qualities of caregivers can determine how such sessions unfold, and how residents respond.

Making use of facilities

Although sessions in a sensory room can provide residents and staff with special moments of togetherness, limited time and staff numbers are a reality. This means that this kind of approach is often difficult to sustain.

It is not uncommon that expensively furnished sensory rooms can become storerooms that are cleaned out and put on show when visitors arrive or accreditation looms. This is a pity. Sensory bathrooms are places that can be used effectively every day. During bathing sessions, nurses have an opportunity to assess residents' skin integrity and many other issues of physical and functional care. Bathing sessions also promote deep relaxation, and provide an opportunity for residents to express their experience of pain or feelings of depression.

However, special sensory rooms, in isolation, do not promote well-being for people with dementia. The sensory and social quality of the everyday lived environment, and the way in which staff value the person-hood of individual residents, are the real determinants of whether people with dementia will experience a rich and meaningful life.

'The way in which staff value the personhood of individual residents, are the real determinants of whether people with dementia will experience a rich and meaningful life.'

Conclusion

The 'kippers and curtains' cultural perspective introduced at the beginning of this chapter is a salutary warning that, regardless of the quality of the built and furnished environment, it is what happens inside the boundaries of that environment that determines the quality of life experienced by people with dementia. The creation of an enriched everyday environment, complemented with special sensory areas, can help nurses to appreciate the real personhood of people with dementia. This enables staff to see these people as sentient and special individuals, and thus facilitates genuine care and concern for them.

By returning to traditional nursing values and enriching the sensory and social environment, nurses working with people with dementia can create a world within which these people can find comfort and pleasure, express their individuality, and rediscover human connection.

Chapter 5

Memory Loss

Jane Hecker

Introduction

Memory loss is a common complaint as people grow older. Memory function involves the ability to perceive something, the ability to register this perception, the ability to encode and store the memory, and the ability to retrieve this information at a later date. As people age, most suffer some decline in memory, especially in their ability to recall recent information, but this healthy ageing does not significantly interfere with normal function in the everyday lives of most people. With increasing age some brain-processing functions become slower, especially the ability to store new information or recall some previously stored memories, but long-term recall and other cognitive processes do not change significantly as people become older. For individuals with dementia, memory loss is more persistent and progressive, and has a greater impact on their daily activities. The speed of their forgetting is usually very rapid, often within seconds, and this can cause great frustration for the people affected and those around them. Other cognitive processes—including language, perception, and problem-solving—are also impaired, and this can lead to confusion and disorientation. The behaviour and personality of the person are also often affected, resulting in impaired insight, reasoning, and judgment.

Classification of memory

Memory can be divided into three major types:
- *procedural memory*—the recall of routine activities and procedures (for example, riding a bicycle or brushing teeth);
- *semantic memory*—memory of facts and figures, and the categorisation or grouping of items; and
- *episodic memory*—memory of events or details specific to a person's life.

The retrieval of facts and information depends on *semantic* and *episodic* memory, and these are the types of memory most affected by dementia. *Procedural memory* includes many deeply learned and semi-automatic activities, and this is better preserved—especially if it is stimulated by appropriate triggers. Information that has some emotional content and relevance is more likely to be recalled. Loss of memory can appear to onlookers to be selective and under voluntary control, and this can produce antagonistic feelings in caregivers, family members, and professional staff. However, an understanding of the process of memory loss can help to avoid such negative feelings.

Memory loss in dementia

Dementia causes an inability to recognise or remember information despite prompting. In addition, the affected person lacks insight into the impairment. Many of the changes in behaviour of afflicted persons can be understood as being a direct consequence of their attempts to make sense of the environment in the face of these losses. These behavioural changes include:
- difficulty with learning new information;
- disorientation in time, place, and person;
- repetitive questioning;
- misplacing items;
- confabulation (that is, making up stories to fit the known pieces of information);
- paranoia; and
- anxiety and agitation due to feelings of insecurity.

An understanding of the origin of these problems can help nurses to acknowledge the validity of residents' feelings, and can enable staff to address the situation more positively. A failure to recognise these deficits—

'Nurses should always be aware that even when a person's capacity for memory and cognitive processing is markedly impaired, he or she still retains a capacity for feeling.'

as can easily occur if the person appears otherwise normal—leads to unrealistic expectations of the person's ability. Nurses should always be aware that even when a person's capacity for memory and cognitive processing is markedly impaired, he or she still retains a capacity for feeling.

Causes of memory loss

Most people in residential care are affected by memory loss. A better understanding of this problem can assist nurses in their efforts to improve management and reduce undesirable outcomes. Accurate assessment and diagnosis of memory disorders is the first step.

The causes of memory loss include:

▶ age-related decline in memory;
▶ cognitive impairment secondary to other medical or psychiatric problems—including delirium, infection, cardiac failure, respiratory failure, hypoxia, traumatic brain injury, depression, anxiety, other psychiatric disorders, and drugs (including prescribed medications and alcohol);
▶ progressive dementing illnesses—including Alzheimer's disease, vascular dementia, dementia with Lewy bodies, fronto-temporal dementia, alcohol-related dementia, and Parkinson's disease.

It is often difficult to distinguish between age-associated memory loss and early dementia. There is overlap between the two, and change is very gradual. A detailed medical assessment, including standardised testing of memory and cognition, is required for the assessment of significant memory loss. Some types of memory loss are reversible, and treatments are now available for progressive memory loss in some diseases, including Alzheimer's disease.

Medical assessment of memory loss

Dementia is less common than age-related decline in memory, and the diagnosis of dementia is based on certain recognised criteria. No single test is diagnostic in itself. Because there is overlap among the signs caused by age-associated changes, mild cognitive impairment, and dementia, diagnosis is based on a combination of the following information:

▶ history-taking—especially from a close contact who has known the person for some time);
▶ physical examination;
▶ formal cognitive testing—for example, the Mini-Mental State Examination Score (MMSE);
▶ laboratory investigation—including blood tests; and
▶ brain-imaging of various types—including (i) scans of brain *structure*, such as computerised tomography (CT) or magnetic resonance imaging (MRI); and (ii) scans of brain *function*, such as single-photon emission computed tomography (SPECT) or positron emission tomography (PET).

There are certain features that help to distinguish memory loss due to early Alzheimer's disease from that due to ageing. Signs of Alzheimer's disease include the following:

▶ a significant decline in the ability of a person to acquire new information (that is, evidence of poor learning across repeat trials);
▶ an impaired ability to recall information after a delay (that is, a rapid rate of forgetting);
▶ a failure to retrieve memories despite prompting;
▶ a significant impact on the person's daily activities; and
▶ associated impairment of other cognitive skills (including language, perception, and the ability to carry out effective practical action).

Differential diagnosis of dementia

Delirium

Delirium can usually be distinguished from dementia. Delirium is characterised by rapid onset and short duration. There is a clouding of consciousness, with reduced awareness and fluctuating alertness. Other features commonly associated with delirium include motor restlessness, hallucinations (especially visual), and sleep disturbance. A specific cause for delirium can usually be detected, although this is not always the case. Common causes include infective episodes (especially chest infections and urinary tract infections), centrally acting drugs, and dehydration.

'Delirium is characterised by rapid onset and short duration.'

There is a large number of medications that can precipitate cognitive decline or delirium, especially those that have anticholinergic properties. Indeed, about half of all cases of so-called 'reversible dementia' result from the effects of drugs or depression, and this should be kept in mind in assessing older people with cognitive impairment. Older people with reduced brain reserves are sensitive to centrally acting agents, including antipsychotics, benzodiazepines, antidepressants, anticholinergics, anti-Parkinsonian drugs, and antihistamines. The cognitive impairment that results from these drug effects might present as a chronic brain syndrome rather than an acute brain syndrome, and improvement following drug withdrawal can take weeks.

Delirium and dementia can co-exist. Although an acute confusional episode on admission might be explained by medical illness or recent surgery, nurses should be aware that this episode might also be an early sign that this person has underlying dementia.

Other psychological disorders

Many psychological disorders can mimic dementia. These include depression, anxiety, mania, schizophrenia, and hysteria. These conditions are frequently called 'pseudo-dementia' and are often treatable.

Depression is the most common cause of pseudo-dementia. However, because the presenting signs and symptoms of dementia and depression are often similar, it can be difficult to distinguish between the two. For example, depression can present with memory loss, poor concentration, apathy, neglect, changes in activity levels (increased or decreased), sleep disturbance, fatigue, changes in eating habits, and changes in weight. All or most of these are also seen in dementia.

'Because the presenting signs and symptoms of dementia and depression are often similar, it can be difficult to distinguish between the two.'

This difficulty in sorting out the presenting signs and symptoms can be compounded by the fact that depression can co-exist with dementia, especially in the earlier stages of dementia when insight is retained. Depression is usually under-treated in the elderly, and a trial of antidepressant therapy is indicated if there is any doubt. However, many elderly people who initially respond to antidepressant therapy can subsequently develop the progressive impairment that is typical of dementia.

Factors that exacerbate memory changes
Checklist

In assessing and managing memory loss, nurses should look for certain factors that can exacerbate memory deficits in the people under their care.

Checklist of exacerbating factors in memory loss

In assessing and managing memory loss, nurses should look for the following in the people in their care. All of the following can easily be overlooked:

* constipation and urinary retention;
* acute illness (especially infections of the urinary tract and chest);
* dehydration;
* pain (especially in those who cannot vocalise or who cannot clearly describe pain and physical discomfort);
* hallucinations and delusional thought;
* poor eyesight (or inappropriate or dirty glasses) and impaired hearing (or hearing aids not worn, turned off, or with flat batteries);
* lack of sleep, stress, depressed mood, boredom, frustration;
* excessive alcohol; and
* effects of medication.

The Box above lists some of the more common exacerbating factors that might otherwise go undetected unless alert staff are aware of their potential to cause memory impairment.

Medications

As noted above (see 'Delirium', page 47), the side-effects of medications are a particular problem in exacerbating memory deficits in the elderly. Older people, particularly those with liver or renal impairment, metabolise drugs slowly. The elderly are more sensitive to the central brain effects of drugs, and these effects are exacerbated in people with dementia or memory loss.

Responsible use of medication is critical in residential-care facilities. Drugs should be used to treat symptoms and improve quality of life for residents, and not for the purposes of chemical restraint.

'Drugs should be used to treat symptoms and improve quality of life for residents, and not for the purposes of chemical restraint.'

Anticholinergics

Many drugs used in treating the elderly block the the brain chemical acetylcholine, and these 'anticholinergic' drugs are especially likely to cause confusion. In addition to those listed below (which have an especially marked anticholinergic effect), many other drugs have a less significant anticholinergic effect, and nurses should therefore be alert to the possibility that other drugs might also cause problems in this regard. Those with an especially marked anticholinergic effect include:

▶ drugs used in the treatment of bladder instability—such as oxybutynin (Ditropan), propantheline (Pro-Banthine), and similar drugs;

▶ anticholinergic drugs used in the treatment of Parkinson's disease and extrapyramidal reactions—such as benztropine (Cogentin), and benzhexol (Artane);

▶ tricyclic antidepressants—such as amitriptyline (Tryptanol, Endep), imipramine (Tofranil), doxepin (Sinequan, Deptran), and dothiepin (Prothidaen, Dothep);

▶ older antipsychotics—such as pericyazine (Neulactil), thioridazine (Melleril, Aldazine), chlorpromazine (Largactil), fluphenazine (Modecate), and trifluoperazine (Stelazine); and the related antiemetic prochlorperazine (Stemetil); and

▶ antispasmodics such as hyoscine (Atrobel, Donnatabs, Buscopan) and dicyclomine (Merbentyl).

Other drugs

Other drugs that have a central brain effect can cause confusion. These include:

▶ benzodiazepines used as anxiolytics (tranquillisers) and hypnotics (sleeping tablets)—such as diazepam (Valium, Ducene), clonazepam (Rivotril), oxazepam (Serepax. Murelax), nitrazepam (Mogadon), temazepam (Normison, Euhypnos. Temaze), and alprazolam (Xanax);

▶ other sedative agents—such as zopiclone (Imovane), zolpidem (Ambien; Stilnox), and buspirone (Buspar);

▶ drugs used in treating Parkinson's disease—such as levodopa (Madopar, Sinemet), selegiline (Eldepryl, Selgene), pergolide (Permax), cabergoline (Cabaser), and entacapone (Comtan);

▶ narcotic analgesics—such as morphine, pethidine, codeine, oxycodone (Endone), dextropropoxyphene (Digesic, Doloxene), and fentanyl (Durogesic); and

▶ various antihistamines.

Treatment of memory disorders
Non-pharmaceutical techniques

Environmental aids and techniques can minimise the impact of memory loss. A balance is necessary between stimulation (that enhances function and provides enjoyment) and over-stimulation (that overwhelms people with activities and causes frustration).

People with dementia lose skills in the reverse order to which they were acquired, and knowledge of this can be used to therapeutic advantage by focusing on retained skills. Creative solutions can often be found to daily problems, and adapting the environment is often easier than attempting to change the person. Creating a sense of usefulness and achievement can be a challenge for nurses in caring for people with dementia. However, it must be remembered that the disease does not remove a person's need for a sense of belonging and importance.

> 'People with dementia lose skills in the reverse order to which they were acquired.'

The following principles and hints are useful in planning activities.

Respecting individuality

- Consider individual interests and needs when structuring activities and daily routine. Knowledge of past habits and interests can aid in structuring a program that has meaning.
- Maintain a positive view of retained skills and qualities rather than a negative approach based on deficits.
- Validate residents' memories and feelings. Allow time for communication and listen attentively. Body language and eye contact can demonstrate empathy.
- Be sensitive to residents' cultural background.

Working as a team

- Work as a team with other staff members, discussing novel approaches and the success or failure of various strategies.
- Communicate with family members and learn from their long-standing knowledge of the person.

General approach

- A calm, gentle, and consistent approach aids in the development of the trust that is essential to successful caregiving. Avoid criticism.
- Focus on participation and enjoyment, rather than achievement.
- Minimise distractions and keep to one activity when performing a task. Concentration is needed to register information.
- Build on retained abilities and strengths. Exploit procedural memory

(which is relatively preserved) because this can enable people with dementia to continue performing semi-automatic and routine activities that can bring pleasure. Examples include singing, dancing, walking, and personal-care activities. Old music and songs, if tailored to an individual's taste, can provide various levels of participation and joy, even in severe dementia.

▶ Keeping to old routines and habits for basic activities can make life easier. Learning new techniques and patterns is far more difficult. Provide meaningful consistent cues. Consistency of staffing is also helpful—people respond better to staff whom they know and trust.

▶ Give choices in appropriate situations to provide people with some sense of mastery and control.

▶ In caring for people with severe dementia, avoid challenging the patient's sense of reality; rather, acknowledge this with empathy, thus fostering a sense of security and trust.

▶ Allow plenty of time and do not overload with planned activities. It is easy to become flustered if under time pressure. Too much or too little stimulation can both result in poor performance.

▶ Communication should be simple, provided at a slow speed, and deal with one concept at a time. Use of gesture can reinforce verbal information. Repetition of information is often necessary. Remember the impact of non-verbal communication including tone of voice.

▶ Adjust expectations to observed abilities—many behavioural problems are due to excessive demands and unrealistic expectations.

▶ People with dementia often tend to perseverate (that is, repeat activities). Providing a simple overlearned procedural task of some meaning to the patient (for example, sweeping, or folding linen) can provide a sense of achievement and distract from other less desirable behaviours.

▶ Keep a sense of humour! We all forget things at times, and making light of it helps to keep things in perspective and reduces anxiety associated with perceived failure.

▶ Remember that enjoyment does not require memory!

Practical hints

▶ Defects in new learning make it difficult to adjust to a new environment. Provision of familiar items in the personal environment provides reassurance. Clothes, furniture, photographs, and personal mementos can help orientate and focus residents. Because recall is focused on the past, the provision of gadgets that fit the past (for example, an old telephone) can help with recognition and function; in contrast new equipment might fail to provoke a response.

▶ In mild impairment, prompts (a good diary, calendar, or notebook) can be useful. Keep a diary of all the person's appointments and social arrangements.

▶ For people who retain the ability to use a telephone, keep a list of important numbers in a prominent place and program important numbers into the telephone for easy dialling.

▶ Orientate in time by prominent clocks and calendars. Newspapers also help to orientate regarding dates and local information. Reality orientation is especially useful in the earlier phases of illness.

▶ Assist orientation to rooms with labelling and other recognisable cues. Leave the toilet door open to provide additional visual stimulus.

▶ Information boards that provide details of activities, recent events, or celebrations are useful. Simple written reminders can be helpful, and pictures can replace written information for people who are unable to read.

▶ Organise belongings. Keep important items (keys, wallets, handbags, bankbooks, and so on) in a consistent place so they do not become misplaced.

▶ Reminiscence helps to preserve identity and self-esteem by recalling past memories and achievements and provides a way to communicate emotion. Use cues or symbols to prompt memories of positive aspects of former life. Old photographs, newspapers, books, magazines, and memorabilia provide useful prompts for reminiscence and help staff to understand the person for whom they are caring. Compiling an album of chronological life history together with photographs provides a basis for discussion with visitors and staff. Celebration of special occasions and festivals or association with music, food, and even odours can provide sensory triggers for reminiscence.

▶ Organising a visitor's book for recording visits by family and friends with details of activities can prompt recall of these occasions. A board or book containing photographs and names of family and friends can also aid recall and discussion.

Pharmacological treatment

Drug treatments for memory disorders have three possible applications:

▶ prevention of Alzheimer's disease;

▶ improvement in cognitive and functional symptoms; and

▶ treatment for behavioural and psychological symptoms
   Each of these is discussed below.

Prevention of dementia

There is no clear evidence that drugs have a role in the prevention of dementia, although research is investigating the potential benefit of certain substances, including the cholinesterase inhibitors, vitamin E, anti-inflammatory drugs, oestrogen (in women), and folate.

Hypertension has been linked to an increased risk of developing Alzheimer's disease. It is already known that high blood pressure causes vascular disease, and the possible link between hypertension and dementia lends further support to the importance of careful blood pressure control. There is also some evidence that people with dementia who have also had a stroke or transient ischaemic attack do better in terms of cognitive performance if they receive anti-hypertensive therapy, even if their baseline blood pressure is not elevated.

Improvement in cognitive and functional symptoms
Cholinesterase inhibitors

Cholinesterase inhibitors are the only approved drug therapy for people with dementia. These drugs include donepezil (Aricept), rivastigmine (Exelon), and galantamine (Reminyl). The drugs are mainly used in the treatment of dementia that is due to mild to moderate Alzheimer's disease. Their use in more severe Alzheimer's disease and their use in dementia due to other diseases (including age-related memory loss) is not yet established. On their initial launch in the UK, the anti-dementia drugs were not available under NHS prescriptions for all patients and there were regional variations as to whether patients were prescribed the drugs by the NHS, depending upon local policy. The position was reviewed by the National Institute for Clinical Excellence (NICE) and since January 2001 the drugs have fallen under national guidelines making them much more widely available.

As noted above (see 'Anticholinergics', page 49), acetylcholine is a neurotransmitter chemical that is important in memory and cognition. Cholinesterase inhibitors block the breakdown of this chemical, and this facilitates neurotransmission. This might help to improve the function of surviving brain cells and pathways, but it does not prevent ongoing neuronal degeneration. Cholinesterase inhibitors do not cure the disease, do not prevent disease progression, and are not effective in all patients. In general, 50–70% of people who are treated with these drugs achieve some symptomatic response. This might be an improvement in cognitive or behavioural symptoms or a stabilisation of disease progression. In view of the progressive nature of Alzheimer's disease, a 'successful' treatment might well be one that simply delays progression of symptoms, rather than actually improving cognition.

Before prescribing cholinesterase inhibitors, certain factors should be carefully checked. The Box on page 55 provides an important checklist.

To minimise side-effects, treatment should commence with the lowest dose. The effects of these drugs are closely related to the size of the dose. Therefore, after starting with the lowest dose, gradual dose titration is undertaken to the maximum tolerated dose.

The cholinesterase inhibitors are generally well tolerated. The most common side-effects are gastrointestinal symptoms. These include nausea, diarrhoea, anorexia, vomiting, and abdominal pain. Non-specific side-effects can include headache, fatigue, insomnia, dizziness, tremor, and muscle cramps. Urinary symptoms, especially urinary urgency and incontinence, have been reported. Some people occasionally develop agitation, hallucinations, and vivid distressing dreams. The dreams can be reduced by administering medication in the morning rather than the evening. All of these side-effects respond to a lowering of the dose (or cessation of the drug if necessary).

The medication should be stopped if:

▶ there are intolerable side-effects;

▶ the person's Alzheimer's disease progresses to a stage where he or she is fully dependent on others for basic living activities;

▶ the ongoing benefit of treatment is deemed questionable by the clinician or family caregiver;

Checklist before starting cholinesterase inhibitors

Before any person is started on cholinesterase inhibitors, the following should be carefully checked:

- a thorough assessment of the person and accurate diagnosis of Alzheimer's disease by a specialist physician or psychiatrist.
- a careful assessment that the person is medically stable, because people with certain systemic illnesses are unsuitable (for example, those with bradycardia, heart block, asthma, and active peptic ulcer);
- a check of other medications being taken by the person and cessation of any anticholinergic drugs (see list of some of these drugs, page 50);
- counselling of the person and family regarding realistic expectations of the benefits and risks, and identifying relevant treatment goals;
- ensuring that careful compliance is guaranteed (administration of medication by a suitable person and adequate verbal and written instructions for administration); and
- careful baseline cognitive assessment using scales such as the Mini-Mental State Examination Score (MMSE), and repeat cognitive testing at suitable intervals to demonstrate improvement on the measurement scales used.

▶ despite treatment compliance, there is the same steady rate of decline as before treatment;

▶ there is acceleration in the rate of decline in mood, cognition, function, or behaviour (not explicable by an inter-current illness).

Other pharmacological therapy

Some other pharmaceutical agents have been suggested as possible treatments to assist in cognitive enhancement. However, the evidence regarding the effectiveness of these agents is either insufficient or contradictory. These possible treatments include vitamin E, gingko biloba, oestrogen, folate, and anti-inflammatory drugs.

Amyloid metabolism is thought to play a central role in the development of dementia, and research is therefore being undertaken into the possibility of using certain drugs in this area.

Effectiveness of treatment

The clinical significance of these treatment outcomes is debated, and research is continuing. A minority of patients treated with these agents do show a significant level of improvement. Commonly reported responses include improvement in attentiveness and alertness, greater involvement in conversation, increased initiation of the activities of daily living, and improvement in behavioural symptoms.

'Commonly reported responses include improvement in attentiveness and alertness, greater involvement in conversation, increased initiation of the activities of daily living, and improvement in behavioural symptoms.'

Additional benefits include a delay in the emergence of behavioural symptoms and sleep disturbance. It also appears that less time is required of caregivers in prompting and assisting people with Alzheimer's disease. There also appears to be a preservation of function in daily living activities. These measurable functions suggest that the general quality of life of Alzeheimer's sufferers is likely to be improved, but this has not been conclusively proven.

Treatment for behavioural and psychological symptoms

Changes in personality and behaviour are common in people with Alzheimer's disease, and can become very significant in the moderate and severe stages of dementia. There are many causes of these behavioural changes. These include:

- neurobiological causes (neurochemical changes and neuropathology);
- psychological causes (pre-morbid personality, response to stress); and
- social causes (environmental change, caregiver factors).

There is great individual variation in both the occurrence and the severity of behavioural symptoms, but they are often extremely disruptive to patients and caregivers. They result in reduced quality of life and increased costs of care.

Research in this area is in its infancy, but there is some evidence that certain neurochemical and neuropathological changes are linked to certain specific symptoms. Symptoms can be related to specific areas of cerebral pathology and to specific deficiencies in brain biochemistry involving acetylcholine, dopamine, noradrenalin, serotonin, and glutamate.

A thorough assessment should include identification of the specific problem behaviour, documentation of relevant antecedent factors, and a careful search for any medical illness or other factors that might be contributing to the behaviour (including physical symptoms, sensory deficits, and drug side-effects or interactions). Agitation and other behavioural symptoms should be assessed carefully for identifiable causes—such as pain, faecal impaction, urinary retention, fatigue, and associated environmental triggers.

Before beginning drug therapy, non-pharmacological approaches should be tried. Extensive training for family and professional caregivers can improve overall function, reduce the frequency and impact of behavioural symptoms, and reduce stress for caregivers. Educational training for staff in residential-care facilities can decrease the use of antipsychotic medication without increasing the rate of disruptive behaviour. Behaviour modification, scheduled toileting, and prompted voiding can reduce urinary incontinence in people with dementia. Graded assistance, skills practice, and positive reinforcement can increase functional independence. Low-level lighting, music (of the persons's preference), and simulated nature sounds can improve eating behaviours and reduce agitation, aggression, and other difficult behaviours. Comprehensive educational training, support groups, and respite services for caregivers can delay the need for placement in residential care.

'Comprehensive educational training, support groups, and respite services for caregivers can delay the need for placement in residential care.'

If a non-pharmacologic strategy is not effective, and if the symptoms remain moderately distressing to the person, family, or professional caregivers, pharmacological treatment can be considered. A set of guidelines for drug treatment of behavioural and psychological symptoms of dementia is provided in the Box below.

When choosing a therapeutic agent, consideration should be given to the side-effect profile of a drug and evidence that the drug is likely to be effective for specific behavioural symptoms. In general, elderly patients with dementia are more sensitive than other people to centrally acting drugs, and the dosages of medication required are therefore significantly lower. It is important to begin treatment with a low dose and to increase the dose slowly. Regular review of both effectiveness and any adverse effects is important.

There is relatively little clinical trial evidence to support the use of antipsychotic agents in the treatment of dementia. The widely fluctuating natural history of these problems means that research into treatments for behavioural symptoms is often inconclusive. It remains difficult to establish whether a medication has actually produced a positive result, or whether this might have occurred anyway.

'There is relatively little clinical trial evidence to support the use of antipsychotic agents in the treatment of dementia.'

Guidelines for drug treatment of behavioural symptoms

In treating any person with medications for distressing behavioural and psychological symptoms of Alzheimer's disease, the following guidelines should be followed:

- identify and evaluate target symptoms;
- exclude other causes (physical illness, drugs, and so on);
- treat symptoms that are distressing and/or dangerous to the person or caregivers;
- treat symptoms that are responsive to drug therapy—delusions, hallucinations, agitation, aggression, depression;
- take into account the fact that people with dementia are sensitive to centrally acting drugs;
- avoid drugs with anticholinergic effect (because of increased risk of confusion);
- start with a low dose (30–50% of usual adult starting dose);
- titrate gradually and allow time for steady state to develop;
- be aware of pharmacology, side-effect profile, and potential drug interactions;
- avoid multiple centrally acting drugs;
- reassess frequently and monitor response; and
- withdraw therapy for trial after 3–6 months (or sooner if no apparent benefit).

Table 5.1 Drugs available for Alzheimer's disease

	Donepezil	Rivastigmine	Galantamine
Structure	piperidine	carbamate	tertiary alkaloid (daffodil derivative)
Mechanism of action	reversible	pseudo-irreversible	reversible
Half-life	70 hours	plasma 2 hours duration action 10 hours	5–6 hours
Elimination	renal and hepatic	renal	hepatic metabolism
Drug interactions	low potential	low potential	low potential
Dosage frequency	daily	twice daily	twice daily
Starting dose	5 mg	1.5 mg twice daily	4 mg twice daily
Administration	tablet	capsule (with food)	tablet (with food)
Maximum dose	10 mg daily	6 mg twice daily	12 mg twice daily
Recommended titration	increase to 10 mg at 4–6 weeks	titration steps every 4 weeks: 3 mg twice daily 4.5 mg twice daily 6 mg twice daily	titration steps every 4 weeks to 8 mg twice daily

Author's presentation

Table 5.1 (above) lists some drugs that can be used in the treatment of Alzheimer's disease.

Conclusion

Changes in memory and cognition are very common in older people, especially in those who are living in residential care. Effective strategies to improve the function and quality of life of these people depend upon an understanding of the nature and cause of the changes, and a careful assessment of their memory deficits and retained skills. It is important to look for causative factors that might be reversed, and to consider non-pharmaceutical techniques to support function in memory loss. A knowledge of the newer drug treatments, including likely benefits and risks, is an advantage in caring for people with memory loss and dementia.

Chapter 6

Nutrition

Mary Marshall

Food is essential to life and is one of life's great pleasures, but eating and nutrition can be problematic and a source of stress to people with dementia and those who care for them. This chapter considers the factors that play a part in this problem, and suggests some practical approaches to alleviating the difficulties.

Every pathway through dementia is different. Each person with dementia is unique, as are those who care for them, and the settings in which they find themselves are all different. No single prescribed approach will be appropriate to every situation, and this chapter therefore makes suggestions, rather than prescribing what to do. The only general injunction that can be made is that there is no substitute for a positive approach and genuine empathy.

This chapter considers the following ten factors that play a part in producing problems with mealtimes:

- communication;
- lack of cues;
- noise;
- stress;
- drugs;
- visual impairments;

- sore mouth;
- brain damage;
- profound disability; and
- staffing issues.

Communication

What are people with dementia trying to say when they refuse food? Behaviour is a means of communication for people with dementia, and it is important to attempt to understand what they are trying to say.

Food refusal can take many forms. People with dementia might turn their heads away, spit food out, refuse to swallow, or throw their food on the floor. Because verbal communication is difficult or impossible, emotions such as powerlessness,

'Behaviour is a means of communication for people with dementia, and it is important to attempt to understand what they are trying to say.'

unhappiness, and anger are being communicated by these behaviours. However, responding to the feelings behind such food refusal is not easy for carers.

Carers can also use food to communicate with people with dementia. It is to be hoped that they communicate love and care. However, when they are busy it is easy for carers to convey messages that these people are a nuisance, unattractive, slow, or irritating. In this way, carers themselves can communicate powerlessness, unhappiness, and anger. Mealtimes can easily become hasty, careless affairs in which neither side is really listening to the other.

There are numerous ways to make people feel more in control. One way is to offer a choice—such as two alternatives on separate plates. Opportunities can also be provided for people to help with food pre-

'Carers can also use food to communicate with people with dementia.'

paration or to set tables. The story of Stan (Box, page 62) illustrates a remarkable transformation.

Recognising unhappiness and offering comfort is the first step towards caring for an unhappy person. Sometimes this might simply mean offering food in comforting ways. The loving care provided to Maisie shows the significance of this simple act (Box, page 62).

Stan

Stan was a big, aggressive man who lived in a long-stay ward. He was perpetually angry; at mealtimes he used to shout and push the table away. He was moved into a small domestic-style unit with an integral kitchen. The staff came to know him better and to understand that he had been an officer in the armed forces who was used to being in charge. He took charge of serving the tea and washing up afterwards. His anger diminished and he became a much-loved member of the group.

Maisie

Maisie's husband died in the nursing home. For several weeks afterwards, Maisie did not seem to understand that he had gone. Then she stopped eating. She would eat only in the arms of her favourite member of staff while warmed mashed food was spooned lovingly into her mouth.

Lack of cues

Many people with dementia need cues before they are ready to eat. As cognition deteriorates, people increasingly rely on their senses to provide appropriate cues for particular activities such as eating, so it is necessary for carers to stimulate as many senses as possible.

Aroma

Appetites are whetted by the smell of food as it is being cooked, or by the aroma of food as it wafts out of the kitchen. However, in many care settings these cues are not available. Food is often pre-cooked before being warmed up in the residential unit, or it might be brought in on trolleys under lids. In many cases, the food itself has very little aroma.

The cue of smell might be an explanation of why many people with dementia enjoy a cooked breakfast more than any other meal—because there are few more appetising aromas than those of freshly cooked toast or grilled bacon.

A residential unit with its own kitchen integral to the unit is helpful in providing appropriate cues (Gresham 1999), as is a unit that has facilities for putting the final touches to meals—such as grilling bacon or warming-up bread. This ability to provide aromatic cues is a strong argument for full kitchens on dementia units. In addition, such kitchens can provide helpful visual cues.

Visual cues

Visual cues can be provided by allowing people to see the food before a meal, especially if they they have watched or participated in its preparation (Knocker 2001). If this is not possible, watching it being served can be helpful.

The appearance of a dining table can provide important visual cues. The table needs to be recognisable as a dining table before the meal is placed on it, thus stimulating anticipation of the meal in those who are waiting to be served.

Indeed, the whole dining room can provide cues. It should look like a proper dining room—perhaps with a dresser with rows of plates along one wall. Cafés are an excellent way of helping some people to 'cue into' mealtimes. Some units have converted an underused room into a café with very good results. Dunwhinny Lodge, a residential home in Peeblesshire (Scotland) undertook such a project (Crombie & Kemp 1999). The lodge asked the local high school to turn an unused lounge into a traditional British café with the décor of the 1940s and 1950s. As well as benefiting residents, this turned out to be an excellent art and craft project for the students. Many of the residents are happy to eat and drink comfortably in the café, whereas these same people struggle in a conventional institutional dining room. Staff members can also adopt roles as customers or as wait staff.

The appearance of the food can also act as a visual cue in stimulating appetite. Unfortunately, the food that is offered in many residential settings is far from attractive, especially in the case of mashed or puréed food. Given the availability of thickeners, there is really no excuse for this.

Touch

Touch can be an important cue for eating. Participating in food preparation can help some people to prepare for a meal. Others can be cued by laying tables, or by the feel of table napkins being unfolded and put on their laps.

Taste

Many people are cued for food through taste. An alcoholic drink before a meal can serve this purpose, as can peanuts, crisps, or olives.

Hearing

Hearing can alert some people to food. The sounds emanating from a kitchen can be important cues. Sounds such as the sizzling and bubbling of cooking food, or the clattering of pans and cooking utensils, can evoke anticipation of food to come. In addition, the sounds of tables being laid, or water glasses being filled, or ice clinking, can all help.

Traditional cups and saucers have many advantages over mugs. One advantage is the noise they make when they are set out. Cups and saucers also provide a familiar touch experience.

The positive effects of these noise cues presuppose that the dining room is quiet enough for these sounds to be heard. Too much noise in the dining room is the third of the factors considered in this chapter.

Noise

'Noise is to people with dementia as stairs are to people with wheelchairs' (Hiatt 1995).

People with dementia are profoundly disabled by noise—especially a confusing variety of noises—and many dining rooms are very noisy. It is not uncommon for residents to be overwhelmed with the noises of rattling trolleys, loud radios, clatter in the servery, shouting staff, chairs and tables scraping on hard floors, and loud vacuum cleaners or dishwashers in the background. This sort of stimulation overload can prevent people with dementia hearing useful cues as they are overwhelmed and stressed by other noises. Reducing such noise can help people to relax.

> 'Noise is to people with dementia as stairs are to people with wheelchairs.'

Calming quiet music might also help. At the very least, such music might assist staff members to be less stressed, even if it does nothing for the residents!

Stress

People with dementia are often stressed and anxious. This is hardly surprising, given that it is very difficult to function if memory, learning, and reasoning are impaired. Some of this stress at mealtimes is caused by noise, and some is caused by the large number of people eating at the same time.

Many people with dementia have lived very quiet lives before coming into a communal setting, and these people have difficulty coping with eating in the company of strangers. Some need to eat on their own, whereas others need to eat in a small familiar group. Few can cope with a large dining room. Some are not able to manage a sit-down meal at all, and these people need food that they can eat while walking about.

Some people with dementia are stressed before they go to the dining room, and it can be very helpful to diminish this stress if possible. A quiet activity before a meal can help. Some might relax with a massage. A quiet personal activity such as going to the toilet and washing hands can be means of relaxing for some people.

Staff can also find mealtimes stressful, and many staff members struggle to conceal their feelings. Some simply hate the whole business. Some find find it personally harassing to help others to eat. Others rush about getting everybody ready, and then continue to rush around throughout the meal. Time constraints add to this stress. If staff members know that they have to get the meal finished in half an hour they will not be relaxing company for residents. Removing time pressures is one of the best ways to cut down on stress for staff and residents alike.

Removing pressures to do other things at the same time can also be helpful. Surprisingly, many residential units administer medications during meals. The justification for this is that some tablets must be taken with food. However, a properly administered 'drug round' needs very careful thought, and doing this at the same time as meals are being served is not best practice.

Disruptions to mealtimes can also be caused by some residents, and it is sensible to make careful seating arrangements that separate the most disruptive people from others.

Other factors that can disrupt fragile concentration at mealtimes include doctors' rounds, cleaning of dining rooms and adjoining passages, and loading of dishwashers.

Drugs

The side-effects of drugs can have a significant effect on appetite. Table 6.1 (page 66) provides a list of commonly used medications and their potential effects on appetite.

Visual impairments

Most older people have some degree of visual impairment. By wearing spectacles and making appropriate compensatory adjustments, most people cope well. However, this is not usually the case for people with dementia. Many people do not understand why they cannot see a plate or perceive the food on a plate.

A first step is to ensure that there is enough light. A useful 'rule of thumb' is that older people need 50% more light than do younger people, and that older people with visual impairments require 100% more light. Many dining rooms are not well lit. Often the walls are lit, rather than the tables.

Table 6.1 Effects of commonly used medications on appetite and food intake

Drug	Possible side-effects
Antipsychotics and sedatives	dry mouth, loss of taste, diminished sense of smell, unpleasant taste, constipation, restlessness, disinterest in food, sleeplessness, restlessness, stiffness, increased appetite
Antihypertensives (some types)	dry mouth, loss of taste, constipation
L-dopa	anorexia
Lithium	dry mouth, metallic taste, nausea, increased thirst, apathy
Tricyclic antidepressants	dry mouth, sedation, restlessness, constipation, increased appetite
SSRI antidepressants	nausea, heartburn, altered bowel habit (constipation or diarrhoea), loss of appetite, drowsiness, restlessness

VOICES (1998); published with permission

A second step is to ensure adequate contrast in the serving of food. The plates should stand out in contrast to the tablecloth, and the food itself should contrast with the plate. White fish in white sauce with potato on a white plate can be very difficult to discern. When buying new china, ensure that the middle of the plate is coloured, and that the edge of the plate has a distinct border to assist people in discerning the outline of the plate.

Sore mouth

People with dementia might be suffering from mouth ulcers, sore gums, ill-fitting dentures, and other mouth problems that make eating uncomfortable. In some cases, long-standing fears of dentistry can exacerbate these problems by discouraging residents from seeking necessary help.

A related problem can be the existence of eating phobias. Some people have had traumatic experiences (such as a fishbone stuck in the throat), and these can cause long-standing aversions to eating. It is important to learn about these phobias from relatives whenever possible.

Brain damage

The most obvious sign of dementia is impaired memory, and this can affect eating in numerous ways.

People can forget that they have eaten, or can believe that they have eaten when they have not. They might forget how to eat. Eating a meal involves a complex sequence of activities, and people can forget how to manage one or more activities of the sequence. They might, for example, forget how to use a knife and fork, or forget how to bring a cup to the mouth.

It can be very helpful if staff members sit down and eat a meal with residents. This provides a model of the required activities for those who have forgotten. Staff members are also able to help at appropriate moments—such as putting a knife and fork into the person's hands. In some places this is difficult to arrange. In some settings (especially in hospitals), occupational regulations forbid the sharing of meals with residents. Sometimes shift patterns mean that there are too few staff members available at mealtimes. Some units have so many people needing help with the whole process that it is impossible to have staff sitting with the more able.

There are many other disabilities resulting from brain damage that can impinge on eating. These include visual agnosia (not recognising objects and their uses) and dyspraxia (an inability to control muscle movement).

Profound disability

Some people with dementia are so impaired, mentally and physically; that food has to be spooned into their mouths. This is a skilled task, but is often under-rated.

To do it well the helper should be positioned below or level with the person being helped. Eye contact should be maintained, and the helper should

---

Mrs Cran's dignified tea

Mrs Cran was no longer able to recognise a cup and saucer, and would sit in front of a cup of tea in bewildered silence.

When staff members recognised the problem, they ensured that one of them was sitting beside Mrs Cran. By hooking her finger into the handle of the cup, and by gently supporting her hand, staff members were able to help Mrs Cran bring the cup to her lips.

Mrs Cran was thus able to share tea with the other residents in a dignified way. She was also able to take some of the fluids she needed.

continuously explain what is being done. Helpers must be aware of the problems that some people have with managing food in the mouth and swallowing it. An experienced helper will know, for example, whether it is helpful to touch the person's lips with the spoon as food is brought to the mouth. If the process is done well, a certain rhythm develops. Conversely, if it is done badly, it is a dreadful experience for both parties.

As a training exercise, it can be very instructive for staff members to help each other to eat. Ice-cream is a good choice of food, and the helped person should not be allowed to move his or her arms. The helped person might even be blindfolded. Such a training exercise should be followed by skilled de-briefing to obtain best results and avoid stressful reactions.

Staffing issues
Lack of ownership
In the past, food and mealtimes were the clear responsibility of nurses. With the passage of time, a variety of other professions took over some aspects of the responsibility. Occupational therapists are competent in some aspects of mealtimes and equipment, speech therapists have knowledge of swallowing difficulties, dietitians know about nutrition, catering managers have an interest in how the food is delivered and served, and health-care assistants are often required to perform the serving and removing of plates. In some settings, the involvement of such a range of people means that no one is actually responsible for the whole experience for any given individual.

'Nurses should reclaim responsibility for the whole eating experience.'

This issue has been fully addressed by Dewing (1996). In the view of the present author, nurses should reclaim responsibility for the whole eating experience.

Education of other staff
A variety of people require education in the needs of people with dementia, and the importance of eating and nutrition.

Those who are in charge of commissioning and planning services require an understanding of the special problems of people with dementia. Difficult routines, poorly designed buildings, inadequate staffing, and inappropriate equipment can all make life difficult for people with dementia and for those who directly care for them.

Catering managers need to understand the importance of food that looks familiar and attractive. There is also a need for 'finger food' that can be eaten while people are walking about (Newton & Stewart 1997). Proper cutlery and crockery should be purchased. The increased costs of buying bone china cups and saucers is not necessarily excessive, and the overall costs of purchasing good-quality crockery might well balance out. The fluid intake of residents will certainly be improved.

Those who are responsible for buildings need to understand the importance of small dining rooms with a domestic ambience. A kitchen within the unit is important so that eating can be a multi-sensory experience.

Education for these various people is not easy to organise. Indeed, there is rarely any recognition of the need. Under-nutrition of residents is usually blamed on the actual care staff. But staff with a variety of roles and responsibilities can certainly benefit from education and the sharing of good ideas.

Conclusion

For many years, food has been considered an obvious and mundane issue that does not require attention. However, a recognition of the levels of under-nutrition and dehydration among residents has stimulated increased interest (Walker & Higginson 2000). The challenges involved in overcoming eating difficulties in people with dementia are worthy of a greater sharing of good ideas and informed practice.

Chapter 7

Wandering

Claudia Lai and David Arthur

Introduction

Wandering is regarded by caregivers as one of the most troubling behaviours of those in their care (Cantes & Rigby 1997), but the occurrence of wandering among the older population is difficult to ascertain. Estimates of the proportion of institutionalised dementia residents who wander have ranged from 11% (Hiatt 1985) to 50% (Hoffman, Platt & Barry 1987; Teri, Larson & Reifler 1988). According to one study, *all* ambulatory cognitively impaired nursing home residents display some degree of wandering behaviour (Algase et al. 1997).

For health-care professionals working in long-term care, the question of how to deal with frail people who wander is a constant challenge. To restrain such people is to take away much of the precious and limited freedom they enjoy in an institution. But to remove restraint and to allow them to wander as they please can lead to accidents, arguments, and disputes among residents.

The outcomes of falls can be serious for those who wander. For other residents and families the intrusive behaviour of wanderers and the loss of personal items is difficult to tolerate. Carers find themselves having to cope with legitimate

---

Annie's day

Annie had just come on duty. The shouting and the arguments from the far end of the corridor sounded familiar. Annie knew immediately that Mrs Smith had again gone into Mr Jones' room. Mrs Smith loved to go into Mr Jones' room every morning. Indeed, Mrs Smith loved to wander into everyone's room.

Then, as usual, Annie heard Mrs Goodman in the adjacent room engaged in a verbal altercation with Mrs Smith.

Annie sighed. Another day in the long-term ward had begun.

---

complaints from other residents and their families, as well as pressure from peers and management. Nurses have to complete incident reports, provide explanations to various people, and cope with a sense of failure when accidents occur on their shifts. In addition, there is always a threat of legal action. Increasingly, nursing homes are being sued by residents or their families who allege that injury, or perhaps even death, occurred through negligence (Frolik 2000).

Types of wandering behaviour

The term 'wandering' has been used to describe diverse patterns of behaviour. These include pacing, trying doorknobs, entering other people's rooms, becoming lost on a walk, and leaving residential accommodation (or attempting to leave). In planning interventions, it is important to recognise that wandering is not just one behaviour, but a group of behaviours.

'In planning interventions, it is important to recognise that wandering is not just one behaviour, but a group of behaviours.'

Ambulation in older people with dementia can be characterised according to its geographical pattern (Martino-Saltzman et al. 1991). Figure 7.1 (page 72) shows patterns of: (i) direct ambulation (straightforward movement to a destination); (ii) random ambulation (haphazard movement without repeating points in sequence); (iii) pacing ambulation (back-and-forth movement between two points); and (iv) lapping ambulation (circuitous movement revisiting points sequentially along a path or track).

For those who wander in a *direct* pattern, functional ambulation is still possible (Algase 1999). A useful strategy is therefore to keep desirable destinations (such as the bathroom) within sight.

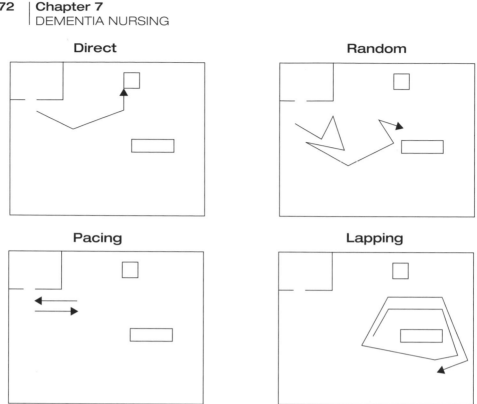

Figure 7.1 Travel patterns of nursing home residents identified as wanderers
Source: Martino-Saltzman et al.(1991); reprinted with permission

Random wandering is the most common pattern (Algase 1999). The frequency and duration of random wandering tends to increase as the day goes on. Because random wandering is often affected by environmental stimuli, rest periods and reduced environmental distractions can help to prevent direct ambulation from becoming random ambulation.

Pacing ambulation does not have a universal pattern. It might be caused by anxiety, agitation, or similar emotions.

Lapping appears to be related to the severity of dementia, and could represent a 'way-finding' strategy or a form of perseveration (Algase 1999). It tends to occur after rest or earlier in the day. Environmental manipulation or strategies to interrupt perseveration might be useful in lapping behaviour.

Causes of wandering

The causes of wandering are poorly understood (Kiely, Morris & Algase 2000). The three main perspectives in understanding the causes of wandering behaviour are: (i) biomedical; (ii) psychosocial; and (iii) person–environment interaction.

Little is known about wandering behaviour from the *biomedical* perspective. Some researchers have suggested that an impaired neural circuit might be the cause (Meguro et al. 1996), whereas others have suggested that hyperactivity is caused by an increased 'drive' to walk as a direct result of brain damage (Hope et al. 2001). Wandering has also been viewed as a motor dysfunction arising from disruption in self-monitoring (Henderson, Mack & Williams 1989; McShane, Gedling, Keene et al. 1998), and becoming lost might therefore be a consequence of faulty navigation due to poor topographical memory.

From a *psychosocial* perspective, wandering expresses a need (Algase, Beck & Kolanowski 1996). Physiological needs (cold, pain, and so on) and psychological needs (looking for company) prompt a person to pace and wander. It is understandable that a confused person seeking to fulfil a need should seek to find something or someone with which to relate. Wandering behaviour could therefore be an indication that a person is lonely and looking for company (Rader, Doan & Schwab 1985) or that he or she is hungry and looking for food. Lifelong patterns of coping with stress (for example, exercise or manual work such as gardening) and previous work roles involving movement (such as a postman or an athlete) might also be psychosocial factors that predispose a person to wandering behaviour (Snyder et al. 1978).

From the perspective of *person–environment interaction*, wandering is a response to various environmental changes. Wandering tends to occur if there is little noise and adequate lighting (Cohen-Mansfield et al. 1991). Most pacing behaviour occurs in the corridor because this provides an open area for such wandering behaviour, and residents pace more often during non-mealtime hours when they are not required to remain in the dining room. These and other environmental circumstances can be playing a part in producing wandering behaviour at certain times and in certain situations.

Determining the exact cause of wandering behaviour is difficult. However, it should never be assumed that wandering is 'aimless'. Rather, it is likely to be purposeful in some sense, and skilled nurses should assess every person from a physical, psychosocial, and environmental perspective in an attempt to determine the likely causes and appropriate interventions.

Positive aspects of wandering

Nurses often associate wandering or pacing behaviours with anxiety, restlessness, and agitation. Such behaviours cause nurses distress. They are understandably concerned that those in their care might become fatigued or wander outside, or sustain injuries, or trespass into other people's space (leading to fights, arguments, and more problems).

However, wandering can be beneficial within a safe environment. Wandering is a form of exercise. It stimulates circulation and oxygenation, and decreases contractures (Heim 1986). Indeed, pacing can reflect good physical health (Cohen-Manfield et al. 1991). It is reassuring to know that wandering has been found to have no relationship with becoming lost (Hope et al. 1994). Elopement, not wandering, should be the real concern of nurses.

Wandering and pacing can be an adaptive or appropriate behaviour for cognitively impaired residents, and should therefore be accommodated by caregivers (Cohen-Mansfield & Werner 1998). The goal in caring for wandering residents is not to prevent all forms of wandering. Rather, the goal should be the provision of a safe level of wandering without putting people at risk of injury (Taft et al. 1993). Strategies to prevent people wandering away outside are discussed below (see 'Management of elopement', page 76).

'Wandering can be beneficial within a safe environment . . . Elopement, not wandering, should be the real concern of nurses.'

Care of the wanderer

It is no easy task to balance the rights of a resident to freedom of movement against the risks of unsafe ambulation. However, if it is undesirable to prevent all wandering and pacing, how can nurses protect those in their care against the hazards of wandering away and becoming lost?

Medication

Sedatives can be useful in decreasing wandering behaviour in some circumstances. For example, alprazolam (Xanax) has been used with some success in decreasing nocturnal wandering (Szwabo et al. 1991). Staff members reported that the wandering behaviour decreased and that residents responded better to other supportive interventions.

Sedatives obviously diminish physical activity and thus tend to decrease wandering behaviour, but the use of sedatives is, in itself, no substitute for individual assessment and care.

Exercise programs and planned activities

Because boredom and a lack of activity might predispose some people to wandering, exercise programs and planned activities have been advocated as a management strategy.

Although such exercise programs do not always influence day-time wandering, night-time wandering behaviour can be significantly reduced (Robb 1985). A wanderer's lounge program with both structured and unstructured time for especially problematic residents with Alzheimer's disease can produce benefits that exceed expectations (McGrowder-Lin & Bhatt 1988).

A walkers' group using volunteers supervised by nursing home staff can decrease the unstructured time of residents and can occupy residents who might otherwise wander if nursing staff are less available to supervise them. Such a program also increases physical and social stimulation (Holmberg 1997).

Behavioural modification

Behavioural modification is another approach in dealing with wandering behaviour (Hussian 1982, 1985; McEvoy & Patterson 1986). Such intervention is based on the principle that all behaviours are learned behaviours, and that they can be reinforced or diminished by appropriate responses.

For example, the reward of wandering for one person might be access to sweet food. For others, the reward might be the sensory stimulation of touching items to their faces or tongues, or the tracing of patterns of the lobby furniture with their hands. If such rewards are provided to these people when they are not exhibiting wandering behaviour, wandering has been shown to decrease by 50–60% (Heard & Watson 1999).

'Behaviour attributed to neurological impairment might nevertheless be responsive to socially mediated approaches.'

However, wandering behaviours return to baseline levels if such rewards are provided when the people wander. Research of this type suggests that behaviour attributed to neurological impairment might nevertheless be responsive to socially mediated approaches.

Enhanced environment

An enhanced environment provides features that maintain connections between residents and previously familiar surroundings, and simultaneously reduces the institutional aspects of the environment (Schiff 1990). Such enhancements can decrease agitated behaviour, restlessness, and wandering, and can increase contentment and positive social interactions—if implemented in association with a program of structured and unstructured activities whereby people can touch or play with objects in the enhanced environment (Arno & Frank 1994).

Simulated scenes (such as a nature scene or a home and people scene) can be constructed using furniture, pictures, and appropriate sounds (such as running water and the singing of birds) and scents (such as flowers and plants). Nursing home residents who spend time in such settings have been observed to decrease their trespassing behaviour. Such an enhanced environment provides a practical alternative for accommodating pacing behaviours and decreases exit-seeking and trespassing (Cohen-Mansfield & Werner 1998). Such environments are easy to implement, and can be done at a low cost.

Management of elopement
Tracking

If residents wander away from the nursing home or other accommodation it is important to find them as quickly as possible. Electronic monitoring of residents by armbands and electronic devices has been used in some facilities (Coltharp, Richie & Kaas 1996), although the use of such tracking devices has been criticised as being degrading and dehumanising. These criticisms have deterred research and development of such tracking devices. However, it can be argued that these devices might result in residents being given more freedom because families and staff will be more relaxed about letting residents wander (McShane, Gedling, Kenward et al. 1998). Such devices might also increase safety by enabling those who have become lost to be found more quickly (McShane, Hope & Wilkinson 1994). Effective monitoring and tracking devices can, at the very least, alert staff to the presence of a resident in a restricted area, and can turn otherwise closed units into open units while maintaining the security of residents (Negley, Molla & Obenchain 1990).

Most current tracking devices utilise the global positioning system (GPS). This is less suitable for tracking people in very large cities, but can be useful in less densely populated environments.

The acceptability of the device by the person at risk of elopement is crucial. Practical considerations include whether the person will continue to wear the device at all times, whether he or she might attempt to take it off, and whether the battery will last should the person be missing for a considerable period of time.

Visual barriers

The rationale behind the use of visual barriers is based on the fact that many people with dementia have difficulties with perception (Schlotterer, Moscovitch & Crapper-McLachlan 1983; Nissen et al., 1985). In posing visual barriers, various designs have been used.

Masking tape laid on the floor can decrease ambulation towards exit doors (Hussian & Brown 1987). This technique is relatively safe, inexpensive, and unobtrusive, and it can be easily modified for used in a private home (Hewawasam 1996).

A visual decoy (such as a full-length mirror placed in front of the door) can be useful (Mayer & Darby 1991), as can cloth panels that conceal doorknobs (Namazi, Rosner & Calkins 1989) or the 'panic bar' of a fire exit (Dickinson & McLain-Kark 1998).

Subjective barriers of this type have not yet been conclusively proven to be effective (Price, Hermans & Grimley Evan 2001), but this does not necessarily mean that the strategies do not work. Nurses are encouraged to continue seeking novel, safe, and economical ways of reducing wandering.

'Nurses are encouraged to continue seeking novel, safe, and economical ways of reducing wandering.'

Bringing back residents

It is not always easy to persuade a resident who has left the premises to return voluntarily. An effective technique is to use two staff members together in search of the resident (Snyder et al. 1978).

Once the person has been located, one of the staff members should approach, and walk or sit with him or her. No immediate attempt should be made to bring the person back, unless initiated by the resident. Rather, casual conversation should be conducted to defuse any potential tension. After a while, the second staff member can approach and ask both the older person and the first staff member to accompany the second staff member back to the home. Often a commitment to return is elicited upon the second staff member's request. If the resident does not want to go back immediately, the second staff member returns to the home, leaving the first staff member and the resident together. If necessary, a third staff member can come by after an agreed time has elapsed.

This rather elaborate approach, although fairly costly, acknowledges the rights of the resident, and allows trust to be developed. If used in combination with a comprehensive staff education program and approaches to wandering that take account of specific causes, the prevalence of 'problem' wandering can be decreased to an occasional incident (Snyder et al. 1978).

Implications for nursing practice

Wandering is not a simple behaviour, and people who wander are not an homogeneous group. No single strategy is applicable to all people, and each situation requires an individualised approach.

In many cases wandering can be healthy and need not be stopped. On the other hand, wandering can have various meanings, and allowing a person to wander unhindered in the belief that this is 'good' for him or her might mean that the person's unrecognised needs and problems are ignored.

A comprehensive nursing assessment is the key to identifying suitable strategies in dealing with wandering behaviour. Table 7.1 (page 79) provides a summary of the elements to be considered and possible strategies that might be implemented.

Even if various strategies have been tried unsuccessfully, nurses should not become exasperated. Quality nursing care implies not giving up on such a person, and nurses should continue to look for clues. There might still be some unrecognised factor that is causing persistent wandering. In particular, nurses should be aware that unstoppable pacing might well indicate a neurological problem (Allan 1994). The Box below relates the story of a lady whose

---

A room with a view

Mrs BD was a 79-year-old lady whose marked wandering behaviour and trespasses provoked frequent altercations between herself and other residents. Staff members had reached the point of contemplating 'extreme measures'. Before doing so, the team observed Mrs BD more carefully.

Much to everyone's surprise, it became apparent that this lady's repeated intrusions into other people's rooms was to get a better view of an outside area that she could not see from the window of her own room. She was also noted to be frequently going into another room to use the mirror in that room.

Having solved the riddle of Mrs BD's behaviour, the team relocated her to a room with a window that looked out into her favourite view and that contained an appropriate mirror. After these changes, Mrs BD's intrusions decreased from 16 times per hour to only twice an hour.

Adapted from Donat (1984)

Table 7.1 Wandering assessment and strategies

	Elements to consider	Strategies and interventions
Basic assessment	Is the person safe and free from harm? Are there any risks of falls or injuries? Can the person recognise risks? Gait, balance, and functional status? What seems to trigger wandering? How often does the person wander? Continuous or sporadic? If sporadic, day-time or night-time, and for how long? How active is the person during the day? Does wandering interfere with other activities of daily living (such as meals)?	Remove to a safe location if behaviour is hazardous. Specially designed facilities allow wanderers to move about safely. Manage risks of falls. Determine possible aetiology of wandering behaviour.
Physiological and/or disease-related factors	Is wandering related to a memory deficit? Does the person forget where he or she is going? Any basic physiological factors that are causing the wandering (such as pain or hunger)? Any neurological symptoms that warrant attention? Any anxiety or psychotic symptoms (hallucinations; irrational fears)? Is the resident more confused than previously? Is confusion caused by acute illness, and/or side-effects of medication?	Non-chemical interventions are first recommendation. Structure environments such that important destinations (e.g. washroom) are visible and convenient. Continuous cueing to maintain orientation. Attend to pain and hunger as indicated. Put fruits, finger foods, and juices along wandering pathways if eating is a concern. If medication is needed, begin with lowest dose and titrate upwards if required. Medical attention and treatment if indicated.

(Continued)

Table 7.1 Wandering assessment and strategies *(Continued)*

	Elements to consider	Strategies and interventions
Physiological and/or disease-related factors *(continued)*	Any altered sleep pattern?	For disrupted sleep pattern: (i) establish a bedtime routine; (ii) structure physical activities in afternoon; (iii) have the resident void before bedtime; (v) ensure room is quiet and conducive to sleep.
Psychological factors	Life history and occupation? Could this be related? Lifestyle pattern in the past? Is the person now seeking solitude, companionship, or a sense of security? Does he or she trail along with someone else? Anxiety about being abandoned? Boredom? Is he or she searching for something of interest? Is the resident looking for a way out?	Promote social interaction through innovative programming. Regular exercise. Music for some wanderers. Promote group activities and personal contact (folding clothes, gardening, supervised walks, cooking activities). Encourage development of relationships. Exercise or gardening if stressed. Identify and eliminate sources of stress (e.g. change routines). Provide opportunities for physical activities. Try to understand what the person wants to do. Promote meaningful activities and a sense of completion. Gently interrupt rummaging, trespassing, or perseverating behaviour by distraction; focus attention on an object (set of keys or wristwatch). Divert attention from elopement efforts; engage in other activities. Disguise doors, use window and door locks (placed out of sight and reach).

(Continued)

Table 7.1 Wandering assessment and strategies (*Continued*)

	Elements to consider	Strategies and interventions
Psychological factors (*continued*)		Interrupt or distract wandering that continues over an extended time or that causes anxiety. Reassure anxious residents that anxiety is understood. Encourage expression of emotion in other ways, and offer comfort. Use music and relaxation techniques (such as paced breathing). Use familiar objects in the environment. Provide opportunities for being alone. Personal stereo for music. Provide materials (pictures and games).
Environmental factors	Does the environment have sufficient cues and signage? Excessive stimulation in the environment? Do noise or crowds distress the resident? Is there a lack of environmental stimulation on the unit?	Environmental cues helpful to those who are alert but who have difficulty locating a specific room. Familiar objects from family home to help orientation and recognition of correct room. Sheltered courtyards and gardens for wandering. Planned activities at various times of day. Keep things simple. Avoid too many guests or activities at one time.

Authors' presentation

wandering behaviour was extremely disruptive until relatively simple problems were recognised and dealt with appropriately.

The key issue is that astute and empathic observations are crucial, together with patience and perseverance in trying various means. Families are a valuable resource in helping to understand the background of residents. Consistency of approach among all members of the team is also very important.

Conclusion

Wandering is a collective term for a complex of behavioural presentations for which there is no magic cure. There is no substitute for astute observation and tender loving care, together with intelligent innovation on the part of staff.

In managing wandering behaviour, the importance of assessment cannot be over-emphasised. Recognition of predisposing or triggering factors enables nurses to devise and implement effective strategies.

For many residents with dementia, wandering is healthy and need not be stopped. If the potential risk of getting away from the premises is high, the use of tracking devices and visual barriers might be useful for some people.

'Because a "cure" is unlikely, nurses have a significant role to play in the effective management of wandering.'

To be effective, care management requires a team approach. Because a 'cure' is unlikely, nurses have a significant role to play in the effective management of wandering. It is up to nurses to take up the challenge of providing quality care for these people.

Chapter 8
Sensory Loss

Wendy-Mae Rapson and Richard Osborn

Introduction

A major presenting sign of dementia is a decline in communication skills. Dementia affects the ability of people both to understand language and to express themselves verbally and non-verbally. In addition, a person who has dementia might also have hearing loss and visual loss. Taken together, these problems can significantly affect a person's ability to communicate effectively and to function independently.

A survey of older Australians living in the community revealed that 57% had hearing loss, 28% had visual loss, and 19% had dual sensory loss (both hearing and visual loss) (Hickson et al. 1999). The prevalence of such problems in residential settings is even higher (Horowitz 1994; Lindeman & Platenburg-Gits 1991; Tesch-Romer 1997). Other estimates of hearing loss in the older population vary between 31% and 87% (Voeks et al. 1993) and estimates of visual loss range from 10% to 25% (Klein, Klein & Lee 1996). The proportion of people with dementia living with sensory loss is likely to be similar.

Appropriate assessment, referral, and rehabilitation of people with both dementia and sensory loss are important factors in preserving the quality of life of these people and in the prevention of further functional decline (Hickson et al. 1999). However, sensory loss is often under-recognised and inadequately managed.

Visual or hearing loss can have a significant impact on a person's life. It can affect his or her ability to hear conversation, walk about safely, read, recognise people's faces, watch television, and listen to the radio. Visual or hearing loss can limit a person's participation in everyday human interactions, and can leave the person socially isolated. Health and safety issues include the safe taking of medication, the risk of falls, and the compounding of existing cognitive difficulties by social isolation. For people with sensory loss and dementia, the ability to receive verbal or written prompts can be compromised by a combination of sensory loss and diminished cognitive ability.

'Visual or hearing loss can limit a person's participation in everyday human interactions, and can leave the person socially isolated.'

Assessment and differential diagnosis

Signs of early dementia can be confused with signs of visual and hearing loss. The confusion and disorientation associated with dementia is also common for some people with sensory loss. Because of the high prevalence of sensory loss in the older population, it is imperative that nurses, doctors, and others engaged in aged care are aware of the importance of appropriate assessment of hearing, vision, and cognition. Ophthalmologists, optometrists, orthoptists, ear, nose and throat specialists, audiologists, and other specialists can assess and treat sensory function and make recommendations for appropriate management. In addition, carers and nursing staff can make a valuable contribution to assessment through their personal observations of people in their everyday settings.

It is important to ascertain whether a person's behaviour is related to dementia or to sensory loss. Possible sensory loss should be assessed by history, examination, and formal testing. It is easy to ascribe certain signs to dementia and to ignore the possibility that the person might be suffering from sensory loss. The Box on pages 86–7 illustrates some examples.

The potential for diagnostic error in the examples given in the Box show that it is imperative to ascertain the underlying cause of a person's difficulty. If the problem is due to sensory loss, a range of options is available to remedy the problem, and these should be incorporated into that person's care plan. If the difficulties are solely related to dementia, other measures are appropriate. The important point is not to overlook something that might be remedied.

Hearing loss
Causes
There are several causes of hearing loss in older people. These include the following.

‣ *Wax occlusion*—cerumen (wax) occlusion of the ear canals is common and easily treated.
‣ *Presbycusis*—this is the most common cause of permanent hearing loss in older people. It is a sensorineural loss for which there is no effective medical or surgical remedy.
‣ *Noise-induced hearing loss*—people who have been exposed to a high noise level through work or recreation might suffer sensorineural hearing loss.

Presbycusis and noise-induced hearing impairment are both sensorineural in nature. In general, sensorineural hearing loss reduces the perception of high-pitched sounds and speech—particularly in the presence of background noise. People with a sensorineural loss often have an increased sensitivity to loud noises and can experience tinnitus (ringing or buzzing in the ears).

Nursing assessment
Many people with significant hearing loss are unaware of the degree of difficulty they experience in understanding what is being said, or are unwilling to acknowledge it. However, an astute nurse might identify a hearing impairment in a person by noting that he or she is:

‣ leaning forward;
‣ cupping an ear;
‣ requesting repetition of words;
‣ responding to conversation inconsistently or inappropriately;
‣ using a loud voice; or
‣ requiring the television or radio volume to be rather loud.

By noting these sorts of behaviours, trained and astute nurses can thus quickly and reliably ascertain whether a person should be referred for a full hearing assessment.

Dementia or sensory loss?

People can present with a variety of signs and symptoms that might imply early dementia. Consider the following examples of people who were initially assumed to have early signs of dementia.

Mrs A

Presentation

Mrs A presents with an inability to follow or understand rapid speech. Is this an early sign of cognitive impairment and therefore an early sign of dementia?

Comment

Further assessment reveals that Mrs A's problems are especially marked in noisy or distracting environments. It is well documented that people with hearing loss have trouble understanding rapid speech, and have trouble understanding speech in the presence of background noise. It is also known that people with visual loss have more difficulty understanding speech in the presence of background noise (Osborn et al. 2000). In everyday listening environments that have significant amounts of background noise, both hearing loss and visual loss might be mistaken for cognitive impairment. Mrs A needs further auditory and visual assessment.

Mr B

Presentation

Mr B is tested for memory and fails to retain a five-item list. Is this an early sign of cognitive impairment and therefore an early sign of dementia?

Comment

Mr B might not have heard the words. Many people with hearing impairment rely on context. But a string of individual test words has no context. Mr B requires proper auditory assessment to determine whether his problem is really due to impaired memory. It might well be due to hearing loss.

Ms C

Presentation

Ms C is reported to have 'difficulty in understanding humour or sarcasm'. Is this an early sign of cognitive impairment and therefore an early sign of dementia?

Comment

Much of our communication is non-verbal. Communication associated with humour or sarcasm is often non-verbal in the form of a wink, a shrug of the shoulders, or even a slight change in facial expression. People with visual loss often report that they have difficulty in understanding humour, jokes, or sarcasm. It should not be assumed that Ms C has a cognitive problem. She might be failing to note subtle non-verbal cues. She requires proper visual assessment.

(Continued)

(Continued)

Mr D

Presentation

Mr D is reported to have 'lost the ability to process language rapidly'. Is this an early sign of cognitive impairment and therefore an early sign of dementia?

Comment

The ability to process language can clearly be related to sensory impairment. People with hearing loss require a greater processing time than their peers with normal hearing because those with sensory impairment rely heavily on context, and this requires time for them to think about what has been said. They often have to guess at what has been said. Mr D's problems might not be cognitive. They might be due to hearing problems and the time required to work out what is going on in a conversation.

Mrs E

Presentation

Mrs E appears to have lost the ability to stay on a topic in conversation. Her words are sometimes inappropriate and she appears to have difficulty in logical thought. Is this an early sign of cognitive impairment and therefore an early sign of dementia?

Comment

People with hearing loss can 'mishear' what has been said, and might therefore respond by speaking about what they believed was said to them, rather than what was actually said to them. Someone listening to Mrs E might wonder about Mrs E's cognitive skills and her ability to maintain coherent thinking on a topic. She might well be misdiagnosed as suffering from early dementia—unless her hearing is properly assessed by formal testing.

Mr F

Presentation

Mr F is reported to be suffering from shortened concentration span. He used to remain alert and involved for long periods, but now he can no longer pay attention to a speaker for more than a few minutes. Is this an early sign of cognitive impairment and therefore an early sign of dementia?

Comment

A person with hearing loss or visual loss has to concentrate intently on a speaker to understand what has been said. This is hard work—especially for an older person. If Mr F has such a sensory impairment, he might tire quickly from the demands placed upon him during conversation. This can be misinterpreted as a cognitive impairment and loss of concentration in a previously intelligent man. In fact, he might merely be finding that conversation is very hard work indeed.

Nursing care

Hearing loss has implications for the everyday care of these people. It affects communication with them, and can limit the activities in which they are able to participate. Each resident's hearing status needs to be considered carefully when planning his or her care and social activities.

For most people, a hearing aid is the most effective means of improving hearing. Unfortunately, many older people who would benefit from wearing such aids do not use them. The most common reasons cited for not wearing a hearing aid include:

▶ problems in inserting the hearing aid or ear mould;
▶ losing the hearing aid;
▶ dislike of amplification of background noise;
▶ difficulty in changing batteries;
▶ hearing aid not working properly; and
▶ a relative or carer having encouraged the person to obtain a hearing aid, but he or she not really wanting it or perceiving the need for it.

Nurses in residential aged-care facilities need to take more responsibility for the care of hearing aids and devices to ensure effective and efficient use. They need to spend time with residents to encourage them to persevere with wearing the aid and to instruct them in how best to manage it. If a nurse is specifically designated to attend to the needs of residents in terms of hearing aid assistance and practice, this will increase hearing aid use and lead to more efficient and effective communication.

> 'Nurses in residential aged-care facilities need to take more responsibility for the care of hearing aids and devices to ensure effective and efficient use.'

For older, frailer people it might be more appropriate to use an amplified listener (or similar device) when required. A carer who is trained to assist can help to manage this. When using the device, the speaker must have the microphone close to and slightly below his or her mouth to ensure that the voice is amplified and that background noise is minimised. One of the advantages of these devices over conventional hearing aids is increased clarity of speech as a result of the proximity of the microphone to the speaker's mouth. A small number of such listening devices in each section of a nursing home or hostel can enable many residents to communicate more effectively. These devices are not expensive, and family and friends who are keen to use them might purchase them for residents. People with dementia and hearing loss often benefit significantly from their use. The devices are easily managed by nurses and family members, but trained and motivated staff members are needed if this approach is to produce optimal benefits. Nurses need to be aware of the availability of listening devices, and staff training in their use is required (Roper 1995).

Group listening devices should also be considered for use in activities. A variety of devices is available for group amplification. These include group FM systems that allow a range of people with differing hearing losses to receive adequate amplification in a group setting (Erber & Osborn 1994). Staff members or volunteers who run groups can readily learn to manage these group devices with confidence.

Devices such as cordless headphones can be very effective for television and radio listening. In addition, the use of these devices means that others are not disturbed by the television or radio.

Visual loss

Causes

Of the people who are diagnosed with 'visual loss', 'low vision', or 'legal blindness', only a small proportion have no useful remaining vision. It is important that nurses identify what residual vision a person has, and the functional capacity this provides.

Most visual loss experienced by aged-care residents is caused by one or more of the following conditions.

- *Age-related macular degeneration* (AMD) is the most common cause of visual loss in older people. It produces a loss of central vision which causes difficulty in seeing detail. This affects the person's ability to read fine detail, recognise faces, and perceive colour.
- *Diabetic retinopathy* produces a loss of patches of the visual field which causes a blurring and patchiness of vision. This affects safe movement, reading, perception of fine detail, and many activities of daily living.
- *Glaucoma* can cause loss of peripheral vision loss which leads to 'tunnel vision'. This affects the person's ability to drive and move around safely.
- *Cataracts* produce a loss of contrast vision which causes blurring and increased sensitivity to glare. This affects reading, safe movement, and face recognition.

There are treatments available for some of these conditions. Ophthalmologists, optometrists, and orthoptists can assess the person's vision and make recommendations about appropriate medical and optical options for treatment and rehabilitation.

Nursing assessment

Nurses can make an informed assessment of the visual function of those in their care by noting their behaviour. Behaviours that indicate visual difficulties include:

▶ inability to recognise the faces of staff and relatives;
▶ inability to follow the movement of an object of interest;
▶ inability to see detail in objects, photographs, and magazines;
▶ inability to see food on a plate;
▶ spilling of drinks or difficulties with pouring;
▶ inability to read;
▶ inability to enjoy television;
▶ difficulty in finding personal belongings (for example, on the bedside table);
▶ withdrawal from activities (such as bingo) that rely on vision; and
▶ rubbing of eyes, red or sore eyes, weeping eyes, and difference in pupil size.

> 'Nurses can make an informed assessment of the visual function of those in their care by noting their behaviour.'

In addition, people might well report their visual difficulties to nurses. However, such self-reporting can be unreliable because many conditions are slow in onset, and people make incremental adjustments to the visual changes they are experiencing. Many people believe that such changes are an unavoidable aspect of old age, and can therefore lack insight into their problems.

In addition to nursing observations of people with visual difficulties, and self-reporting from these people, functional tests of visual function can also be used in making assessments. These include the use of standardised reading cards, assessing the person's ability to read magazines and newspaper articles (headlines and text), and asking people to identify people and objects in photographs.

Visual handicap scales have also been used to identify severe visual difficulties in older people (Horowitz, Teresi & Cassels 1991). However, assessment on the basis of accurate observations by experienced nurses is more effective in identifying these problems.

Nursing care
Buildings and environment

Marked visual loss is common among people in residential care. For these people, the following should be addressed:

▶ modifying the built environment of nursing homes and other accommodation;

▶ improving lighting for such tasks as reading and sewing;

▶ using increased contrast—both in general surroundings and in facilities and equipment used in everyday activities;

▶ reduction of glare; and

▶ increasing the size of signage and notices.

Advice from various sources is available on the appropriate design of buildings and environments. This advice should be sought from relevant local authorities and experts.

Personal nursing care

It is important during conversation to face the person at a distance of no more than one metre (Erber & Osborn 1994). It also is important that the nurse faces any light source so that direct light is on the nurse's face. This provides a person with visual impairment an opportunity to perceive cues and ensures that he or she does not have to cope with excessive glare.

'It is important during conversation to face the person at a distance of no more than one metre.'

Care planning in sensory loss

Residential-care facilities should focus on sensory loss as a priority. These problems are very prevalent among residents and the difficulties can be alleviated through the use of aids and targeted strategies.

Many activities of daily living require that a person can both hear and see adequately. Instructions and explanations routinely given to residents by staff can be difficult for a person with sensory loss to understand. Activities might have to be modified and groups formed more carefully to ensure that residents are able to hear, see, and participate fully. Adaptive devices (such as individual and group listening devices, and tactile game boards) can enable residents to participate more fully in all activities.

Care planning for communication should focus on:

▶ the recognition of difficulties and the making of a diagnosis;

▶ referral of residents to specialists (if appropriate);

▶ the use of adaptive devices (such as hearing aids, assistive listening devices, low-vision aids, talking books and so on); and

▶ clear communication strategies to maximise the quality of life of residents and their access to activities.

The individual communication needs of all residents must be viewed as an integral part of all other aspects of their care.

Appropriate referral to audiologists, optometrists, and speech pathologists is important in the management of sensory loss. Detailed assessment by these professionals improves nurses' understanding of the capabilities of residents, and provides guidance for interventions to enhance the quality of life of those in their care.

'The individual communication needs of all residents must be viewed as an integral part of all other aspects of their care.'

The case study of Cathy (Box, below) illustrates many of the matters discussed in this chapter.

Conclusion

A significant proportion of older people with dementia also suffer from sensory loss. Nurses must be skilled at identifying people in whom sensory loss might be affecting their capacity, and must plan for their care accordingly.

Many relatively simple solutions to the problems produced by visual and hearing loss are available. Organisations with expertise in visual and hearing disorders can provide assessment, guidance, and training for staff.

The ultimate aim is to identify and treat sensory losses in residents with dementia so they can attain optimal independence and quality of life.

Cathy

Cathy, a 75-year-old woman, had recently been admitted to a nursing home with diagnoses of dementia and age-related macular degeneration (AMD). Her hearing was described as 'fair'.

In the nursing home, Cathy became becoming increasingly egocentric, withdrawn, and socially isolated. She enjoyed one-to-one contact at certain times but, at other times, became verbally aggressive towards certain people. Cathy was often confused and disorientated with her new surroundings and complained that 'everyone looks the same'. Although she had previously been able to find her way around her home environment, Cathy now had difficulty reading the signs that indicated individual rooms, the lounge room, and the dining room in the nursing home. She increasingly called out for attention from nurses.

Cathy's relatives became concerned that her behaviour had worsened since her admission, and requested that staff reassess her.

(Continued)

(Continued)

As part of the reassessment, staff members noted that Cathy had difficulty hearing when background noise was present. Her television was too loud for others who were nearby. It was apparent that she communicated more effectively when people spoke clearly and deliberately. Relatives reported that Cathy's hearing had not been checked for some time.

Otoscopic examination revealed that Cathy's ears were blocked with wax. Her general practitioner prescribed ear drops to soften the wax, and subsequently removed the wax. Cathy's hearing then improved to a certain extent, although she still had difficulties with quiet conversation. Nurses then arranged for softly spoken staff members or relatives to use an assistive listening device (ALD) when talking to her.

Nurses also observed Cathy for signs of increased visual difficulty. It was noted that she did not seem to see people who were standing directly in front of her, but that she was able to find her way around without bumping into furniture. Good lighting improved Cathy's ability to read large print signs. Her relatives advised that Cathy's vision had also not been checked for some time, and an appointment was therefore made for Cathy's ophthalmologist to assess the progression of her AMD.

After this assessment, nurses rearranged Cathy's room to make best use of natural light. They also made a point of introducing themselves before initiating conversation with Cathy.

To decrease her calling out, the staff did two things. First, they left the ALD with Cathy while she was alone. With the ALD picking up her own voice, Cathy was able to monitor her loudness and soften her voice levels. Secondly, nurses clearly marked the call bell so that it contrasted with the surrounding environment. Each time that Cathy called out, the staff reminded her that she calling rather loudly, and asked her to use the call bell. This significantly decreased Cathy's calling out.

As a result of these measures, Cathy became more settled. It was apparent that the deterioration in her general behaviour had been largely due to her sensory problems, rather than her dementia. Even if Cathy's dementia does progress, the use of appropriate communication strategies and assistive devices will continue to be of assistance to her.

Chapter 9

Communication

Jane Crisp

Introduction

Effective communication plays a crucial role in all caregiving, especially in the provision of care to people with dementia. This is not only because of the day-to-day communication problems that can be caused by dementia, but also because of the broader obligation to maintain the quality of life of those receiving care.

Communication involves more than inducing cooperation in some caregiving task, such as bathing. In practice, activities such as bathing involve not only task-oriented communication but also a substantial amount of social and supportive interaction between nurse and resident (Gibb 1990). These social and supportive components help to accomplish the task smoothly and help to meet the psychological needs of the resident. The caregiving of social interaction is as important as the caregiving of the task itself.

'The caregiving of social interaction is as important as the caregiving of the task itself.'

Supportive social interactions are especially important in meeting the needs of those who have dementia. The behaviour and attitudes of nurses and carers towards these people can have an effect for good or ill. Negative feelings about dementia can prevent carers from seeing the person behind the symptoms. As a result these people can be ignored, excluded, or treated as infants, thus robbing them of a valid social identity (Kitwood 1997). In contrast, by taking a positive approach in all interactions with a person with dementia, nurses and carers can help him or her to maintain a sense of well-being. The underlying goal of interactions with people in care is to make them feel valued as persons.

Good communication involves interaction and is a two-way process. Good communication is therefore not restricted to strategies for communicating something *to* people with dementia. Just as importantly, it is about strategies for achieving a better understanding of what they are communicating to others.

Everything that is said or done by nurses communicates something about their attitudes to those in their care. By passing through a room and ignoring the residents in it, a nurse is sending a clear message to them. Nurses need be aware of the impression that they are giving, and ensure that their attitude and demeanour helps effective communication.

> 'Everything that is said or done by nurses communicates something about their attitudes to those in their care.'

Good communication takes time. The strategies presented in this chapter will assist nurses to make more efficient use of the time they spend with the people in their care, but will not reduce that time significantly. If staffing levels, work loads, or priorities in time allocation do not allow nurses sufficient time to meet the special social and emotional needs of these people, nurses should raise this as an issue with colleagues and management. Good communication is the key to dementia care and worth the time spent on it.

Principles of good communication

Good communication, especially with people who have dementia, involves:
- engaging in social interaction as well as achieving set tasks;
- providing support for the person's sense of identity and worth;
- ensuring that exchanges are a two-way process by listening and responding to one another;
- being aware that any communication involves the communication of an attitude of concern and care;
- allowing enough time for communication to achieve these broader goals.

Strategies for better communication
Before making contact
Before approaching a person with dementia, nurses should take stock of what they know about this person and his or her present environment. What factors can be turned to advantage, and what problems can be anticipated? The following should be considered:

▶ the person's cultural, social, and personal background;
▶ the person's name, and how he or she prefers to be addressed;
▶ whether the person has any problems other than dementia;
▶ the person's daily routine and the present time of day; and
▶ the immediate environment, and how it might help or hinder interaction.
   Each of these is considered below.

Cultural, social, and personal background
The form of address and gestures used, how close the nurse stands to the person, and the possible topics of conversation should all be appropriate to the person's culture and background. A person who has been used to commanding or instructing others might well prefer a more formal approach. Similarly, knowing that someone spent his or her life farming allows the nurse to turn a passing comment on the weather into a more significant comment that acknowledges the person's special interests and expertise. For example, someone who had once farmed in a drought-prone region of Australia might welcome the advent of rain in a way that would not be understood by a person from a different background.

Name and preferred mode of address
The type of relationship that a nurse has already established with the person is relevant. The use of personal names and familiar names might be appropriate from favourite carers, but being called by these names by an unfamiliar person can seem false or inappropriate.

Problems other than dementia
The person might have other problems, and the nurse might need to compensate for these. If the resident has trouble with sight or hearing, nurses should check whether glasses or hearing aids are available and functioning properly. For example, assisting someone at the meal table is easier if the resident is wearing the right glasses, and if these are clean.

Daily routine and time of day

Nurses should consider whether the resident is likely to be refreshed and ready to respond, or whether he or she might feel tired or disturbed. If the nurse has a potentially difficult task to accomplish, it is helpful to consider the best time of day to undertake this.

'The use of personal names and familiar names might be appropriate from favourite carers, but being called by these names by an unfamiliar person can seem false or inappropriate.'

The immediate environment

Sometimes it is appropriate to move to a quieter area, or to a setting with more suitable seating. The presence of a comfortable-looking sofa can be used to encourage acceptance of an invitation to sit and chat. Similarly, the sight of the toilet reinforces a question about whether the person needs to use this facility. For example, if it is planned to take a person for a walk in the garden, it can be useful to 'save' a question about toileting until actually passing the toilets.

Making an approach

The success of an interaction frequently depends on getting off to a good start. How a person is approached, and what is conveyed to him or her are important. The following points are important in making an approach:

- giving time to register a new presence;
- being alert to how the person is feeling;
- giving a sign of wanting to speak;
- using standard greetings and greeting rituals;
- providing a simple, clear, and tactful introduction;
- being alert to what posture and stance suggest; and
- making the other person feel 'at home'.
  Each of these is discussed below.

Giving time to register a new presence

It is important for a nurse to provide the person with sufficient time to register a new presence. He or she needs to see the nurse approaching, rather than suddenly having an unannounced person speak from behind.

Being alert to how the person is feeling

As the nurse approaches, it is important to be alert to any clues as to how the person is feeling. These clues are provided by posture and other body language.

Is the person drowsy, alert, agitated, content, miserable, or perhaps under the effects of sedation? This tells the nurse how best to proceed.

Giving a sign of wanting to speak

A smile, a nod, or a routine greeting shows that the nurse wants to speak to the person—and indicates that the nurse is friendly!

Using standard greetings and greeting rituals

Nurses can exploit the fact that memory for social rituals and other routines tends to survive the effects of dementia better than other types of memory (such as memory for facts and figures, or memory for specific episodes in the past). Nurses will therefore find that standard greetings and greeting rituals usually trigger an appropriate response.

Providing a simple, clear, and tactful introduction

Nurses should introduce themselves simply, clearly, and tactfully. If this is the first meeting with this person, the same 'rules' apply as on meeting someone who does not have dementia. The person needs to know the nurse's name, and the nurse should use the form of name that he or she wants the person to use. The nurse should also state his or her role. Time should be allowed for this information to 'sink in'.

> 'If this is the first meeting with this person, the same "rules" apply as on meeting someone who does not have dementia.'

If this is not the first meeting, it should not be assumed that the person will remember the nurse. If he or she does need reminding, this should be done tactfully. People with dementia often try to 'cover up' their memory failures—just as people who do not have dementia try to 'cover up' when they do not immediately recognise someone who seems to know them. It is kinder to help the person remember, rather than draw attention to the memory problem. For example, a nurse might begin by saying: 'Yes, it's me again—Mary who looks after your feet. I did enjoy the chat we had last time I was here'. In introducing herself in this way, Mary is speaking as if the person *does* know who she is. At the same time, Mary is providing key information about her identity and previous meetings with the person.

Even if the person does not immediately recognise the nurse with precision, he or she is likely to recognise the nurse's 'general identity'—that is, that this is a 'known person', even if precise identity is difficult to recall. A person with dementia might therefore greet a visitor with: 'How lovely to see you. How is your family?'. This is a courteous attempt to conceal the fact that the person is not precisely remembered, but is recognised as someone who 'should be known'.

Being alert to what posture and stance suggest

As the nurse approaches, it is important to be aware of how posture and stance can make an impression.

If the nurse is tall and the person being approached is sitting down, the effect can be rather intimidating. Sitting by a person is more friendly than standing over that person. Sitting at right angles to each other makes interaction easier.

Making the other person feel 'at home'

Nurses should remember that they are interacting with this person in the place where he or she lives. The nurse is in this person's home, and should act accordingly.

Although it can be comforting to be in hospital if really ill, no one chooses to live permanently in a hospital atmosphere. Whatever they say and do, nurses should make the person with dementia feel 'at home'.

> 'The nurse is in this person's home, and should act accordingly.'

Dealing with a hostile reception

Even if a nurse happens to know a person well, the nurse might sometimes meet a hostile reception. In these circumstances, it might be wise to leave. It is important to realise that the problem that has triggered the hostility could be temporary. Try again later. The nurse might well find that the person then greets him or her warmly. Alternatively, it might be appropriate to ask another staff member to take over.

This is not a situation in which 'blame' should be attached to the nurse or to the person with dementia. If the person is in a bad mood, he or she might be projecting negative feelings onto people who are usually appreciated. In some cases, the person's background might explain the problem. Past experiences and deep-rooted prejudices can trigger an unexpected reaction. Such 'gut' responses should not be held against someone with dementia.

Beginning individual communication

Time should be taken at the start of any task or activity to respond to the other person as an *individual*. By smiling and greeting the person personally, and by using the person's preferred name, the nurse is immediately showing that the person is recognised as an individual in whom the nurse is interested. This impression can now be reinforced, drawing on what the nurse knows about the person and what can be gathered about his or her present mood.

The nurse should recognise and validate the person's current feelings before introducing the activity or task. This is especially important if the person is agitated or upset. Hearty cheerfulness can be quite offensive in such circumstances. Even if the anxiety or fear of the person is quite unfounded, this does not make the emotions any less real or painful. It is inappropriate to argue, or to attempt to 'jolly them out of it'. The emotion should be recognised with words such as: 'I'm sorry to see that you are feeling sad'. The person should be given an opportunity to express his or her feelings. The nurse's sympathy will help to comfort and reassure.

> 'Even if the anxiety or fear of the person is quite unfounded, this does not make the emotions any less real or painful.'

If the person is already in a positive mood, this sense of well-being should be reinforced. Respond to it, and share in the person's mood. A cheerful person might even show it by singing an appropriate song—for example, 'Oh what a beautiful morning'. The nurse can admire the singing, and perhaps join in.

If the person is neither especially happy nor especially sad, the nurse can draw on knowledge of the person's past interests or activities to make a comment that addresses him or her personally. The person's body language and the tone of any verbal response will indicate whether the nurse has 'hit' on a suitable topic.

Another way of validating someone as a person is to ask for his or her help or advice. Everyone dislikes feeling 'useless', and this also applies to people with dementia.

Obviously a request for advice or opinion needs to be suited to the person and his or her level of capacity. Asking someone for help or advice makes the person a partner in the activity and encourages him or her to cooperate in it. Indeed, this technique can be used by a nurse to lead into any specific activity that is the reason for approaching a resident.

Working together

A deliberate policy of 'working together' will help the nurse to maintain a friendly and cooperative atmosphere throughout the task or activity.

The technique of seeking advice is not only applicable to making an initial contact, but also can be used to introduce an activity. For example, the person

Seeking advice and asking opinions

A nurse in a care facility successfully used the communication strategy of seeking advice in dealing with a resident who often wanted to leave the place. She knew that the man had always been a keen gardener and enjoyed pottering about the grounds, so she would ask him for his advice about an aspect of the garden.

'Don't go just yet. I really want your advice about this plant over here. Come and see it and tell me what you think.'

Such a request not only turned the man's attention away from thoughts of escape, but also made him feel that he had a worthwhile role and identity in the care facility.

---

could be asked if he or she would mind holding or carrying something for the nurse—such as a hairbrush or a towel. Or the person might be encouraged to move towards the dining room by asking for his or her opinion on an aspect of the forthcoming meal or the arrangements in the dining room.

It is useful to deal with the task or activity in simple steps. Taking one step at a time, and keeping instructions simple, help to decrease confusion.

There are various ways in which each step of the activity can be reinforced. Repeating key words and phrases in conversation can be useful—especially if this is done in an encouraging and supportive way—'That's right, lift your arm. Is it comfortable for you to lift your arm?'.

Miming gestures and props can also be helpful. For example, holding a hairbrush and making brushing gestures reinforces what the nurse is saying about wanting to brush a person's hair.

The environmental context also reinforces communication about activities. The sight of a toilet can reinforce a question about whether a person needs this facility. Similarly, a comfortable sofa invites a person to sit and chat, and the sight of a garden outside suggests going for a walk together.

It helps to have a routine and to stick to it. Memory of regular, repeated activities tends to survive the effects of dementia. Indeed, people with dementia can often learn new routines. It is helpful if nurses establish a suitable routine that all colleagues follow in certain activities (such as toileting of residents). This might also include set phrases for introducing each step in the process.

Throughout the activity, nurses should make friendly, supportive comments. Emphasising the social aspect of an activity not only makes it more pleasurable, but also improves effective communication.

However, nurses should not be 'over-helpful'. The person should be allowed time to do for himself or herself whatever can still be done. This ensures that people with dementia continue to function normally for as long as possible, and helps to foster their self-esteem.

Strategies for listening
Active listening

Being a good listener helps nurses to get to know the people in their care and understand their feelings and needs. It also helps people to feel valued because they will be made aware that they are still worth listening to. Even if it is difficult to make sense of what is being said, it is worth making the effort to listen with care.

Nurses should always assume that whatever is being said or done by those in their care *does* have meaning—whether or not nurses can immediately grasp it. This is a much more productive attitude than automatically attributing everything to the effects of dementia.

> 'Nurses should always assume that whatever is being said or done by those in their care *does* have meaning—whether or not nurses can immediately grasp it.'

However difficult it might be to understand what a person with dementia is saying, the person's tone of voice and body language can help nurses to grasp the feeling behind the words. 'Listening' to body language helps nurses to frame an appropriate response (for example, 'I'm so sorry that you are feeling sad').

Looking for an explanation

Contrast the following reactions of two attendants to a resident who was shouting angrily.

'They've been at my pockets,' claimed the angry man.

One attendant merely commented: 'He's delirious again'.

The other asked herself why the resident would think someone had 'been at' his pockets. Something he had expected to find there must be 'missing'. She asked the man what he was missing, and then explained: 'No . . . You've changed your trousers. That's why you don't have your handkerchief.'

The man immediately calmed down.

Adapted from Toucheboeuf (1987); present author's translation

By making encouraging murmurs and nods, and by repeating key words and phrases, the nurse can demonstrate active listening.

Making sense of misnamings and verbal fragments

Dementia gradually affects a person's ability to speak normally. People can use the inappropriate names for people and objects, and can speak in fragments rather than in complete sentences. However, the language systems of people with dementia do not simply fall apart. Rather, they work differently. Nurses who listen carefully will recognise that a large proportion of the 'wrong' word choices have a connection with the 'right' word, and the proportion is even higher if nurses know the person well. These connections can be used to develop a set of strategies for working out what the person is trying to say (Crisp 2000).

Nurses might recognise a 'wrong' word as making sense if they look for possible links or likenesses. People with dementia often use a specific word for a much broader range of similar items. A person might use the word 'dog' to refer to a variety of other small dog-like animals (Schwartz, Marin & Saffran 1979). The word 'bear' might be used for all the toy animals or real animals of which the person is fond. In effect, the person is saying that these toys are 'like' a favourite teddy bear. By prefixing the word 'like' to a misnaming, nurses can often grasp what the person means.

As the 'bear' example shows, the link might be an emotional link. Nurses should ask themselves what feeling the misnaming might express.

A 'wrong' word often makes sense if nurses look for verbal links. Which word or words are frequently spoken with this one? Looking for such verbal links can help nurses to complete fragments of standard phrases. If someone is talking about a baby, and gets stuck on 'their first . . . their first', the nurse can look for words that might complete this phrase for the person.

Making sense of statements that seem confused or untrue

A knowledge of the effects of dementia can be used to make sense of statements that might otherwise be dismissed as confused or simply untrue. For someone with dementia, events from long ago can seem more real than what happened yesterday. In addition, people with dementia often cannot distinguish between what actually happened and what they have imagined, read about, or seen on television. Everything in their minds can be equally real to them.

Nurses should therefore ask themselves whether a statement makes sense if it is related to the past. A statement that is false in the present might be perfectly valid if applied to the person's past. A person who has certainly never moved the rocks in the residential garden, might make comments about such an activity that are true of other gardens that he or she has made in the past. Similarly, a person's comments might relate to something that he or she used to do regularly at a particular time of the day—such as going to work at this time, or picking up children from school.

Nurses can also ask whether a comment makes sense if applied more broadly. In the previous example the hospital garden and all the gardens from the person's past are stored together in his or her memory. The claim that the person has moved the rocks in the residential garden becomes valid if nurses apply it more broadly to 'gardens that this person has known'. A nurse can then respond: 'Yes, you've made some wonderful rock gardens'.

Items stored together in memory often become combined in this way. Some of the unlikely things that a person says can make sense if this is understood. For example, a person might comment that Willie, a pet sheep, is sitting on his or her lap. Such a comment makes sense if it realised that Willie represents a composite figure made up of other pets, including a small dog or cat that might have sat on the person's lap. Nurses should ask themselves whether the person is talking about several items or events as if they were one.

'People with dementia are extremely vulnerable to exploitation and abuse—not least because any complaints they make can be dismissed as examples of disorientation or paranoia.'

Nurses should always allow for the possibility that what the person is saying is true. People with dementia are extremely vulnerable to exploitation and abuse—not least because any complaints they make can be dismissed as examples of disorientation or paranoia.

Listening sympathetically to stories

A common sign of dementia is pseudo-reminiscence or confabulation. People might tell stories about themselves in which they improbably mix up fact and fantasy. For example, they might speak of amazing wartime exploits, thanks to 'a gift of guns from the people at Buckingham Palace'. Listening sympathetically to such stories is a challenge, but the following strategies can help nurses to recognise the purposes that such stories serve and allow appropriate responses to be made (Crisp 2000).

It should be recognised that plausible but untrue stories are sometimes a means of saving face. People are covering up the fact that they have forgotten something that they would normally be expected to know—such as what they did yesterday. This is especially common in early dementia. If it is really necessary to correct their version of events, nurses should try to do it tactfully: 'I think that was last week. Didn't you go for a drive with your family yesterday?'

In some cases, the person might be making a bid for sympathy. Presenting oneself as useless or as a victim can be an indirect way of asking for comfort and reassurance. Alternatively, the person might be seeking attention and respect. Boasting about wartime exploits might be an example of this.

This might also be an attempt to compensate for present handicaps. People who are powerful and active in their wartime stories might thus be compensating for their current difficulties.

Some stories are like daydreams, giving people the successful career, large family, or social importance that they wish they had.

A story might also give concrete form to a general problem or general anxiety. For example, a story of someone or something awful creeping up on a person might be expressing a general anxiety about his or her condition. Similarly, a story about searching for the lost pieces of a mother's embroidery might reflect a struggle to regain the missing fragments of memory.

Nurses should listen—even if they cannot make sense of the story. The story is important to the person who is telling it, as is the fact of being able to tell it to a sympathetic listener. Nurses should show that they are listening and trying to understand by nods, encouraging murmurs, and the repetition of key phrases.

Nurses should bear in mind that people are not lying, however fantastic the story. The distinction between truth and lies has been lost, and the stories seem true to them. Nurses should take the stories at face value, and respond to the broader truths or needs that they express.

> 'Nurses should bear in mind that people are not lying, however fantastic the story.'

Communicating to the very end

When a person's dementia is very advanced, it is easy for nurses to wonder whether there is any point in trying to communicate. However, it is still possible to have worthwhile interaction, even though the person can no longer speak or respond as he or she once did.

Nurses should continue to speak with these people as they did when they were still able to respond. The communication might well be 'getting through'. At the very least, a friendly and caring presence will be communicated. This is standard procedure in caring for unconscious patients in intensive-care wards, and the principle applies equally well in caring for people with severe dementia.

Any response should be valued, however minimal. When words fail, a grunt, body movement, or hand pressure from the person communicates that he or she is aware and responding.

The essence of communication is human contact. Continue to reach out to people and give them a chance to reach out in response.

Chapter 10

Restraint

Carole Archibald

Introduction

> I'm held a prisoner here; my sister has stolen my life;
> Now I'm old I'm put away; and expected to dream my time away;
> But I want a natural life where I can see my forebears
> And enjoy the fruits of my labour
>
> KILLICK (1994, P. 4)

The above quotation of an elderly man in a nursing home is quite profound, and provides insights into how it is for some people with dementia. This quotation is pertinent in terms of restraint. The man speaks of being 'held a prisoner' and feels 'expected to dream [his] time away'. But he wants a 'natural life' in which he 'can see [his] forebears'.

The use of restraint is a contentious and emotive issue. Some argue that restraint should never be used, whereas others suggest that, in certain circumstances, it might be the only means of keeping a person safe. The premise of this chapter is that the effects of restraint should largely be seen as adverse.

It is widely accepted that person-centred care is the best approach for quality care, and a person-centred approach includes restraint only when other options have been tried. However, nurses are faced with challenging and difficult decisions to make about older people in their care. These decisions must often be taken with few guidelines and in an environment that eschews risk-taking. Often, it seems, the concept of 'person-centred care' does not extend to staff members, but their needs and safety also have to be considered. How the needs and concerns of residents and staff members can be reconciled with regard to risk-taking and restraint requires further exploration.

This chapter addresses what is meant by restraint, why it is used, and who are the people who tend to be restrained. The adverse effects of restraint are explored, as is the question of why other options should be considered first. Nurses' anxieties regarding risk-taking are addressed, and the chapter suggests that there is a need to develop a philosophy and policy on risk and restraint in every residential/nursing home. The chapter emphasises a multidisciplinary approach, rather than an approach in which decisions are made on an *ad hoc* basis by individual nurses, with the personal anxieties that this involves. If restraint is decided upon as a course of action, this should be based on a full assessment of the person involved, and the decision to use restraint should include family members and a multidisciplinary team.

> 'The decision to use restraint should include family members and a multidisciplinary team.'

Types of restraint

Restraint has been defined as 'anything which interferes with or stops, a resident doing what they appear to want to do' (Clarke & Bright 2002, p. 14). Restraint can be explicit and intentional, or it can be subtle. It can even be unwitting. The Box on page 109 lists some examples of restraint.

Although physical restraint is reported to be widespread, different criteria are used to define the term (Gallinagh et al. 2002). The most commoin form of restraint appears to be the use of bedrails (Retsas 1997; Retsas & Crabbe 1997, 1998).

Reasons for restraint

The most commonly reported reason for the use of restraint is to prevent resident harm. However, the use of restraint often results in the very problems that it is

Some examples of restraint

Restraint can be explicit and intentional, or it can be subtle. It can even be unwitting. Examples of restraint include:

- tagging;
- locks on doors;
- chairs with tables;
- bedrails;
- tight bedclothes;
- harnesses;
- manipulating furniture to keep the resident in one area;
- camera surveillance; and
- chemical restraint—use of sedatives and anti-psychotic drugs.

Mr Andrews

Mr Andrews, a big strong man, had been moved to a nursing home from an acute hospital setting. He had been reported to be aggressive by hospital staff and, in the nursing home, he caused significant injuries to the wrists of several nurses while they were attempting to carry out personal care.

The charge nurse explored the reasons for Mr Andrews' behaviour and discovered that nurses in both the hospital and the nursing home, fearful of their own safety, had held Mr Andrews firmly by the wrists to restrain him while carrying out his personal care. He reacted violently to this restraint. It appeared to the charge nurse that, in grabbing the nurses whenever they came near, Mr Andrews was attacking nurses as a form of self-defence.

The charge nurse worked out a care plan for Mr Andrews in consultation with staff. Nurses who felt able to work with Mr Andrews did so, whereas others who were less confident cared for other residents. According to the plan, nurses suggested to Mr Andrews that he wash his hands in the sink in the bathroom. While he was doing this, a nurse attended to his continence needs. Because no one held him by his wrists, Mr Andrews remained calm, and was more willing to cooperate in his own care.

supposed to overcome (Gallinagh et al. 2002). The Box above provides an example of how the use of restraint can be counter-productive.

In the United Kingdom, the use of restraint is allowed under various Mental Health Acts for specific purposes—provided that its use can be shown to have been the only way of preventing harm to the individual or others (RCN 1999). Any nurse who applies restraint must be able to justify its use. These legal requirements make the casual use of restraint less likely. Nurses have a duty of care to act only in the best interests of the person, and obtaining consent from people who have complex mental-health needs (including people with dementia) is a complex process (RCN 1999).

This is made more difficult by organisational matters and other issues with which nurses have to cope in their daily work. Low staffing levels and heavy workloads can mean that full attention cannot be given to all residents. It is sometimes necessary to direct nursing care to protection, with the focus being on restraint, rather than having a focus on care and responsibility. This work climate can make nurses anxious, and can lead to over-control—which can reinforce and escalate violence (RCN 1999).

People who are restrained

According to a study by Gallinagh et al. (2002), the people most commonly restrained by physical means were those who were more dependent on nurses to meet their needs, particularly those with cognitive impairment. This group of people received more drugs than those whose mobility was not restricted. The common rationale of nurses for the use of restraint was to prevent wandering and to protect people who were confused. Those who were physically restrained were also more likely to be chemically restrained. There was also an increased use of diuretics in those who were restrained. It can be speculated that these residents might have been restrained due to their increased restlessness and distress levels resulting from their need to find the toilet, especially if there were few environmental cues and if nurses were slow to respond to the needs of these people.

People with dementia who have associated sleep disorders and general restlessness are at increased risk of falls, and are therefore more likely to be physically restrained. Poor cognitive status makes a person more likely to have falls. Arising from a bed safely involves mobility skills and memory skills. However, bedrails can frighten these people and increase their confusion. They are more likely to suffer entrapment, and death has been reported in some cases (Gallinagh, Slevin & McCormack 2001). Most deaths have occurred when the person has tried to get out of the restraint. Bedrails are rarely appropriate, except in situations in which the person is somnolent or sedated, or unless the person has suffered a stroke and the bedrails are there to prevent the person from rolling out of bed (Clarke & Bright 2002).

Restlessness, wandering, and aggression are common in nursing homes, and are associated with increased use of physical and chemical restraint (Opie, Doyle & O'Connor 2002). However, behavioural signs such as these are usually an indicator of need. As such, these signs require a behavioural analysis. This is explored later in this chapter (see 'Considering other options', page 115).

Adverse effects of restraint

Physical restraint can have a number of adverse results—including pressure sores, constipation, dehydration, incontinence, muscle loss, deep venous thrombosis, and decreased pulmonary and cardiac capacity. Psychologically, people can feel 'caged', hurt, angry, humiliated, and helpless. The use of restraint can also cause confusion, depression, and loss of self-esteem (Molassiotis 1995). Restraint undermines autonomy. It emphasises the power of staff and the powerlessness of residents (Clarke & Bright 2002).

There is an increased risk of injury associated with the use of bedrails. Serious injury can occur as a result of residents climbing and falling from the elevated side (Gallinagh, Slevin & McCormack 2001).

'Restraint undermines autonomy. It emphasises the power of staff and the powerlessness of residents.'

The effect of chemical restraint is inconsistent, and its use commonly worsens confusion and increases the risk of falls. In addition, many residents in nursing homes are often on at least one inappropriate drug, other than those used for chemical restraint (Furniss et al. 2000). These drugs often have side-effects, such as restlessness and agitation, that can provoke the use of restraint. Assessment should therefore aim to reduce the number of inappropriate prescribed drugs (Furniss et al. 2000).

Risk assessment and restraint

When caring for people with dementia who lack insight into what constitutes a risk for themselves or other residents, some form of distraction or diversion is necessary to keep the person safe. However, this need to keep the resident 'safe' can be overstated, and can result in physical or chemical restraint being used inappropriately. To some extent, this is understandable. Risk assessment needs to be seen within a social context, and nurses are being held increasingly responsible for the risks they take. This can produce a climate of defensiveness in which risk assessment becomes defined by an attitude of 'better safe than sorry' (Kemshall 2002).

In such a climate, if an accident occurs, someone must be to blame, someone must be held to account, and someone must pay (Douglas 1992). Nurses are not only at risk of criticism, but also at risk of public blame and legal liability. In these circumstances, person-centred care, and its central concept of the facilitation of personal choice for the person receiving care, are significantly undermined.

However, risk-taking is advocated by user groups who challenge the restraining practices of professionals that lead to overprotection and increased dependency (Kemshall 2002).

Resolving the tensions between nurses' fear of litigation and the need of residents to take some risks requires the development of a policy on risk and restraint. Such a policy provides a philosophy of care within the service and practical guidance for staff members—thus informing both policy and practice.

The existing philosophy of a unit influences the use of restraint (Marangos-Frost & Wells 2000). A philosophy informed by a medical model—whereby behaviour is considered as a sign of an illness to be controlled—legitimises the use of restraint. In contrast, if the philosophy is more psychosocial—whereby behaviour is perceived as an expression of need—restraint is likely to be used only after other options have been carefully considered. Moreover, any restraint that is used will then be closely monitored.

Individual nurses can, in principle, carry the consequences of any decision not to restrain. However, the views of colleagues can make it more difficult to take that decision (Hantikainen & Silvia 2000). In the absence of a clear policy, to restrain or not often depends on individual staff members, rather than the consistent application of a clear policy.

Family members should be involved in the decision-making process, but this worthy recommendation can be fraught with difficulties. The demands of the family might be in conflict with those of the resident. The family often wants to keep a relative safe at all costs. Family members can collude with nurses in keeping the person safe, washed, and tidy—rather than contemplating considered risk-taking that would enhance the person's quality of life (Clarke & Bright 2002). Nurses can feel a sense of responsibility to the family that overrides responsibility for the resident. For those nurses who want to allow a certain freedom for the resident, the question arises as to how far they can go without neglecting their responsibilities for ensuring safety. The case of Mrs McSorley (Box, page 113) illustrates the dilemma.

> 'Nurses can feel a sense of responsibility to the family that overrides responsibility for the resident.'

The case study of Mrs McSorley highlights the issue of potential conflict between the needs of a resident and those of the family. There is clearly a need

Mrs McSorley

In a support group for family members whose relatives were living in a long-term care facility, a daughter of a woman with dementia—who had recently fallen and fractured her hip in the unit—provoked a lively discussion with regard to risk-taking.

The woman who had fallen and fractured her hip, Mrs McSorley, was now close to death. The trauma of surgery, the pain, and other aspects of the treatment process had all contributed to her poor physical state. In the residential unit Mrs McSorley had been allowed to walk about, rather than being confined to a chair. There had been risks attached to this, but nurses had considered that Mrs McSorley's quality of life would have been severely compromised if she had been restrained.

This group of twelve family members was asked whether, if Mrs McSorley had been their relative, they would have preferred the staff to manage the situation differently.

The relatives formed themselves into two extreme positions. Six wanted their relative to be protected at all costs, even if it required the person to be confined in a chair. The other six felt that quality of life was paramount, and that their relative should be allowed to wander in relative freedom.

to have a policy in place that is based primarily on the needs of the resident, albeit in consultation with the family.

In drawing up such a policy, it needs to be recognised that nurses do not necessarily make decisions that are based on rational choice. Decision-making is often based on the internalised moral values and routines of the service. These factors shape the information that is gathered, how it is processed, the inferences that are drawn, the options that are considered, and the making of the final decision itself (Etzioni 1992). Staff members need to be aware of how their perceptions are formed, and recognise the effect of these perceptions on attitudes to restraint (Hantikainen & Silvia 2000).

The Box on page 114 summarises the various influences that play a part in decision-making on risk-taking and the use of restraint.

Policy guidelines

In developing policy guidelines the basic principle should be the use of the least restraint possible. The decision-making process should include, if possible, residents, families, and the interdisciplinary team.

A physical restraint assessment should be undertaken and documentation of approved devices should be made. More detail is provided below (see 'Documentation', page 114).

Influences on risk-taking and use of restraint

Various difficulties and subtle factors can play a part in determining policies regarding risk-taking and the use of restraint. These include:

- the views of individual staff members;
- the views of other staff members;
- the demands of the family;
- the fact that nurses do not always make decisions based on rational choice; and
- the internalised moral values and routines of the service.

To ensure safety and appropriateness, the nurse's responsibility for checking the device before and during its application should also be documented.

Chemical restraint should be used only as a last resort.

Overall care-planning for physical restraint should be undertaken within the context of stringent guidelines (Gallinagh et al. 2002).

Having developed a policy on the basis of the above principles, there should be patient-centred educational programs for staff combined with organisational consultation to help nurses to reflect on and use behavioural measures, as opposed to using physical restraint. There is also a need to consider environmental cues and layout, bed and chair alarms, and diversional activities.

'Chemical restraint should be used only as a last resort.'

Assessing the need for restraint
Documentation

In the principles outlined above, it was noted that every person should be individually assessed and that such assessment should be properly documented.

Figure 10.1 (page 116) provides an example of such a risk-assessment form. This can be used in deciding whether to use restraint or to look at other alternatives. A risk-assessment form of the type shown in Figure 10.1 ensures that a full assessment takes account of the person (including his or her physical and psychological needs) and includes due recognition of family members, other residents, and staff.

Restraint is situation-specific and should not be seen only in its negative sense (Hantikainen & Silvia 2000). Whether benefits are likely to outweigh adverse effects depends on the situation, and this needs to explored and documented with all options considered.

Principles of policy development

In developing a policy on restraint and risk-taking, the following principles should apply:
- the least possible use of restraint;
- involvement of residents, families, and interdisciplinary team in the decision-making process;
- physical-restraint assessment undertaken and documentation of approved devices;
- specification of a review period;
- checking of devices before and during use for safety and appropriateness;
- full documentation of the purpose of restraint; and
- chemical restraint only as a last resort.

Considering other options

In any assessment process, options other than restraint must be discussed. A person-centred approach looks at the situation from the perspective of the resident and his or her particular needs. Although it might seem to be quicker and easier simply to apply restraint, it can be far more satisfying for nurses to explore why the person is behaving in this way. Nurses should note when the behaviour is occurring, and look for patterns. This will help to identify possible reasons for the behaviour. The following steps are useful:

▶ What form did the behaviour take?
▶ When did it occur?
▶ Where did it occur?
▶ What else is happening?
▶ Are other people involved?
▶ What was the response? (For example, more attention?)

The assessment process needs to consider any physical problems that might lead to behavioural disturbance—such as dehydration, hunger, pain, delirium, infection, and paradoxical drug reactions. If these factors are identified, appropriate steps can be taken, and restraint might not be necessary.

By adopting this sort of reflective process staff can better assess the behaviour and its consequences, and thus make more apropriate assessments of the actions that might be taken. The actions might include a certain type of restraint, but this reflective process ensures that the behaviour is properly assessed and that alternatives are considered.

Risk-assessment form

Describe activity:
....
....

Risks for resident:
What risks could the activity cause the resident?
Risk 1:
Description ....
Assess risk (low, moderate, or high risk of serious harm): ....
Risk 2:
Description ....
Assess risk (low, moderate, or high risk of serious harm): ....

Positive outcomes for resident:
What positive outcomes might there be for the resident in carrying out the activity?
....
....

Risks for other residents and staff:
What risks might the activity cause for other residents and staff?
Risk 1:
Description ....
Assess risk (low, moderate, or high risk of serious harm): ....
Risk 2:
Description ....
Assess risk (low, moderate, or high risk of serious harm): ....

Current situation:
Is the risk suitably controlled? Yes/No ....
If yes, what precautions are already in place to help reduce the risk? ....
If no, what further action is necessary to control the risk? ....

Actions needed:
Actions needed following risk assessment:
Action (1): ....
Who will take the action? ....
Date the action must be carried out by: ....
Action (2): ....
Who will take the action? ....
Date the action must be carried out by: ....

Resident's view:
....
....

Relative's or representative's view (where relevant):
....
....

Signatures:
Resident ....
Date: ....
Relative or representative (if relevant) ....
Date: ....
Manager ....
Date: ....

Date for future review:
Date of review ....

Figure 10.1 Suggested format for risk-assessment form
Adapted from Clark & Bright (2002)

Conclusion

This chapter has explored what is meant by restraint, the difficulties that can accrue as a result of its use, and a reflective process that facilitates other ways of addressing residents' needs in a creative way. Several other chapters in this book explore creative alternatives to restraint, especially Chapter 7 Wandering (page 70), Chapter 13 Falls Prevention (page 142), and Chapter 16 Aggression (page 184).

Although there might be a few specific circumstances that merit the use of restraint, the adverse physical and psychological effects on the person require nurses to look for alternative therapeutic ways of addressing needs. It is necessary to explore ways that allow residents to take risks while remaining as safe as is possible.

'It is necessary to explore ways that allow residents to take risks while remaining as safe as is possible.'

Chapter 11

Quality Use of Medicines

Jill Beattie

Introduction

The use of medicines to treat and prevent disease has enhanced the health and well-being of people throughout the world. However, medicines can also cause harm, and there has been increasing concern about the overuse, underuse, and misuse of medicines and their effects on the well-being of individuals, as well their social and economic costs.

In the 1980s the World Health Organization (WHO) adopted a strategy for the rational use of medicines and called on governments throughout the world to implement national drug policies. By the end of 1999, approximately 80 countries had a national drug policy, and were implementing various strategies for the quality use of medicines (WHO 2001).

This chapter focuses on the meaning of the term 'quality use of medicines' (QUM) in the care of people with dementia. It explores some of the factors that influence clinical decision-making and some of the challenges to QUM. Real-life examples from residential aged care are used to highlight what is actually happening in some aged-care facilities and how nurses can play a crucial role in influencing QUM.

The meaning of QUM

QUM involves:

▶ judicious selection of management options;
▶ selection of the most appropriate medicine; and
▶ safe and effective use of medicines.
Each of these is discussed below.

Judicious selection of management options

Management options for people with dementia can be pharmacological or non-pharmacological. Sound clinical judgment based on up-to-date knowledge and experience should be used to decide the best treatment option for people with dementia. The best treatment option might well be non-drug therapies.

'The best treatment option might well be non-drug therapies.'

Selection of the most appropriate medicine

Once it has been decided that medicines are the best management option, it is necessary to select the most appropriate medicine from those available. This requires a consideration of the person's clinical condition, the risks and benefits of using a given drug, the length of treatment, therapies already in use, monitoring requirements, and the financial cost to the person, the person's family, the community, and the health system as a whole.

Safe and effective use of medicines

The safe and effective use of medicines requires nurses to be clear about the goals of treatment, and the documentation of those goals. It also requires nurses' ensuring that these goals are being achieved by monitoring and documenting the outcomes of the use of medicines. Appropriate monitoring of the person's health and well-being, and noting early signs of any adverse effects, decrease the likelihood of overuse, underuse, and misuse of medicines. This enables prompt action to be taken to resolve any medication-related problems, or lack of response to the medicines prescribed (DH&A 2002).

The above requirements represent a logical and rational approach to QUM. However, in managing the well-being of people with dementia in the real world of aged care, doctors, nurses, pharmacists, people with dementia, and their relatives often have different views of what is entailed in QUM.

Interests affecting clinical decision-making

Nurses often feel powerless to influence QUM because, in most residential aged-care facilities, nurses do not have prescribing rights. However, the actions of nurses, pharmacists, other carers, relatives, and the residents themselves all influence the prescribing patterns of doctors. Nurses should be aware that they *do* influence both the initiation and the discontinuation of medicines.

> 'Nurses should be aware that they *do* influence both the initiation and the discontinuation of medicines.'

Nurses also need to recognise that their 'worldview' about appropriate intervention options (both pharmacological and non-pharmacological) affects their clinical judgment and decision-making—just as other members of the medication management team (doctors, pharmacists, residents, and relatives) are affected by their particular 'worldviews'. These 'worldviews' can be categorised as a focus on:

- science and medicine;
- benevolence;
- medication administration;
- economic rationalism; and
- organisational factors.

Each of these is discussed below.

Science and medicine affecting decision-making

A scientific medical worldview values medicines as a primary management option. Although there is no doubt that some medicines can prolong lives, decrease disease, and enhance the well-being of residents, relying on medicines to 'fix' the majority of problems often leads to the inappropriate use of medicines. This often occurs at the expense of a consideration of non-drug options. This worldview is reflected in the words of a nurse who observed:

> Doctors prescribe it readily. We ask for it readily. We look at it as a fix for everything.
>
> AUTHOR'S PERSONAL SOURCE

The following comments of a doctor emphasise this reliance on medicines, and reveal a dilemma:

> The nurses can growl at you all [they] like about [people] having multiple drugs, but every time they call you, they want you to do something. They

call the doctor to do something. When they call you, it's very hard not to do something, because you feel that you're being dismissive of their concerns if you provide nothing in the way of drugs. So, that's a major problem for both sides to recognise—that you *can* do something without prescribing a drug.

AUTHOR'S PERSONAL SOURCE

The words of another nurse highlight the dilemma when a person relies on medicines to sleep:

A lot of residents depend on sleeping tablets. They won't sleep until they know that their tablet is right there.

AUTHOR'S PERSONAL SOURCE

If members of the medication management team focus on medicines as a way of managing the signs and symptoms of a disease, their actions centre on finding the best drug to treat a *problem*. In contrast, if the focus is on the quality use of medicines for the *well-being of the person*, the emphasis is on finding the best available intervention option from among non-pharmacological therapies, as well as from pharmacological therapies.

Benevolence affecting decision-making

'Benevolence' in decision-making is the basing of decisions on what is thought to be in the best interests of the person receiving treatment. However, who is to decide what is in the best interests of the person? This is a difficult question to answer, especially when caring for people with dementia.

> 'Who is to decide what is in the best interests of the person . . . is a difficult question to answer, especially when caring for people with dementia.'

From the perspective of residents and relatives, a commitment to benevolence is expected. Residents and relatives place their trust in health-care professionals and assume that nurses, doctors, and pharmacists act in the person's best interests. This is illustrated by the following comment made by a resident:

. . . they prescribed them for me. They must have thought they were the best type of tablets to give me.

AUTHOR'S PERSONAL SOURCE

However, each member of the medication team has different interests that drive his or her understanding of what is in the best interests of the person. For example, a relative or primary carer knows the person intimately, and is aware of his or her likes, dislikes, and nuances. However, relatives might demand medicines inappropriately—for example, in demanding antibiotics for viral infections. Conversely, relatives might request the discontinuation of medicines if they are concerned about adverse effects. This is illustrated in the following example:

> I kept telling them, kept telling them. In the finish I had to say that if they didn't change [a medication], I would get another doctor. And finally they did change the drug, and my wife came good as soon as they took her off the tablet. Came good, just like that.
>
> AUTHOR'S PERSONAL SOURCE

Nurses might consider that the distress that is experienced by some people during the administration of medication is not in the person's best interests. The nurse in the following example voices the frustration that nurses can feel when relatives insist on medicines:

> I think that medication is, at times, totally inappropriate . . . the lady over here, she's having multivitamins . . . and she's on death's door . . . and [we are] pushing all this stuff into her. At this stage of her health, she really needs quality care . . . [But she's getting] calcium tablets like big eggs . . . and multivitamins. She can't even swallow them.
>
> AUTHOR'S PERSONAL SOURCE

A doctor might consider that the best interests of the person are served if he or she receives the latest drug treatment based on the latest knowledge of the disease with which the person presents. Doctors are professionally responsible for determining the best available treatment, and this has legal ramifications in that the doctor can be considered negligent if he or she does not prescribe according to current practice. This issue was raised by a nurse in the following terms:

> Because the resident has a certain condition, the doctors are very reluctant to actually take them off the drug, because they say . . . they need it and they will be negligent if they just [take] them off this drug—[whether it is] for Parkinson's, or cardiac problems, or whatever. So they can't take them off it, because they will appear to be negligent.
>
> AUTHOR'S PERSONAL SOURCE

Although communicating with people who have dementia can be challenging, people with dementia do communicate many of their needs. A nurse who had to cope with several people who refused medication made the following insightful observation:

> And [I] say to the resident: 'Open your mouth . . . please, now come on, this is for you'. [But] it's not for them at all really, is it?
>
> Author's personal source

> 'Although communicating with people who have dementia can be challenging, people with dementia do communicate many of their needs.'

The answer to this nurse's question is that the resident's interests are *not* driving the administration of these medicines. The doctor might have ordered the drug because it was the best treatment at the time, or because a relative felt that it was 'best' for the resident. The nurse believes that she has to administer what is ordered—that is, she is coming from a worldview of medication *administration*, rather than a worldview of medication *management*. The person with dementia, in attempting to refuse the medication, is certainly communicating his or her interests—not to have the medicine.

In supporting QUM, nurses need to collaborate with doctors, pharmacists, residents, and relatives to weigh the *demonstrated* benefits of administering medicines, as well as the risks. In the example above, there is a risk in forcing administration. This coercion provokes distress, not only for the resident but also for the nurse.

Medication administration affecting decision-making

Much of the time of nurses is spent administering and managing medications. However, this is only one aspect of nursing care. Focusing on medication administration can lead nurses to act in ways that do not support QUM in the interests of the well-being of the persons in their care. If nurses allow a worldview of medication administration to drive their actions, they focus on getting the drug into the person at all costs. This is highlighted in the following example.

> Sometimes the resident is actually woken up to be given their sleeping tablet. And I think . . . 'What is the point?'
>
> Author's personal source

A medication administration worldview focuses on spending time and energy on working out various ways of getting a drug into the person, often without success. This is illustrated by a nurse:

> GPs always prescribe them, but the residents spit them out. They refuse
> them. They don't take even half of the drink that they're in. They're
> getting only about 50% of the drugs, yet they manage quite well.
>
> AUTHOR'S PERSONAL SOURCE

To administer medications to people with dementia, nurses spend much of
their time crushing medicines, disguising medicines in food and fluids, and
coercing residents to take medicines. All of this is time-consuming and focuses
on the drugs—not on an assessment of the residents' well-being or the possible
discontinuation of inappropriate medicines. This raises issues of ethics and issues
of appropriate use of resources.

Economic rationalism affecting decision-making

The economies of many countries are modelled on economic rationalism,
which aims to produce efficient systems with reduced waste and increased
profit. This is achieved by taking a logical approach that considers the
advantages and disadvantages of using particular means with finite resources
to achieve stated ends. Many residential aged-care facilities are run as
businesses and must sustain a profit to remain viable. Health care in many of
these facilities has thus become quantified, with funding being allocated
to various tasks. The available time to complete these tasks has also become
a commodity.

If nurses focus on tasks to be completed and remunerated, the time available
for the care of people and QUM is often limited, and nurses can feel that they
never have enough time to care for people. In these circumstances, the use of
medicines as a 'quick fix' often predominates. As one doctor put it:

> I worry sometimes that the medication is more for the institution than the
> person because the resident might be . . . more disruptive than is liked and
> there are not enough staff to manage this.
>
> AUTHOR'S PERSONAL SOURCE

The focus in the example above is on keeping the person quiet so that staff
members can carry out the tasks to be completed. In contrast to this approach,
time should be spent on assessment of the person's needs, education of staff in
the management of people with 'disruptive' behaviours, and strategies to
decrease these behaviours.

Economic pressure is felt by all members of the team. Doctors are aware of
how little time it takes to write a script, and how long it takes to communicate.
For example:

> . . . it takes two minutes to write the script and two hours of
> communication not to, and if you've had all that communication and
> anything goes wrong, you're the donkey.
>
> AUTHOR'S PERSONAL SOURCE

When health-care professionals are driven by an economic rationalist
worldview, it is often difficult for them to take the time to reflect upon their
practices and see that their actions actually support the inappropriate use of
medicines. The doctor in the following example recognises this dilemma:

> Sometimes, when you've got someone in long-term care, what happens
> is that their drug treatment is just continued, rolled over, and con-
> tinued without often really [determining] is this really necessary, is that
> really necessary?
>
> AUTHOR'S PERSONAL SOURCE

Furthermore, in their haste to administer medicines, nurses can be providing
inappropriate care for people. In some instances, this places relatives in
compromised positions. This is illustrated by the following words from a relative.

> I was there one Friday and she had mashed fish and vegetables, and she
> was just starting to eat it and looked like she was really enjoying it.
> Someone came up and said: 'Right, here's your medication', [and] stuck it
> in her mouth . . . She immediately spat the whole lot out. I thought I
> should really do something and say something, but . . . time just gets away
> and you've got other things going on.
>
> AUTHOR'S PERSONAL SOURCE

In this example the relative also felt constrained by a form of economic
rationalism in making an allocation of personal time and resources.

Organisational factors influencing quality use of medicines

Although quality-improvement programs and accreditation processes in
residential aged care are rigorous, questions have been raised about the emphasis
in many of these programs on fulfilling documentation requirements, rather than
on sustained improvements to the well-being of residents.

Several organisational factors have been identified that impede QUM in
residential aged-care facilities:
- a lack of collaboration among pharmacists, doctors, nurses, residents,
  relatives, and government bodies;
- inappropriate personnel, unqualified staff, and inappropriate staff skill mix;

- poor staff-to-resident ratios;
- inadequate continuing education (about medicines and about dementia and other diseases);
- ineffective communication systems (for residents, their relatives, and health-care professionals); and
- lack of continuity of care (between the person's home and the facility, and between a hospital and the facility).

Some facilities do not provide appropriate structures and environments for quality care, including QUM and the special care needs of people with dementia. Nurses who work in these facilities can feel that they are unable to carry out their duty of care, and many of these nurses have consequently left the aged-care sector.

Unfortunately, the response of some proprietors and managers of facilities has been to lobby for less-qualified staff to carry out tasks, rather than provide the environment and conditions for appropriately qualified nurses to manage the complex processes involved in the quality use of medicines. However, many facilities *are* providing appropriate environments for quality residential aged care, and these organisations are attracting qualified and experienced staff.

Towards best practice

Collaborative decision-making processes

The specialised expertise of each member of the medication management team is crucial for QUM. But without collaborative decision-making, QUM cannot be achieved. The following words of a pharmacist illustrate this:

> I had a call [from a nurse] the other day. Mrs So and So's drug chart [was] now four pages [long]. That's too many. And I had a look at her medications, and I spoke to her doctor . . . She's a very difficult case, and she's going to stay on four drug chart pages.
>
> AUTHOR'S PERSONAL SOURCE

This decision to continue four pages of medications was made by the pharmacist and the doctor during a telephone call. The decision-making process did not include the nurse or the resident, and did not involve a review of the documentation of the woman's condition and her response to the medicines. In this case, the woman had actually been refusing the majority of the medications prescribed—a fact that the pharmacist and doctor did not apparently know because they failed to consult with other members of the team.

Involvement of residents and relatives in the decision-making process is crucial. Unfortunately, relatives sometimes have to 'beg' for their voices to be heard:

> He's been tried on [anti]psychotic and sedative drugs, and each time he [has become] bombed out. Dad said that he thought he was dying. He felt so bad . . . I said: 'Doctor, please, I beg you, I beg you, please reduce the dose' . . . I was able to rectify it in conjunction with the doctor and the senior nurse. We were able to discuss it. He hardly has any doses now.
>
> AUTHOR'S PERSONAL SOURCE

Nurses enabling QUM

QUM requires judicious selection of management options—including non-pharmacological interventions. QUM also requires that appropriate medicines are chosen, and that medicines are safe and effective. To achieve these requirements, appropriate evidence must be available and communicated within the medication management team.

Gathering evidence

The primary role of the nurse is to monitor and manage the care and well-being of residents. With respect to QUM, nurses must be skilled in:

▶ monitoring the effects of non-pharmacological and pharmacological interventions by frequent observation and assessment of the person's clinical condition and well-being;

▶ frequent communication with other nurses, residents, relatives, and other care workers; and

▶ accessing up-to-date knowledge through doctors, pharmacists, specialists, and the literature.

Communicating evidence

Quality care and QUM cannot occur unless all the members of the team have access to evidence to guide their decision-making in the best interests of the resident. Nurses therefore also need to ensure that they:

▶ access documented evidence of the resident's health status;

▶ document evidence of the resident's response to medicines, including early recognition of any adverse effects; and

▶ notify the doctor promptly of the resident's response (or lack of response) to medicines prescribed, including early recognition of any adverse effects. Nurses should document repeated refusal and partial administration of medicines. They should also notify doctors and pharmacists if residents require medicines to be crushed because of swallowing difficulties. Many medicines are not designed to be crushed and can have an unpleasant taste if this is done.

If multiple medications are being crushed and concealed in food because of refusal, a case conference is required to determine the real needs of the person with respect to prescribed medications. Actions then need to be taken to address any issue identified in such a conference.

Medication review

Nurses in residential aged care coordinate the care of residents in collaboration with other members of the team. There should therefore be regular review of the medicines prescribed and the medicines actually taken by the resident—perhaps at intervals of 6–8 weeks.

Facilities should establish a medication advisory committee—including a doctor, nurse, pharmacist, resident, and relative. The aim of such a committee is 'to develop, promote, monitor and evaluate activities which foster the quality use of medicines in residential aged care facilities' (APAC 2000). In practice, such a committee is difficult to maintain unless adequate funding is allocated. Nurses should raise this issue with management, proprietors, and government funding bodies.

'As required' medications

The ordering of medications to be administered 'as required' ('prn') is common practice in aged-care facilities. These medications are administered at the discretion of a nurse, based on sound clinical judgment. However, the clinical judgment of a nurse is often affected by the nurse's worldview and the organisational constraints under which he or she must practise.

> 'The clinical judgment of a nurse is often affected by the nurse's worldview and the organisational constraints under which he or she must practise.'

The most common drugs ordered on this basis are tranquillisers and other psychotropic medicines, aperients, and analgesics. Evidence suggests that (Beattie 2003):

▶ tranquillisers and other psychotropic medicines are overused;
▶ aperients are overused; and
▶ analgesics, especially in the care of people with dementia, are significantly underused.

With respect to psychotropic medicines, non-pharmacological therapies can decrease the use of these drugs. In managing constipation, if increased attention is given to activity, nutrition, fluids, and the minimisation of medicines that have constipating effects, the use of aperients is decreased. With regard to the use of analgesics, assessing pain in people with dementia is a challenge for the assessment skills of nurses. Nurses need to refine these skills, and recognise that they have a role in acting as advocates for people with dementia who are in constant pain.

Nurses in residential aged-care facilities *do* influence the use of medicines. In the case of medications that are administered 'as required', nurses have the sole power to determine the appropriate use of medicines.

Conclusion

Nurses are uniquely placed to encourage the quality use of medicines. Every drug that is administered to people with dementia should have a clearly documented rationale, and should be monitored and evaluated carefully. Nurses provide continuity of care and can act to enhance the quality use of medicines to improve the health and well-being of people with dementia and their families.

Chapter 12

Incontinence

Mary King

Introduction

Incontinence has serious implications for people with dementia, and is often the main reason for admission to a residential aged-care facility. Fonda et al. (1994) reported that, in Australia, 50–70% of people suffering from incontinence live in residential aged-care facilities. In a later study, Fonda et al. (2002) referred to the increased number of older people with incontinence, and noted that this 'demographic imperative' will impose significant demands on future health-care resources. However, in residential aged care there is not always a direct correlation between dementia and incontinence. Although a person with dementia might have significant memory loss, confusion, and disorientation, and although these can cause incontinence, it is important to recognise there are many other causes of incontinence.

Continence management calls for skilled nursing interventions based on the best evidence available. Continence management for a person with dementia must also be based on a nurse's sensitivity towards that person's feelings about incontinence and the individual responses that ensue. For example, one of the major causes for restlessness in a person with dementia is a frustrated desire to visit the toilet. If that person does not have the cognitive ability to link the desire to visit the toilet with a meaningful action, the result can be restlessness that escalates to aggressive behaviour which is distressing to all concerned. When an experienced nurse is able to identify the person's needs, negative responses can often be avoided.

'When an experienced nurse is able to identify the person's needs, negative responses can often be avoided.'

Urinary incontinence
Types of urinary incontinence
There are four main types of urinary incontinence, and each responds to different treatments. (For more on this, see 'Treatment of urinary incontinence', page 136.)

Stress incontinence
Stress incontinence is characterised by leakage of small amounts of urine during or after coughing, sneezing, laughing, or brisk walking. Stress incontinence is often related to weak pelvic floor musculature and/or an ineffective urethral sphincter. This type of incontinence is more common in women, but it can occur in men after prostatic surgery.

Urge incontinence
Urge incontinence is characterised by leakage of urine after an urge to pass urine. There are two main types of urge incontinence:
▶ *Sensory urgency incontinence* is the loss of small amounts of urine before getting to the toilet. This has been called 'key-in-the-front-door' urgency because of the feeling that, if the toilet is not accessed immediately, urine leakage will occur.
▶ *Motor urgency symptoms* are usually characterised by the loss of a larger volume of urine, and often occurs when the person is getting up from a chair or bed. The leakage of urine is typically described as 'running down my legs and I can't control it'.
  Causes of urge incontinence include:
▶ cystitis due to urinary tract infections or other causes;
▶ brain pathology (such as a tumour or stroke) preventing the sending of a nerve message to the bladder to 'hold on';

- alcohol, caffeine, and certain prescription medications—for example, diuretics and some non-steroidal anti-inflammatory drugs (NSAIDS);
- atrophic changes in the bladder and urethra due to hormone deficiency;
- anxiety causing hypersensitivity and inappropriate bladder contractions; and
- constipation and faecal impaction pressing on the bladder.

Residents who complain of symptoms of urge incontinence and who have a family history of renal stones or bladder cancer should be referred to a specialist urologist to exclude other pathology.

Overflow incontinence

Overflow incontinence is any involuntary loss of urine associated with over-stretching of the bladder due to urinary retention. The most common signs and symptoms are frequency of micturition, constant dribbling of urine, straining to void, hesitancy, dribbling after passing urine, and increased urge to void.

Overflow incontinence can easily be misunderstood in people with dementia who might continue to pass urine even after rising from the toilet. This is due to confusion related to positional retention.

Persistent urinary tract infections can follow urinary retention. If not treated, reflux of urine to the kidneys can eventually cause kidney damage.

The most common causes of overflow incontinence are:

- obstruction due to enlargement of the prostate gland;
- urethral obstruction due to stricture or other causes;
- nerve damage from spinal surgery, injury, or spinal pathology from osteoporosis; and
- atonic bladder or diminished bladder function that affects the bladder's ability to contract and empty effectively.

Functional incontinence

Functional incontinence occurs when a person loses the ability to pass urine or awareness of the urge to pass urine. Functional incontinence is often seen in association with the other forms of incontinence, and is commonly due to immobility or cognitive dysfunction. A person with this form of incontinence needs to be fully assisted to maintain all levels of personal hygiene—including toileting, showering, and dressing.

The aim of continence management

The aim of continence management for a person with dementia is to identify the most effective treatment program to lessen the incontinence—based on the particular needs of that person at the time. The aims are to maintain the resident's dignity (especially if that person has little awareness of being incontinent) and to keep the resident's skin clean and dry. In the context of dementia, the nurse's skilled management is fundamental to the resident's comfort and well-being.

Skilled continence management in dementia requires a thorough under-standing of dementia as well as a thorough understanding of inconti-nence in all its manifestations.

In many cases a nurse will not be able to rely on a resident's ability to

> 'The aims are to maintain the resident's dignity . . . and to keep the resident's skin clean and dry.'

comply with a program, or on a resident's ability to learn new skills. This calls for the utmost patience on the part of the nurse, together with a readiness to be adaptable and flexible, responding with a 'trial-and-error' approach if required. It is also important that a nurse focuses on what capacities are retained by residents, rather than focusing on their deficits. For example, identifying clear, specific, and attainable goals, and accompanying this with regular prompting, can result in a resident visiting the toilet appropriately. As Resnick and Fleishell (2002, p. 93) observed: 'Residents with cognitive impairment can often identify simple goals that, if repeated frequently, can help sustain motivation'.

The most important component of continence management is compre-hensive assessment—both at the time of a resident's admission and as that person's condition changes.

Assessment of urinary incontinence
Initial assessment

Initial assessment of a person with dementia on admission to residential care depends on the involvement of family members or other carers who can provide an accurate history of the person's incontinence. This initial assessment includes the following:

▶ discussion with the resident and/or carer to identify whether incontinence is a new problem or whether it has been present for some time;
▶ identification of the extent of the problem and whether the person experiences urinary incontinence or faecal incontinence (or both);
▶ a thorough understanding of what the incontinence means to the person (in terms of identified responses) and how the family responds to the problem;
▶ establishing the person's (and the family's) level of understanding of incontinence, its causes, and its treatments;

▶ gaining information from the person and the family about the resident's previous management of the problem—for example, whether a toileting schedule has been established or tried, and whether continence appliances have been used (and to what effect); and

▶ identifying medical reasons for the incontinence—for example, past medical conditions or surgical interventions.

Further assessment for urinary incontinence

Following the initial assessment, further detailed assessment is required. This should be carried out frequently—depending on the nature and extent of the problem. Further assessment might include the following.

▶ Urinalysis of a midstream specimen of urine (MSU) should be performed to check for infection. If infection appears to be present, the urine should be sent for microbiological analysis to identify the microorganism and its sensitivity to antibiotic therapy.

▶ If incontinence continues after infection has been treated, further investigation is warranted. Some infections require more than one course of antibiotic therapy.

▶ The person's post-voiding volume of residual urine should be checked by bladder palpation or percussion, or by ultrasound scan if this is available. This is helpful in assessing effective bladder emptying and identifying bladder dysfunction.

▶ Any bladder dysfunction thus identified might respond to medications or to a toileting program.

▶ The resident's fluid intake and output over a 72-hour period should be established by accurately recording all details. This should include the time and amount of each void, together with descriptions of episodes of incontinence.

Depending on the resident's cognitive abilities, it can be difficult for nurses to obtain the above information accurately. It can also be difficult to obtain a urine specimen because this depends on the resident's ability to cooperate. If the person is able to initiate voiding in an appropriate location, a suitable receptacle can be placed in the toilet.

Past medical or surgical history

A full review of the person's medical and surgical history should be undertaken.

For a female resident, this includes an examination of the vulva and vagina to detect any atrophy and to assess any prolapse of the bladder, cervix, or bowel. A gynaecological history should include details of previous surgery such as a hysterectomy or repairs of prolapse of bladder or bowel. A detailed obstetrical history might also be relevant, and should include any history of forceps delivery or vacuum delivery.

For a male resident, it is important to identify signs and symptoms of prostatic disease—including hesitancy, poor stream, dribbling, or evidence of prostatomegaly. It is also important to document any relevant past urological history—such as prostatic surgery or dilatation for urethral stricture.

In both sexes, the following should be checked:

▶ any past history of pelvic irradiation;
▶ past history of tumours of the bladder, pelvis, or genitalia;
▶ any evidence of constipation (especially rectal impaction)—because this can diminish bladder emptying and increase urgency;
▶ evidence or past history of diabetes mellitus—because high blood sugar can increase urine output and precipitate incontinence in a person with small bladder capacity;
▶ evidence or past history of peripheral neuropathy (as a result of diabetes or alcohol excess for example)—which can affect bladder emptying;
▶ history of stroke or Parkinson's disease; and
▶ medications that might affect continence—including sedatives, tranquillisers, diuretics, anti-hypertensive drugs, opiates, and other analgesics.

Other contributing factors

In persons with dementia, several other factors can contribute to incontinence, and a proper assessment includes the following.

▶ *Mobility:* Is the resident able to access the toilet without assistance? If not, what assistance is required?
▶ *Cognitive function:* Is the person able to identify a need to go to the toilet? What planning ability or motivation is evident? Can the resident identify the toilet and then remember how to get there next time, or is direction needed on each occasion? Is the resident aware of the need to manage his or her clothing and appliances, or is assistance required? What particular signs are evident that the person is seeking assistance with toileting?
▶ *Dignity and social issues:* Does the resident pass urine or faeces in inappropriate places?
▶ *Dexterity:* Is the resident able to adjust clothing and satisfactorily manage the changing and disposal of an appliance; or is assistance required?
▶ *Safety and risk factors:* Is the resident in danger of slipping or falling when attempting to reach the toilet?

> *Fluid intake:* What is the resident's desired and recommended fluid intake? What past influences affect fluid intake? The Box below describes a common misconception about the relationship between fluid intake and incontinence.

Treatment of urinary incontinence

As noted above, there are four main types of urinary incontinence, and each responds to different treatments. In most cases, a treatment program can be successful in decreasing the episodes of incontinence, even when the person has impaired mental function

Stress incontinence

The selection of appropriate therapy for *stress incontinence* depends on the person's degree of cognitive impairment. For example, encouragement to undertake frequent pelvic-floor exercises is appropriate only for a person who has the ability to understand the procedure.

There are several non-surgical techniques for stress incontinence—including the use of oestrogen creams and pessaries, and the use of disposable and reusable intravaginal support devices. All of these products need to be fitted by a trained health professional—because sizing is required before fitting. Use of such devices is dependent on the person's cognitive functioning and the ability to cooperate in their use. A containment product for this type of

---

Maintain fluid intake

Many people misunderstand the relationship between fluid intake and incontinence in the elderly. When asked about her mother's fluid intake before her admission to a nursing home, Mrs A told nurses:

'I make sure she has only small amounts to drink and nothing at all after 4 pm. She worries so much when she wets her pants or wets the bed, so I always restrict her drinking for that reason.'

Nurses are in a position to educate other staff and family members that a decreased fluid intake actually reduces the bladder's holding capacity. A low fluid intake also increases the risk of constipation—thus causing increased urinary incontinence and the possibility of faecal leakage.

A healthy fluid intake should be about 1500 millilitres a day, unless otherwise contraindicated. Some types of fluid, especially caffeine or citrus drinks, can heighten sensation of urgency and increase the frequency of micturition. These fluids should therefore be kept to a minimum.

urine leakage is a small disposable pad (or washable pad) with a capacity of 80–100 millilitres.

Surgical interventions are not the treatment of first choice, and assessment by a specialist surgeon is required before such surgery is recommended.

Urge incontinence

Treatment and selection of appropriate interventions for *urge incontinence* depends on the person's ability to understand a program and the nurse's willingness to participate in managing the program. Most treatment programs consist of teaching the person to 'retrain' the bladder to hold more by deferring the urge to void. Medications can be used to dampen the urge to void. However, these drugs can also increase confusion, so they should be used with caution. Surgical options are available, but the success rate is better with non-surgical interventions.

Containment products recommended for this type of incontinence depend on the amount of leakage and the ability of the person to respond to a toileting program. Referral to a nurse continence adviser is recommended.

Overflow incontinence

Treatment of *overflow incontinence* includes estimating the residual amount of urine after voiding by a post-voiding bladder scan or an 'in–out' catheter. If an elderly person has no symptoms of incontinence, a post-voiding residual volume of 300–350 millilitres is acceptable. If the person has a higher than recommended fluid intake, reducing the fluid intake to 1500–1800 millilitres per day might decrease the high residual amount. Teaching the person the technique of 'double voiding' (as described below) has been shown to help. For people with dementia, this requires nurses' reinforcing the technique every time voiding occurs.

For females, 'double voiding' involves the passing of urine normally. The woman then stands up, walks forward or turns, and then sits down again. She then tries to pass further urine. For males, the technique involves standing in the normal manner to pass urine, then sitting down and trying to pass urine again. If a male resident is unable to stand, the technique described for females is recommended.

Urinary catheterisation should be considered only as a last resort—due to the inherent problems associated with this procedure.

Containment products recommended for this type of incontinence

'Urinary catheterisation should be considered only as a last resort—due to the inherent problems associated with this procedure.'

depend on the sex of the person and the volume of leakage. A nurse continence adviser is the best person to assess the options.

Functional incontinence

Treatment of *functional incontinence* depends on a thorough assessment, together with open and honest communication with the resident and family about the best method of decreasing or containing the incontinence.

Containment products recommended for this type of incontinence vary according to the resident's willingness to wear a product and the volume of urine leakage. If it is considered appropriate to use a containment product for a person with dementia, it is advisable to discuss all the options with a continence adviser. Frequent review and ongoing assessment will determine when other options need to be considered, particularly in response to any decline in the resident's cognitive capacity.

Faecal incontinence

Faecal incontinence is a very distressing problem for residents with dementia and for their carers. Many of the principles outlined above also apply to faecal incontinence. Successful treatment depends on an accurate diagnosis of the underlying problem, and the resident's cognitive ability to cooperate with interventions. In most cases, 70% of the incontinence can be managed effectively.

Principles of bowel management

Success in decreasing episodes of faecal incontinence depends on nurses understanding the principles of bowel management, including the following.

- *Dietary requirements:* for an older person with dementia, it can be useful to encourage smaller, more frequent meals, rather than three large meals per day.
- *Fluid intake requirements:* the myth that reduced fluid intake will reduce incontinence should be dispelled. On the contrary, decreased fluid intake increases the risk of incontinence, urinary tract infections, and constipation. The volume of fluid intake should be determined in consultation with the resident's doctor and should take into account such factors as cardiac and renal function. The majority of the fluid should be taken early in the day—approximately one cup per hour from eight in the morning until midday—with the intake then being reduced to a lower level in the afternoon.
- *Exercise:* Exercise and the relationship between general mobility and bowel evacuation should be evaluated.

▶ *Use of laxatives:* Daily aperients are not recommended because they interfere with normal bowel movement and make it ineffective

▶ *Side effects of medications:* If the resident's medications include codeine or other morphine derivatives, aperient usage needs to be adjusted accordingly.

▶ *Regularity of bowel movement:* Residents with dementia might be encouraged to have a bowel movement on a regular basis—for example 30–40 minutes after a meal. Whether to expect bowel movements daily or less frequently depends on the person's past habits, volume of food intake, mobility, and ability to respond to a toileting program.

▶ *Bowel regimen appropriate to each resident's needs:* If a resident with dementia requires assistance with bowel evacuation it might be more effective to establish a pattern by the use of suppositories twice per week or every fourth day, rather than daily. This regimen assists with bowel training, establishes some predictability, and is less intrusive than daily or second-daily interventions.

Assessment of faecal incontinence

As for urinary incontinence, assessment of faecal incontinence begins with a thorough understanding of the resident's past history and attitudes towards bowel management, together with a comprehensive medical assessment to identify factors that might be contributing to the problem.

Specific assessment includes accurate documentation of the resident's bowel actions for a period of five days.

As well as this accurate recording, which includes details of all bowel actions, further assessment might be required to establish the reasons for the documented descriptions. These reasons include:

▶ faecal impaction—leading to frequent watery stools ('overflow incontinence' or 'spurious diarrhoea');

▶ anal sphincter relaxation or damaged mucosa—leading to production of mucus or fluid;

▶ decreased bowel motility resulting from poor mobility;

▶ side-effects of medications—such as morphine or codeine; and

▶ previous history of bowel problems or bowel surgery.

A plain abdominal x-ray might be required to check for evidence of high faecal impaction if the rectum is found to be empty on digital examination.

Developing a plan for faecal incontinence

As with urinary incontinence, following a comprehensive assessment of all the related factors, a plan to address the problem of faecal incontinence is developed by the care team, resident, and family representative. Stated objectives can include:

▶ achieve continence by promoting changes in diet and fluid intake;
▶ facilitate bowel emptying by establishing a routine of place and time; and
▶ contain incontinence with an appliance recommended by an appropriate adviser.

Social containment

This term applies to the management of incontinence that cannot be otherwise controlled. The aims of this form of management are to maximise the resident's independence and to maintain personal dignity—both for the resident's own satisfaction and for the social environment.

Social containment is facilitated by the following.

▶ *A regular toileting regimen:* This is usually identified from the continence chart, but generally should not be any less than at two-hourly intervals. The toileting program involves the nurse prompting the resident to visit the toilet, or the nurse fully assisting the person in the whole procedure.
▶ *Providing helpful signs:* Providing helpful signs assists residents with dementia to access the toilet. This can include the use of sensor light for night-time use.
▶ *Bedside commodes, urinals, or over-the-toilet chairs:* The use of such equipment should be based on comprehensive discussion with the resident and/or family member to ascertain what is the most comfortable and dignified practice for a person with dementia.
▶ *Adaptable clothing for easy removal for toileting.*
▶ *The use of containment products and or urinary drainage systems (for men).*
▶ *Products to prevent skin damage:* Appropriate products can prevent skin damage from incontinence, maximise comfort and dignity, and minimise odour. The type of product should be decided in consultation with a continence adviser and the family, according to the needs of individual residents.
▶ *Pad or containment product:* A pad or containment product can be used—in liaison with nurse continence adviser.
▶ *Use of washable or disposable bed-protection appliances.*

Nurses must be aware that the application of a continence appliance does not obviate the need to assist residents with frequent toileting. Providing residents with a frequent opportunity to visit the toilet (or to use a bedpan or commode) helps to maintain the residents' dignity and to maximise independence for as long as possible.

Conclusion

In summary, the key factors for nurses in addressing the complex issue of incontinence and dementia are:

◗ a comprehensive assessment that includes the resident's past responses and coping strategies;

◗ involvement of family or representative in all aspects of care planning and review;

◗ frequent review and ongoing assessment in response to the resident's changing physical and cognitive status;

◗ acknowledging that each resident is unique and requires an individualised, personalised plan of care;

◗ teamwork—whereby the skilled nurse imparts his or her knowledge to other team members;

◗ referral to a qualified continence adviser for advice on products and management strategies; and

◗ support and encouragement for the resident, family, and the whole care team.

The management of incontinence demands the expertise of nurses whose knowledge base, both for dementia and incontinence, is derived from the best evidence available at the time. This knowledge is used to improve the quality of life for the person with dementia, who is dependent on the nurse for the maintenance of his or her dignity and independence.

'The quality of life for the person with dementia . . . is dependent on the nurse for the maintenance of dignity and independence.'

Chapter 13

Falls Prevention

Keith Hill, Robyn Smith, Dina LoGiudice,
and Margaret Winbolt

Introduction

Falls among older people in aged-care settings are common, with up to 60% of residents experiencing one or more falls during a 12-month period (Tinetti 1987). Although falls can often be related in part to the age and frailty of older people, there is considerable research evidence that falls can be reduced among older people in aged-care settings (Rubenstein et al. 1990; Ray et al. 1997).

This chapter provides a review of the range of activities that can be implemented to reduce falls among older people with dementia. Many of the commonly used falls-prevention strategies are more difficult to implement with people with dementia. However, as with all falls-prevention practice, the processes of thorough falls risk assessment and development of an individual management plan that considers the multiple needs of the individual in the context of the environment provides the best chance of reducing falls and the consequences of falls. The National Service Framework for Older People (DoH 2001) clearly highlights the impact of falls on the lives of older people.

Standard 6 of the Framework emphasises the cost to both the individual and the healthcare system of the consequences of an individual falling. The need for the development of strategies to reduce the risk of falling is made a key priority for all care staff.

Circumstances and consequences of falls

The annual incidence of falls among people with dementia is estimated to be as high as 80% (Van Dijk et al. 1993), although accurate data collection is limited because many falls that are not witnessed or do not cause injury are not reported. In one study, there was an average of four falls per resident per year (van Dijk et al. 1993). One in four older people with dementia who fall suffer a fracture (Oleske et al. 1995; Buchner & Larson 1987)—a significantly higher serious injury rate than for elderly people in the community. Of visits to emergency departments from nursing homes in the United States, 9% are due to falls, and 11% of these result in hospital admission (Ackermann et al. 1998). It is apparent that there is a high incidence of falls by older people with dementia in aged-care facilities, and that these are associated with major health consequences.

A high proportion of falls among older people with dementia occur in the first weeks after admission to a residential facility, or transfer to a new facility (Friedman, Denman & Williamson 1995; van Dijk et al. 1993). This appears to be a time of increased confusion and agitation, and a time when staff are becoming familiar with new residents and their routines. Strategies are needed to improve safety during this time—such as increased surveillance and detailed handover from families (regarding resident routines and preferences that influence behaviour).

> 'The annual incidence of falls among people with dementia is estimated to be as high as 80%.'

The most common activities at the time of a fall for older people in aged-care facilities are (Tinetti 1987):

▶ getting in or out of bed (29%);
▶ walking (27%);
▶ getting up from sitting (16%); and
▶ reaching, bending, and performing activities of daily living (12%).

The most common causes of falls by older people with dementia in aged-care facilities are (Van Dijk et al. 1993):

▶ material, slipping (over urine), stumbling (17%);

▶ gait and equilibrium disturbances (16%);
▶ sitting down incorrectly (11%);
▶ urge to walk in spite of physical inability to walk safely (6%);
▶ fatigue (5%); and
▶ agitation, confusion, and irritation (4%).

In 22% of falls, the cause is unknown, and approximately 30% of the falls are considered preventable (Van Dijk et al. 1993). Agitation and behavioural problems are common among older people with dementia, and these might be factors in a proportion of falls in which the cause is unknown.

Documenting falls incidents

There have been several suggested definitions of what constitutes a 'fall'. One of the more commonly used definitions is (KIWG 1987):

> . . . an event which results in a person coming to rest inadvertently on the ground or other lower level, and other than as a consequence of the following: sustaining a violent blow, loss of consciousness, sudden onset of paralysis as in stroke, or an epileptic seizure.

All nurses should be familiar with the agreed definition of a fall, to ensure the accurate documentation of all identified incidents. There is considerable variation in the amount and type of information recorded in the documentation of falls. A standard incident report form should be completed for all incidents. Such a form can be used to identify factors that might prevent future falls by the same resident, or other residents in the same situation. For this reason, nurses should complete all details on the form. An example of an incident report form developed for use in aged-care settings is shown in Figure 13.1, page 145.

Risk factors

Falls

Risk factors for falls can be classified as extrinsic or intrinsic.

Extrinsic factors

Extrinsic risk factors are hazards in the environment, including:
▶ uneven or slippery surfaces;
▶ poor lighting;
▶ inappropriate placement of frequently required items (for example, a drink being placed on a table out of reach); and

Falls Incident Report

Resident's name:

| Date of fall: | Time of fall: |

Name of witness(es):

Brief description of the fall:

Activity at time of fall: ○ walking   ○ getting in or out of chair or bed   ○ other

Place where fall occurred: ○ bedroom   ○ bathroom   ○ common room
○ toilet   ○ outside   ○ dining room   ○ other

Fell from: ○ bed   ○ chair   ○ wheelchair   ○ commode   ○ toilet
○ other   ○ not applicable

Was the resident using a walking aid at time of incident?

Any environmental hazards identified:

Were there risk factors identified **before the fall** (in terms of the Falls Risk Assessment and Management Form)?

Is it clear how the fall might have been prevented?

Immediate impact of fall: ○ no injury   ○ bruising (where?) ....
○ pain (where?) ....   ○ laceration/skin tear (where?) ....
○ possible fracture (where?) ....

Nursing interventions: ○ transfer to hospital   ○ attend first aid treatments
○ refer to general practitioner for immediate review
○ refer to general practitioner on next visit
○ alteration to medications   ○ alteration to nursing care
○ alteration to environment   ○ discuss fall with patient
○ discuss fall with family

Date to be reviewed:

Signature of staff member: Date:

Figure 13.1 Falls incident report form
Shanley (1998); © Commonwealth of Australia, published with permission

▶ poorly stored items in walkway areas that might be tripped over (such as stands or cleaning equipment).

Intrinsic factors

The major intrinsic risk factors include age-related functions involved in balance—such as reduction in eyesight, sensation in legs, muscle strength, and coordination—as well as medical conditions that affect these functions. Dementia and other causes of impaired cognition are another risk factor.

Other intrinsic falls risk factors include:
▶ history of previous falls;
▶ acute health problems (for example, pneumonia, urinary tract infection);
▶ polypharmacy and specific medications (such as antidepressants and psychotropics);
▶ incontinence; and
▶ orthostatic hypotension.

Fractures

In addition to the risk factors for falls, there are other risk factors for fracture. These include:
▶ osteomalacia (softening of the bones without change in bone structure, usually related to lack of vitamin D and calcium); and
▶ osteoporosis (softening of the bones together with loss of bone structure, more common in older women than men).

Older people in residential aged-care facilities have been shown to have low levels of vitamin D (Stein et al. 1999).

Risk assessment and care-planning

Risk-assessment tools and care plans

Falls are usually due to a combination of two or more of the risk factors described above. A falls risk-assessment tool can help staff to identify the major risk factors, and to determine an appropriate care plan. There are several such tools available, although none has been well validated or widely implemented in residential aged-care settings. An example of a falls risk-assessment tool developed for use in such facilities is shown in Figure 13.2 (page 147).

There are several decisions to be made regarding the use of such a falls risk-assessment tool. These include:
▶ When should it be completed?
▶ Who should complete it?
▶ Who is responsible for developing a care plan based on the results?

Falls Risk Assessment and Management Form

Name of resident:

Problem or issue	Assessment	Yes or No	Management options (tick which ones you suggest)
Medications	• Does the person take 4 or more medications in total? or • Does the person take one or more psychotropics (tranquillisers, antidepressants or sedative/hypnotics)?		• Allocate to high-risk group • Review by GP to try to reduce medications or dosages
Acute illness	• Does the person have any sign of acute illness eg. altered behaviour, confusion, pain, malaise, fever, cough, urinary symptoms		• Review by GP to ensure appropriate treatment
Mental state	• Is the person confused and/or disoriented and/or wandering?		• Refer to GP to exclude treatable causes • Allocate to high-risk group
Ongoing medical conditions	• Does the person have: — CVA? — Parkinson's disease? — Osteoarthritis in knees/hips? — Dementia? — Postural hypotension? — Depression? — Dizziness?		• Allocate to high-risk group • Review by GP to ensure optimum treatment • Refer to physiotherapist for possible treatments
History of previous falls	• Has the person had: — one fall in past year which requires treatment or — more than two falls not requiring treatment in past year?		• Allocate to high-risk group *(Continued)*

Figure 13.2 Risk-assessment tool

Shanley (1998); © Commonwealth of Australia, published with permission

Falls Risk Assessment and Management Form

Name of resident:

Problem or issue	Assessment	Yes or No	Management options (tick which ones you suggest)
Poor balance	• Is the person unsafe when asked to stand from chair, walk 3 metres, turn and return to chair independently (even with walking aid)?		• Allocate to high-risk group • Refer to GP for assessment • Refer to physiotherapist for assessment
Use of walking aids	• Does the person use or need aids to mobilise?		• Allocate to high-risk group • Assess use of aids according to guidelines in this manual • Refer to physiotherapist for specialist assessment and treatment
Bowel or bladder problems	• Does the person have urinary or faecal incontinence, or urgency during the day or night?		• Institute appropriate nursing care • Refer to GP for assessment • Allocate to high-risk group
Visual problems	• Does the person (while using their normal glasses) have problems reading headlines in the newspaper, making out figures on the TV or seeing objects alongside them?		• Refer to GP and ophthalmologist to exclude cataracts or other treatable disease and review glasses • Refer to optometrist for revision of existing glasses • Allocate to high-risk group if there is poor vision which cannot be corrected
Hearing problems	• Does the person have problems hearing you with normal speech?		• Refer to GP for checking of ears and hearing • Refer to audiologist for hearing aid assessment • Ensure hearing aids are working and being used correctly • Allocate to high-risk group if there is poor hearing which cannot be corrected *(Continued)*

Figure 13.2 Risk-assessment tool *(Continued)*

Shanley (1998); © Commonwealth of Australia, published with permission

Falls Risk Assessment and Management Form

Name of resident:

Problem or issue	Assessment	Yes or No	Management options (tick which ones you suggest)
Feet problems	• Does the person have corns, ingrown toenails, ulcers, deformities or infection of the feet?		• Institute appropriate nursing care • Refer to podiatrist for treatment • Allocate to high-risk group if problems cannot be successfully treated
Footwear	• Does the person have unsafe footwear, according to guidelines in this manual		• Correct problems, according to guidelines in this manual

Signature of staff member: **Date:**

Figure 13.2 Risk-assessment tool (*Continued*)
Shanley (1998); © Commonwealth of Australia, published with permission

❱ How is falls risk and the associated care plan communicated to all concerned?
Each of these questions is considered below.

When should it be completed?
Falls risks can vary over time, and assessments should therefore be repeated intermittently. A common approach is to complete the falls risk assessment on admission, after any acute event (such as pneumonia or urinary tract infection), and at regular intervals (for example, every six months).

Who should complete it?
Nursing staff usually have this responsibility, although it can also be undertaken by other health professionals (such as physiotherapists). Policies should clearly identify responsibilities.

Who is responsible for developing a care plan?
This role is usually undertaken by the staff member who completes the falls risk assessment, with the input of others as needed.

How is falls risk and care plan communicated?

The risk assessment and care plan must be communicated to all concerned (including the resident, family, and staff). Strategies are required to facilitate communication so that all staff, not just those involved in direct resident care, are aware of an individual's falls risk and the strategies to minimise this.

Environmental hazards

Environmental hazards frequently contribute to falls. All staff members have a responsibility to rectify or report any environmental hazards observed during daily routines. In addition, staff should undertake a regular audit of all areas to review potential falls hazards and to develop ways to address these. All areas should be reviewed—including residents' rooms, bathrooms and toilets, corridors, kitchen and dining areas, recreation and therapy areas, entry and exit points, and the outdoor environment. An example of an environmental hazard checklist is shown in Figure 13.3 (page 151).

'All staff members have a responsibility to rectify or report any environmental hazards observed during daily routines.'

Environmental hazards should be considered in the context of the people who most commonly use the areas. For example, seating in an individual resident's rooms should be appropriate to the resident's height, and ease of sit-to-stand transfers. Higher chairs reduce the difficulty of standing up—even a few centimetres can make a significant difference. In contrast, seating in communal areas (such as along corridors) needs to be of an intermediate height that is suitable for most residents. An occupational therapy assessment might be necessary to identify the best options to meet individual needs.

The impact of the environment on vision also warrants consideration. Sudden changes in lighting should be minimised—such as bright sunlight to dim interior lighting. In addition, sharp contrasts in floor surfacing can be perceived as a change in level of floor surface by people with dementia, causing them to alter their walking in these areas. Observation of residents' mobility, in conjunction with an environmental audit, is likely to identify key areas to be addressed.

Dementia and increased risk of falling
Specific features of dementia

In addition to the falls risk factors described above, a number of features associated with dementia and related conditions increase the risk of falling.

GENERAL ENVIRONMENTAL HAZARD CHECKLIST:

To be completed via general audit of facility.

Flooring	Indoors		
	Non-slip surfaces	Yes	No
	Absence of raised edge	Yes	No
	Good condition	Yes	No
Circulation	Absence of clutter	Yes	No
	Adequate storage for equipment	Yes	No
	Adequate space for mobility aids	Yes	No
Visibility	Walls contrasting colour to floor	Yes	No
	Handrails contrasting colour to walls	Yes	No
	Rails contrasting colour to background	Yes	No
	Steps edges contrasting colour	Yes	No
	Absence of glare from windows	Yes	No
Lighting	Well light hallways and rooms (75 watts)	Yes	No
	Stairs well lit? day and night	Yes	No
Bathroom	Non-slip flooring	Yes	No
	Step-less shower base	Yes	No
	Room for seat near to shower	Yes	No
	Room for seat in shower	Yes	No
	Free of clutter (storage of equipment)	Yes	No
	Rail in shower / near toilet	Yes	No
	Lightweight door / easy to use	Yes	No
Bedroom	Adequate space for frame access	Yes	No
	Bedspreads clear from floor	Yes	No
	Call button within reach	Yes	No
Rails	Handgrips along walls in all areas	Yes	No
	Handrails on all steps	Yes	No
	Beside toilet	Yes	No
	In shower	Yes	No
Signs	Clear/Adequate signs throughout	Yes	No
Outdoors	Absence of potholes	Yes	No
	Even pathway	Yes	No
	Sufficient width for two people (inc. one using frame)	Yes	No
	No overhanging branches	Yes	No

(Continued)

Figure 13.3 Environmental hazard checklist

Falls Prevention Service, Peninsula Health Care Network (1999); published with permission

GENERAL ENVIRONMENTAL HAZARD CHECKLIST:

To be completed via general audit of facility.

Outdoors	Paths clear of shrubs, bushes	Yes	No
	Regular removal/sweeping of leaves on paths	Yes	No
	Non-slip steps and step edges	Yes	No
	Steps in good condition	Yes	No
	Sufficient number of outdoor seats for regular rest	Yes	No
	Outdoor seating secure/sufficient height	Yes	No

ACTION/S REQUIRED: BY WHOM

_____

_____

_____

Assessed by .... Date ....

Figure 13.3 Environmental hazard checklist (*Continued*)
Falls Prevention Service, Peninsula Health Care Network (1999); published with permission

Table 13.1 Dementia and falls risk

Factors associated with dementia	Implications for falls
Memory loss	impairs ability to learn and maintain safety measures (for example, forgetting to use walking frame)
Dyspraxia	disturbance in perception of body in space, and perception of depth and distance
Language impairment	inability to express desires or understand verbal and written cues (for example, signs or directions)
Impaired executive function (planning and organisational capacity, and mental flexibility)	diminished ability to initiate, monitor, and stop certain actions (for example, wandering or repetitive behaviour)
Diminished insight into ability	poor monitoring of safety issues and performance of unsafe actions

Authors' presentation

Table 13.1 (page 151) lists some of the clinical features of dementia that can lead to increased risk of falls.

Other clinical features often associated with falls among residents with dementia include:

▶ behavioural and psychological symptoms associated with dementia; and
▶ delirium (acute brain syndrome).

Behavioural and psychological symptoms associated with dementia include agitation, hallucinations, anxiety, depression, and delusions. All of these can contribute to falls. Anxiety and agitation can diminish a person's capacity for concentration, attention, and interpretation of their environment. Hallucinations and delusions can be distressing and frightening, and can affect a person's sense of reality and lead to inappropriate responses.

Delirium is characterised by fluctuating confusion and is associated with diminished attention and concentration. It can be associated with vivid hallucinations and delusions. Delirium is often caused by an underlying acute medical condition such as infection, hypoxia, metabolic disorders (such as unstable diabetes), or medications (see below). If so, the underlying cause requires urgent identification and treatment. Any sudden change in status warrants a prompt medical review to identify any potentially reversible cause of the cognitive impairment.

Other health conditions

Other health conditions can increase the risk of falls among older people with dementia. Table 13.2 (page 154) lists some of these medical problems.

In residential aged-care facilities, responsibility for medical care usually remains with the resident's general practitioner. Effective communication between staff and the general practitioner is essential to ensure that optimal care is provided. Both staff and the general practitioner need to adopt a proactive approach to communication that fosters teamwork and resident-centred care. This includes:

▶ notification of changes in status at an early stage, before the problem progresses;
▶ regular medication reviews; and
▶ developing a care plan that considers potential problems for the resident, and institutes a preventive program.

Medications

Many medications can lead to increased confusion, postural hypotension, and increased rigidity—all of which can cause falls. These drugs include

Table 13.2 Other medical conditions and falls

Health condition	Balance systems affected	Issues to consider
Stroke	motor, sensory, central integration	physical abilities can deteriorate, especially if relatively inactive; can benefit from physiotherapy, walking, or exercise
Parkinson's disease	motor, and motor planning	should have regular medical review; might require medication review; might benefit from physiotherapy, walking, or exercise
Meniere's disease, vestibular neuritis, benign paroxysmal positional vertigo	vestibular system	dizziness requires medical assessment; some causes of dizziness are treatable by simple measures
Musculo-skeletal problems (arthritis, joint pain, muscle weakness)	motor, skeletal systems	medical review for any change in joint pain or function; might benefit from physiotherapy, walking, or exercise; consideration of aids to reduce pain
Glaucoma. cataracts, macular degeneration	visual system	eyesight review at least every two years; note signs of increased visual difficulty
Peripheral neuropathy (especially with diabetes)	somato-sensory system	diminishes ability to feel feet; causes weakness in muscles that clear foot from floor when walking

Authors' presentation

benzodiazepines (for example, oxazepam, temazepam), antipsychotics (for example, haloperidol, olanzepine, risperidone), antihypertensives, anti-Parkinsonian medications, and antidepressants (for example, amitriptyline, doxepin).

All medications should be reviewed frequently, and the lowest effective dose maintained. Withdrawal of these medications can, in some cases, be difficult (such as withdrawal of benzodiazepines), and this should be undertaken in a staged manner (Foy 1993). Reduction of such psychotropic medications has been shown to result in a large reduction in falls (Campbell et al. 1999).

The total number of medications is also a risk factor for falls. Rationalising the number of medications being taken by a resident is an important goal of regular reviews.

Toileting

Toileting is a significant risk activity for falls. Indeed, 38% of falls among residents in one residential aged-care facility were identified as being related to slipping on urine on the floor (Meddaugh Friedenberg & Knisley 1996). Other aspects of the toileting process have also been implicated in falls—including problems in recognising the need to go to the toilet, getting safely to the toilet, removing clothing as appropriate, re-dressing, and returning to the place of origin.

Table 13.3 (page 156) lists some of the common problems, and some potential solutions. The risk of falling can be reduced if nurses are aware of the toileting needs of individual residents, especially the timing of administration of diuretics, aperients, and enemas. A prompted voiding program can reduce agitation in cognitively impaired older people (Schnelle et al. 1995). Treaded slippers fitted on residents' feet at night time can also reduce falls from slipping on urine (Meddaugh, Friedenberg & Knisley 1996).

Restraint

The use of restraint has often been a first response in managing residents with high risk of falls, especially for those with dementia. Restraints include physical restraints (such as bedrails, vests, wrist ties, belts, and chair tables positioned to limit movement), and chemical restraint (pharmaceutical management to limit movement). It is becoming generally accepted that restraint is not the strategy of choice in the prevention of falls.

Falls can and do occur even when restraint devices are in place, and the removal of physical restraint does not necessarily lead to an increase in falls (Capezuti et al. 1998; Neufeld et al. 1999). When restrained, confused residents are at

> 'Falls can and do occur even when restraint devices are in place, and the removal of physical restraint does not necessarily lead to an increase in falls.'

Table 13.3 Toileting issues and falls

Issue	Strategies
Clothing (undoing fasteners such as zips, buttons, and belts can cause difficulties standing or holding rails)	loose fitting clothing; minimal or modified fasteners (buttons, zips)
Constipation (discomfort, frequent trips to the toilet, and confusion)	comprehensive bowel assessment; bowel management program; increased fluid intake; adequate diet (including adequate fibre); increased walking or other physical activity; review of medication and potential drug interactions
Bowel incontinence and urgency	raised awareness of impact of aperients and enemas; prompted voiding program; prompt response by staff to requests for toileting post aperients and enemas; use of bedside commode; increased monitoring of at-risk residents; use of chair or bed alarm; privacy
Urinary incontinence and urgency	comprehensive continence assessment and referral to specialist if necessary; prompted voiding program; use of appropriate continence aids; review of medications that affect micturition; prompt staff response to resident request for assistance; use of a bedside commode; increased monitoring of at-risk residents; use of chair or bed alarm
Diuretics	raised awareness by staff of effects of diuretics; staff responding to more frequent requests for toileting; review of medications that influence micturition; prompted voiding program

Authors' presentation

risk of harming themselves, especially when attempting to get up or remove the restraint. The use of restraint devices can cause extreme distress and can pose risks greater than the risks involved should a resident fall.

Bedrails are often used in the belief that they are a safety device to prevent falls from bed. However, they can increase risks to residents who can become entangled or climb over the rails and fall from a greater height.

A prospective study that used an education program for staff on strategies to reduce restraint use resulted in a 90% reduction in restraint use in the participating facilities, and a significant reduction in moderate and severe injuries (Neufeld et al. 1999). Alternatives to restraint include:

▶ placing high-risk residents in high-surveillance areas during daytime;

▶ regular visual observation checks overnight;

▶ the use of bed or chair alarm systems that alert staff to a resident attempting to get out of the chair or bed; and

▶ the use of high–low beds that lower down to floor level.

In addition to the above measures, communication with family members regarding previous home routines can identify reasons for increased agitation which, in some instances, can be addressed by changes in the routine or the environment.

There can be instances in which restraint is deemed to be the only strategy available. Such a decision should be made only after a comprehensive assessment and evaluation of other management strategies. Any restraint that is used should abide by existing restraint protocols for observation, monitoring, and review.

Resident and family involvement

When making decisions about falls-prevention strategies, particularly the use of restraint, it is essential that the resident be involved if able or, alternatively, the resident's relatives. This involvement includes discussions relating to:

▶ assessment and development of appropriate fall-prevention and injury-minimisation strategies;

▶ risks posed by the use of restraint versus the risks if a fall were to occur;

▶ explanation of alternative falls-prevention measures; and

▶ consent to restraint.

Feet and footwear

The effect of foot problems and footwear is often overlooked as a risk factor for falls (Menz & Lord 1999). Important factors to be considered include the following.

▶ Foot pain can impair balance and functional ability, and any foot pain should therefore be investigated and the cause treated if possible. This might include adequate pain control. Adequate footcare is essential and should include frequent examination of the feet (skin condition, nails, sensation, circulation) by nurses, with referral to a podiatrist as required.

▶ Correct fitting and supportive shoes (with a high collar at the back of the heel) will improve balance. Flat shoes are recommended because high or narrow heels can reduce balance.

▶ Older people often prefer to wear slippers inside but these are often ill-fitting or slip-on, and this can increase the risk of falling. Residents should be encouraged to wear appropriate shoes instead of slippers. If the person continues to wear slippers, these need to be a good fit with a supportive heel and a non-slip sole.

Mobility and walking aids

Appropriate use of a prescribed walking aid increases stability. Table 13.4 (page 159) lists various walking aids and the support and limitations associated with their use.

Before using a walking aid, a physiotherapy assessment should be undertaken to determine whether other management programs (such as exercise) might improve balance and walking. If a walking aid is to be used, the physiotherapist can advise on the most appropriate aid, and provide instruction and training regarding correct use. Inappropriate or incorrect use of a walking aid is one of the most common extrinsic factors associated with falling among older residents (Tinetti 1987). If a walking aid is used incorrectly, it can cause more risk of falling than walking without it.

> 'If a walking aid is used incorrectly, it can cause more risk of falling than walking without it.'

The hand grip of a walking aid should be at approximately the height of the distal wrist crease when the resident is standing upright. Residents with dementia can have difficulty learning to use a new walking aid, and remembering to use it. However, if it is considered appropriate, repeated prompting and correction regarding use can gradually result in improved use.

Physical activity

Muscle weakness, reduced balance, and unsteadiness during walking and turning are common problems for older people. Formal exercise programs have been shown to improve a range of functions in older people (Hill et al. 2000), even in frail, cognitively impaired people.

Group exercise programs are often performed to music, and can involve sitting or standing exercises. In conducting such groups for frail residents with dementia, there is a need for increased staff-to-resident ratio due to the reduced attention span and compliance of these people. Shorter, more frequent sessions can be helpful. Physiotherapy exercise with individualised treatment programs can also improve balance and function for older people.

Table 13.4 Use of walking aids

Walking aid with use	Amount of support	Potential problems with use	Care of the walking aid
Single-point stick	least supportive	stick should be in opposite hand to weak or painful leg; stick should be on ground when opposite leg is on ground	check stopper is effective
4-point stick (quad) or 3-point stick (tripod)	intermediate support	stick should be in opposite hand to weak or painful leg; stick should be on ground when opposite leg is on ground	check stoppers are effective
Pick-up frame	moderate support	frame should be on the ground when stepping with either leg; frame should be placed on ground when stepping while turning, or reversing back to a chair difficult to use on stairs if more than one step needs to be negotiated	check stoppers are effective
Crutches	moderate support	difficult to coordinate (rarely used for older people)	check stoppers are effective
Wheelie frame	moderate support	some frames have wheels on the front that go only straight; can make turning difficult or unsafe; if negotiating slopes, ensure frame can be used safely in these situations	ensure braking mechanism working effectively
Forearm support wheelie frame	maximal support	unable to go up or down steps	check stoppers and slides are effective

Authors' presentation

Walking also has benefits for residents with dementia. These include improved walking endurance, and reduced agitation and improved sleep. Walking programs aimed at promoting functional mobility in frail residents who require assistance to walk can reduce behavioural problems and falls (Koroknay et al. 1995; Rolland et al. 2000). Volunteers can support staff during such walking programs.

Another strategy that has been demonstrated to lead to improvements in physical performance, as well as reduced agitation, is a program called 'functional incidental training' (FIT), in which residents are encouraged to perform a small amount of additional functional activity (for example, walking or transfers) after regular prompted voiding (Schnelle et al. 1995). This approach requires minimal additional nurse contact time, and emphasises the importance of routine physical activity, in addition to the benefits of group or individualised exercise programs. Although this type of program also has potential to reduce falls, this outcome was not investigated in the study.

Injury minimisation

Even in the presence of a range of falls-prevention strategies, some people will continue to have falls. In these circumstances, strategies to minimise the severity of injury, in particular hip fracture, can be instituted.

Hip protectors can be worn in special undergarments to dissipate or absorb the impact of a fall. Although a hip fracture can still occur when wearing hip protectors, the use of hip protectors reduces the risk (Parker, Gillespie & Gillespie 2001; Lauritzen, Petersen & Lund 1993).

As with falls-prevention strategies, injury-minimisation strategies require the compliance of residents, and efforts must be made to involve residents in accepting and wearing such protective devices. Some hip-protector undergarments can accommodate incontinence pads.

Another strategy to reduce the likelihood of fractures among residents is the use of vitamin D and calcium supplements. These slow down the loss of bone density, thereby reducing the likelihood of fractures (Chapuy et al. 1992).

Organisational environment

It is important that there is a consistent approach to falls prevention that becomes part of routine nursing care. Achieving this is extremely difficult if only one or two nurses are involved in falls prevention. Falls prevention needs to be integrated into standard assessment, care planning, and ongoing management if it is to be effective and sustainable.

It is important to develop staff knowledge and skills in falls prevention. This should lead to modifications of nursing practice, with nurses receiving supervision and support in applying their knowledge and skills.

Barriers and facilitators to the successful implementation of falls-prevention programs also need to be considered and addressed. Engaging and empowering staff members is an effective way of fostering reflective practice. It is important that this complex area of falls prevention in older people who have dementia is addressed using a team approach that involves all staff within the organisation. An approach whereby staff work with management, residents, and carers is likely to lead to the successful development and implementation of best practice (Lindeman et al. 2002).

Conclusion

Falls among older people with dementia represent a common and significant problem, but a range of strategies can be effective in reducing such falls. Nurses have a key role in identifying an individual resident's risk, determining appropriate management and referral strategies, and implementing a tailored program.

'Nurses have a key role in identifying an individual resident's risk, determining appropriate management and referral strategies, and implementing a tailored program.'

Chapter 14

Pain Management

Susie Kerr and Lynn Chenoweth

Introduction

Illness, disability, and pain are not easy to accept, particularly when they disrupt peoples' lives for long periods. This is particularly relevant for older people because pain signifies that time is moving on for them and that their life goals are in need of review. Unfortunately, the presence of an ageing skin and the disabilities associated with dementia can cause others to ignore or neglect older people's health needs in certain areas (Oliver 1996; Madjar & Higgins 1996). Pain management is one such area.

Providing comfort to people who are in distress involves the creation of a sense of ease for the person, satisfaction of his or her bodily wants, and relief of pain and associated anxiety. Whether pain is well managed in a person with dementia can make the difference between experiencing a satisfying lifestyle or a life controlled by debility. Assessing such elderly residents' pain is an important nursing responsibility and is now recognised as the 'fifth vital sign' to assess when determining a person's health status (Victor 2001).

Experiencing pain in older age

Many people are now living well into their 80s or 90s. Although most of these people are living independent and fulfilled lives, others experience pain and other discomforts associated with physical or social decline. Increasing age is associated with increased frequency of chronic illness and disability, including musculoskeletal and joint disorders, sensory loss, heart and blood vessel disease, endocrine disorders (such as diabetes), and neurodegenerative diseases (such as dementia and Parkinson's disease). Unless they are well managed, many of these conditions give rise to pain and discomfort. Inadequate management is more likely to occur if a person has dementia and is unable to express his or her symptoms.

Pain syndromes that are more common in older people include:

▶ lower back disorders;
▶ arthritis;
▶ spinal canal stenosis;
▶ post-herpetic neuralgia (shingles);
▶ facial pain;
▶ polymyalgia rheumatica;
▶ temporal arthritis;
▶ diabetic neuropathy;
▶ painful legs;
▶ throbbing vaginal pain; and
▶ painful mouth conditions

What is pain?

The International Association for the Study of Pain (IASP) (1979) defined pain as 'an unpleasant sensory and emotional experience associated with actual or potential tissue damage'. However, pain is an intensely subjective experience, and this has led to definitions of pain that emphasise the idea that 'pain is what the patient says hurts' or, as McCaffrey (1968, p. 95) so memorably put it, pain is 'whatever the experiencing person says it is, existing whenever he or she says it does'. McCaffery's definition poses problems in caring for people who are less able to speak about the pain—such as those who have experienced a stroke, those with limited English, or those who with cognitive impairment, including dementia.

> 'Pain is whatever the experiencing person says it is, existing whenever he or she says it does.'

Complications of pain

When pain is not relieved, complications are more likely to arise in older people—such as an inability to take deep breaths and cough, thus predisposing them to pneumonia. Other complications of pain can include prolongation of illness, impairment of the immune system, social isolation, and a need for expensive treatments (Victor 2001).

Effective management of pain in older people is therefore important for maintaining their health, well-being, social activity, and relationships with others.

Barriers to effective pain management

The sensory and emotional experiences of pain are subjective, complex, and multidimensional. In people with dementia, an important barrier to effective pain management can be an inability to describe the extent, effect, and sometimes even the location of the pain. Pain arising from one cause can be experienced differently from time to time because of contextual factors, and a person's expression of his or her pain is influenced by developmental, cultural, familial, environmental, and emotional factors.

The various ways in which individuals express their pain must be understood and respected by nurses (Landi et al. 2001). For various reasons, some older people mask quite severe pain, and infection or other disease can remain un-detected until serious health problems become evident. Others will express their feelings of pain in ways that help them to relieve it. People with dementia might not be able to tell nurses that they have pain, but the pain can become evident in other ways. They might resist being touched, groan, cry, hit out when handled, show agitation, refuse food and fluids, or become withdrawn.

'People with dementia might not be able to tell nurses that they have pain, but the pain can become evident in other ways.'

Acute confusion superimposed on pre-existing dementia is a common presenting feature of unresolved pain, and a sudden change in mental state might therefore be an indication of unde-tected pain.

Poor pain management can result from the misconception that pain sensation decreases with ageing, from a belief that cognitively impaired people do not experience pain, and from the unfounded fear that pain-relieving medication will cause addiction and other health problems (Ferrell 1995; Zalon 1997; Victor 2001). Unfortunately, if nurses maintain these misconceptions and do not look for physical and emotional signs of pain, the person might continue to suffer in silence.

Pain thresholds increase in older age (Gibson & Schroder 2001) because the afferent nerve pathways are slower to conduct and the nerve receptor sites become altered. For example, the pain of a heart attack is often experienced quite differently from that experienced by younger adults.

It is also worth remembering that pain is not merely physical in origin. It can be associated with losses of many kinds—loss of good health, reduced ability to self-care, difficulty in making decisions, poor memory, impaired mobility, loss of home, lack of close loving relationships, and a general loss of meaningful living. The loss of physical, sensory, or cognitive function can lead to depression, particularly if the need for comfort is neglected and pain is badly managed. Nurses have an ethical responsibility not only to assess and manage pain effectively, but also to act sensitively with respect to the distress associated with these losses. The story of Mrs Youssef (Box, page 166) is an example of how several factors can play a part in providing barriers to effective pain management.

> 'It is also worth remembering that pain is not merely physical in origin. It can be associated with losses of many kinds.'

In the case of Mrs Youssef, she might have been fearful that her pain would never be relieved, or that if there was relief today the pain might still return tomorrow. Isolation from the safe environment of her home and the closeness of family might have added to this anxiety, and the combination of factors might have interfered with her pain control. In these sorts of circumstances, people can develop a sense of powerlessness regarding their ability to control pain and its impact on their lives. This fear can be reinforced if past pain events have not been handled well.

Additional problems that make pain management more difficult in older people such as Mrs Youssef are the chronic disease itself, the taking of multiple medications, age-related effects on the brain's chemistry (including reduced levels of endogenous opiates), and a tendency to delirium superimposed on dementia as a result of inflammatory illness such as arthritis (Helme 2001).

Assessing pain in people with dementia

To assess pain in older people with dementia it is essential that an experienced practitioner conducts a comprehensive physical examination and functional

Mrs Youssef

Mrs Youssef was a 78-year-old woman with dementia who had recently become resident in a nursing home. She had been admitted three times to a major public hospital in the past 18 months because of flare-ups in her various medical conditions and her inability to self-care. Because of her dementia and language difficulties, communication with nursing staff was difficult.

Mrs Youssef's husband had died two years ago after a long and painful illness. Her daughter lived 20 kilometres away and relied on public transport to visit her mother. She was therefore able to visit only on weekends. Mrs Youssef's daughter-in-law lived closer, and had supported her over the past ten years with shopping, food preparation, and some cleaning. However, her daughter-in-law communicated very little with the staff.

Mrs Youssef had recently begun to develop painful, hot, and swollen joints in many areas of her body, including her spine and jaw, and this made it difficult for her to eat, change her position, and sit out of bed for more than an hour at a time. Although she was unable to verbalise her pain to staff, it was clear from her appearance and behaviour that she was experiencing fatigue and anxiety. Her temperature had been elevated intermittently for three days, and she had a dry mouth. At times Mrs Youssef appeared to be confused, and she had become increasingly agitated despite the nurses' attempts to provide comfort.

Mrs Youssef's general practitioner asked staff to continue the treatment commenced in the hospital, including partial bedrest, assistance with all activities of daily living, warm packs to her painful joints, salicylate therapy, two-hourly pressure relief, lambskin bootees and underblanket, and mineral and vitamin supplements to her diet.

Nurses were finding some aspects of this treatment schedule difficult to achieve, and Mrs Youssef had lost the ability to assist them in maintaining her activities of daily living.

assessment. The person's pain-related behaviour should be observed at different times to determine the site and intensity of pain, its duration, and the factors that cause, reduce, or eliminate the pain. Quality of life should also be evaluated and charted.

Assessment and measurement

The difference between assessment and measurement is an important distinction to make in pain management.

Assessment of a person's pain refers to an overall examination of multiple aspects of pain and the various factors that affect the pain experience. This includes the site and type of pain, the effect of the pain on the person, and the factors that cause or eliminate pain.

Measurement of pain refers to assigning a specific number or value to one dimension of pain—such as its severity (intensity) or quality (burning, throbbing, and so on). In most circumstances, assigning a value to the intensity or quality of pain is dependent on the person being able to articulate how severe it is, where the pain is felt, what brings it on, and what relieves it.

Importance of direct observation

Direct observation is sometimes the only way of determining whether pain and other discomforts are present. This includes recording all changes in behaviour and mood, and identifying possible causes by speaking with people who are most familiar with the resident's usual demeanour. Families are often a great help in this respect.

Because people with significant cognitive dysfunction might not be able to communicate their pain verbally, nurses must look for non-verbal cues, such as those outlined in Table 14.1 (page 168). Because expressions of pain are socially and culturally determined, some of the cues listed in the table will differ among different cultural and social groups, as well as among individuals.

> 'Direct observation is sometimes the only way of determining whether pain and other discomforts are present.'

Pain scales

Pain scales and evaluation charts can also be very useful,. including verbal description scales, behaviour rating scales, visual analog scales, and numerical rating scales of various types. Pain-relief scales are also very useful. However, many of these scales require a person to see, read, and speak the language depicted on the scale.

Non-verbal analog pain-intensity scales allow the person to point to a number or words that indicate the intensity of their pain. Faces scales, which show a range of expressions from a happy smile to a grimace, can be useful for people with language difficulties, but they are not as likely to reveal a clear indication of pain intensity in a cognitively impaired person. It has been found in many studies that the perception of meaning of the facial expressions can be influenced by the context in which the faces are presented, and that they can therefore be misunderstood (Herr et al. 1998; Scherder & Bouma 2000; Chibnall & Tait 2001; Hicks et al. 2001).

Whatever scales are used, they need to be in very large print for older people, and nurses must ensure that eye glasses and hearing aids are available (and used) for people with sight and hearing impairments.

Table 14.1 Non-verbal cues to pain

Cues to look for	Related pain behaviours
Vocalisations	Sighs, moans
Facial expressions	Grimacing
Motor activity	Extremely slow movement
Disposition	Irritable
Verbal reports	Questions: 'Why did this happen to me?' Requests for help in walking
Body postures, gesturing	Limping or distorted gait Rubbing or supporting affected area Shifting posture frequently Sitting with rigid posture
Behaviours to reduce pain	Taking medication Using health-care system Reduction of tasks or activities Using protective devices, cane, cervical collar
Functional limitations	Lying/sitting for extended periods of time Moving in guarded or protective manner Stopping to rest when walking

Adapted from Turk (1993); published with permission

Additional cues in chronic pain

If pain is chronic, additional cues might be apparent:

- dry skin;
- immobility or reduced physical activity;
- certain movements and favoured ways of doing things;
- social withdrawal;
- eating disorders;
- insomnia or excessive sleeping; and
- anxiety and despair.

Interviewing skills in caring for people with dementia

In assessing pain in people with cognitive impairment, questions should be simple and specific about how the person is feeling right now. It might be necessary to ask questions that require a yes or no answer: 'Do you have any burning?' or 'Do you have an ache?'.

Nurses need to speak calmly and at a pace the person can cope with. A caring and patient manner should be maintained. The nurse should maintain eye contact and keep checking whether the person is comprehending what is being asked. If it is necessary to repeat a question, the same words should be used to avoid confusion.

'Nurses need to speak calmly and at a pace the person can cope with. A caring and patient manner should be maintained.'

It is important to assess the person in a quiet and safe environment. For a resident from a non-English speaking background the services of accredited translators should be used (if available), and help should be sought from relatives who are able to give accurate information.

Pain management
Principles of pain management

Managing pain starts with prevention. Nurses should strive to prevent infection and trauma. Urinary tract infections, fractures, pressure ulcers, bruising, and skin tears should be prevented as far as possible by employing safe-handling techniques and proactive care practices.

'Managing pain starts with prevention.'

Comprehensive assessment, close monitoring, and prompt reporting of the resident's physical and emotional health are the next steps in minimising and eliminating pain.

When pain is present, systematic evaluation of the effectiveness of pain-relieving strategies is needed. Most pain problems in older people can be managed with the careful use of medications and effective non-pharmacological treatments. Using both pharmacological and non-pharmacological means results in more effective pain control and less reliance on medications that can have major side effects in older people.

The following well-tested principles of management are recommended:
- maintaining close liaison with the person's medical practitioners;
- identifying and treating organic causes of pain;
- addressing functional impairments and psychological factors; and
- identifying the person's wishes and the family's views on preferred pain-relieving strategies.

Types of medications

Analgesics continue to be the mainstay of therapy in pain management. To achieve effective pain relief, nurses must understand the basic principles of analgesic administration. Three types of medications are commonly used for older people: (i) non-opioid analgesics; (ii) opioid analgesics; and (iii) adjuvant drugs.

Aspirin and other nonsteroidal anti-inflammatory drugs (NSAIDs) are useful in musculoskeletal pain, but they have some unwanted side-effects, including gastrointestinal upsets. Paracetemol might be an appropriate non-opioid alternative in many cases.

Opioid (narcotic) analgesics, such as morphine, work by attaching to specific opioid receptors in the brain and are useful for severe pain. However, these drugs can produce unwanted side effects, such as constipation, respiratory depression, nausea, and vomiting. Careful management of these side-effects by the appropriate use of anti-emetics, laxatives, and other medications can facilitate the effective use of opioids for a person with dementia. As Ebersole and Hess (1998, p. 333) have wisely observed: 'Narcotics may be used safely in the elderly. Although elderly patients may be more sensitive to narcotics, this does not justify witholding narcotics and failing to relieve pain.'

'Although elderly patients may be more sensitive to narcotics, this does not justify witholding narcotics and failing to relieve pain.'

The adjuvant drugs are not strictly analgesics, but they can be used alone or in conjunction with analgesics to enhance their action. Adjuvants are primarily recommended for chronic pain. Examples include antidepressants and anticonvulsants.

The examples in the Box (page 171) give an indication of two management regimens utilising various combinations of these types of medications.

Principles of medication management

The analgesic needs of people vary, but the following general principles provide helpful guidance in medication use in the elderly (Castonguay 2001).

▶ Pain should be prevented by regular analgesia.
▶ Long-acting analgesics should be used to provide longer duration of comfort.
▶ Short-acting analgesia should be prescribed for breakthrough pain associated with physical activities such as toileting, bathing, physiotherapy, and recreation programs.

Examples of two pain regimens

Nociceptive pain

Nociceptive pain is caused by damage to an organ or tissue, while leaving the nerves intact (for example, the pain from pressure ulcers).

Suggested management:

- regular simple analgesics—for example, paracetamol;
- opioids (for example, morphine) at half or quarter the dose given to younger adults;
- topical analgesic ointments—lignocaine 1% mixed with morphine jel 0.1% or 0.3%.

Neuropathic pain

Neuropathic pain is caused by damage to the nerves, spinal cord, or brain (for example, phantom limb pain and shingles). In most cases, neuropathic pain is not responsive to opioids.

Suggested management:

- use regular analgesia and add a tricyclic antidepressant—for example, nortriptyline (Allegron) 1mg/kg;
- if inflammation is present, add an NSAID—for example, piroxicam (Feldene) or celecoxib (Celebrex) (the latter being better for patients at risk of peptic ulcers);
- if 'burning' pain, continue tricyclic antidepressant; if 'stabbing' pain, use anti-convulsants—for example sodium valproate (Epilim) or carbamazepine (Tegretol).

◗ Treatments should be simplified so that night-time monitoring requirements are minimised.

◗ If possible, only one drug at a time should be prescribed.

◗ Analgesics should begin with a low dose.

◗ Side-effects such as postural hypotension, sedation, and confusion should be monitored.

◗ Analgesia should be continued for a sufficient length of time.

◗ Drugs that can cause confusion (for example, anticholinergics and antispasmodics, should be avoided if possible).

◗ Constipation should be prevented through diet, exercise, and judicious use of laxatives.

Non-pharmacological strategies for relieving pain

Many nurses are afraid of producing addiction when treating people for chronic pain, and they therefore tend to give only the minimum doses ordered, which might not be effective. Education of staff can assist in changing this behaviour, and nurses can also improve pain control through non-pharmacological care techniques used in conjunction with analgesic or adjuvant drugs.

Various programs have been found to improve pain management and quality of life (Ferrell, Ferrell & Rivera 1995). Physiotherapy, including the use of heat, cold, and massage, is very useful for some types of pain, as are therapies directed at stretching, strengthening, and relaxing muscles and joints. These can reduce muscle spasm and enhance functional activity. Another treatment is transcutaneous nerve stimulation—which is particularly useful for shoulder pain, bursitis, and fractures. Biofeedback, acupuncture, acupressure, behavioural modification, hypnosis, meditation, and prayer, or a combination of these modalities, have also been found to be beneficial for older people. However, because many of these modalities require relatively high levels of cognitive function, they might not all be suitable for people with cognitive impairment (Helme 2001; Luggen & Gladden 2001). Every person's needs and capacities should be considered individually.

For people with dementia, nurses can prevent and relieve pain through measures such as quietly talking with the person, gently stretching, massaging or repositioning a painful area, and using pillows or other devices to relieve pressure on bony points. Pain can be minimised by the use of special mattresses and pillows, through gentle handling and touch, by allowing people to move at their own pace, and simply by avoiding knocking the person's chair or bed. If assessment is accurate and the person is listened to with care, anxiety can be controlled and interventions will prove more effective.

Encouraging residents to involve themselves in regular, gentle activity can also be helpful. This is a form of distraction from the pain, and also helps with weight-bearing and exercise tolerance. Music can help to make these physical activities enjoyable. It is important to find activities that are acceptable and well tolerated—to improve quality of life and reduce anxiety, depression, and despair. Use of analgesics in conjunction with an activity is often necessary for someone in constant pain. Providing understanding and emotional support is one of the most effective ways of gaining a person's cooperation and increasing activity levels.

Conclusion

The uniqueness of pain and the difficulties that older people with dementia can have in expressing their pain can make pain a solitary experience. Non-verbal signs and symptoms of pain can easily be overlooked. If this happens with older people who have chronic health conditions that are painful and unremitting, their quality of life, health, and well-being can be significantly reduced. Nursing staff can change this situation in a number of ways.

The first is to reduce or eliminate the factors that give rise to pain by adopting gentle and safe handling techniques when attending to the person's daily care needs. Nurses can learn to assess and monitor pain by using pain charts and scales. The careful use of analgesic and adjuvant drugs, combined with some of the other therapies and treatments described in this chapter, can provide good relief.

Nurses can work with the person's doctor in assessing the drugs and other treatments that are likely to be most effective for individual residents, and nurses can ensure that these are prescribed and reviewed as often as necessary to achieve effective and ongoing pain relief.

> 'Nurses have an ethical and legal obligation to do everything possible to provide comfort and effective pain management for those in their care—especially those who suffer in silence.'

Finally, the express wishes of the resident and family need to be taken into consideration when drawing up plans of care and review. Nurses have an ethical and legal obligation to do everything possible to provide comfort and effective pain management for those in their care—especially those who suffer in silence.

Chapter 15

Depression

David Arthur and Claudia Lai

Introduction

Most psychiatric textbooks use several terms that are related or linked to the term 'depression'. For example, terms such as 'psychotic depression', 'major depression', and 'biological depression' are used, as well as terms such as 'the blues' and 'neurotic depression' or 'reactive depression'.

The terms can be confusing, but behavioural scientists understand these various sorts of 'depression' in terms of a response to a changed situation. When people experience loss, or change, or trauma, a common response is to feel sad. With this feeling of sadness there is a tendency to slow down physically and to experience physical and psychological discomfort and a decreased inability to relate socially. This is mild reactive depression.

It also seems that people have an in-built mechanism, perhaps genetic and metabolic, which, when triggered can slow thinking, feelings, and physical responses. This might represent a way for people to cope physically with environmental stress—such as famine or extremes of climate. This might be a primitive genetic mechanism that has now become relatively redundant, but which, in some people, is triggered by stress. In much the same way as an animal hibernates, some people become severely depressed to the point that they have trouble thinking and acting. They become emotionally numb. Their bodies slow down, their metabolism decreases, and their appetite, bowel movements, and associated processes are diminished. This is a rare and very severe form of depression called 'biological' or 'psychotic' depression, and the cause might be deep within the person and difficult to explain. More commonly, however, depression is a less severe response to stress that is explicable in terms of a reaction to the environment.

'In much the same way as an animal hibernates, some people become severely depressed to the point that they have trouble thinking and acting.'

To help explain 'depression' it is useful to place it on a continuum, as shown in Figure 15.1 (below). On this continuum, the severe maladaptive depression described above in terms of extreme 'hibernation' is at one extreme, with less extreme forms, often considered 'adaptive', towards the other end of the continuum.

For example, imagine what it would be like to have your world changed, your partner gone, and your physical agility and strength depleted. Then, imagine what it would be like to be forced to move out of your home, possibly against your will, into a strange environment in which you are surrounded by people you do not know and would not choose to know in normal circumstances. How would you respond?

People respond to such changes in life circumstances in many ways, but many become depressed. This is a form of depression called 'reactive depression'. Another example of this type of depression is observed in response to physical illness. Many people with severe illnesses go through phases of despair, anger, and remorse. This is easy to understand following major

'Many people with severe illnesses go through phases of despair, anger, and remorse.'

Most severe	→	→	**Least severe**
major depressive disorder (psychotic depression)	reactive depression	grief reaction	'blues'

Figure 15.1 A continuum of depression
Authors' presentation

trauma, such as road accidents. However, it can be less easy to recognise and understand if the change is less dramatic. In elderly people depression can be a reaction to the process of ageing or a reaction to the progressive development of dementia, chronic obstructive lung disease, heart failure, malignancies, or stroke.

Depressive signs and symptoms can also be caused by physical illnesses such as Parkinson's disease, hypothyroidism, and malnutrition. Certain drugs can produce similar signs and symptoms. These include anti-hypertensive agents, sedatives, steroids, anti-Parkinsonian drugs, and opioid analgesics (Johnson, Sims & Gottlieb 1994).

The signs and symptoms of depression can thus be caused by a severe psychotic illness, reactive depression of various degrees, certain illnesses, and certain drugs. For nurses who are caring for old people with dementia, it is easy to see how 'depression', dementia, and physical illness are often mixed up, and why it is important to attempt to differentiate among them. Understanding this is one of the crucial elements of good nursing in caring for these people.

Causes of depression

Why do some people become depressed and not others? For example, why do some soldiers return from world wars (often regarded as one of the most stressful experiences in life) and not experience major problems, whereas others become incapacitated with depression for life? The answer probably lies in the interaction between an individual's personality and coping devices and the degree of stress experienced in the environment. Figure 15.2 (below) shows a model for nursing that relates these predisposing and precipitating factors to the continuum of depression (previously shown in Figure 15.1).

People are born with a genetic complement and then develop personalities in response to other people in family, society, and peers (predisposing factors)

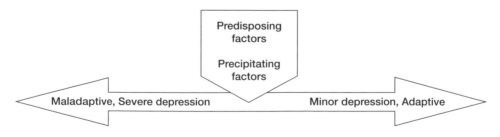

Figure 15.2 Influences on depression
Adapted from Stuart & Laraia (2001)

and in response to the way that they manage the environment (precipitating factors). This determines the way that they behave. Although this description is necessarily simplistic, it provides a useful model for understanding the development of psychiatric disorders.

The clinical presentation of a person with depression is that of a person who has come from a family, who has lived in a community, who has developed a personality as a result of these influences, and who has a certain physical make-up and ability to cope with illness. All of this is woven into the complex presenting picture. Proper assessment and management must be based on this sort of holistic understanding of the person within the context of his or her environment.

Prevalence of depression

The lifetime risk for a major depressive disorder is 10–30% for women and 5–12% for men (APA 1994; Steffens et al. 2000; Stuart & Laraia 2001). The proportion of people at any time with a major depressive disorder is 5–9% in women and 2–3% in men (APA 1994).

Depression is a problem in elderly people, and estimates of depression in chronic care settings vary from 15% to 20% (Cooper 1994). About 20% of people with Alzheimer's disease also have major depression (LaBarge 1993).

Dementia, delirium, and depression are the three most prevalent mental disorders in the elderly (Johnson, Sims & Gottlieb 1994), and patients with major depression are commonly misdiagnosed as having dementia (Draper 1999). The converse problem also exists—making a diagnosis of depression in a person with established dementia (Draper 1999). The problems of misdiagnosis are highlighted in this comment by Cooper (1994, p. 45):

'Dementia, delirium, and depression are the three most prevalent mental disorders in the elderly . . . and patients with major depression are commonly misdiagnosed as having dementia.'

> Those who are experienced in clinical management of the elderly know that, often, what seems to be senile dementia of the Alzheimer's type . . . really isn't. Rather, the resident is experiencing a transient dementia caused by a reversible pathology or outside factor . . . perhaps most common of all, drugs.

The biochemical explanation of depression, and the reason that antidepressants are often effective, is that there is a change in levels of neurotransmitters such as serotonin. Neurotransmitters are complex chemicals that conduct nerve impulses across nerve synapses. Irrespective of the cause, these neurotransmitter levels are altered in depression, and the complex interplay between these changes in neurochemistry and the associated pathology (such as nerve cells atrophying) is a possible explanation as to why depression is more likely to occur in association in dementia.

Assessing depression
Criteria and assessment tools
A major depressive illness includes the following:

▶ depressed mood;
▶ loss of interest or pleasure;
▶ weight loss or gain (5% in a month);
▶ insomnia;
▶ agitation or retardation;
▶ loss of energy;
▶ feelings of worthlessness or guilt;
▶ difficulty thinking or concentrating;
▶ thoughts of death or suicide.

According to the diagnostic criteria of the DSM IV TR (APA 2000) a major depressive episode should have five or more of the above signs and symptoms present for two weeks (including one of the first two—that is, depressed mood or loss of interest or pleasure). In addition, to meet the DSM criteria, the signs and symptoms should: (i) cause significant psychosocial dysfunction; (ii) not be caused by physical means; and (iii) not be accounted for by bereavement.

Several assessment instruments using short questions and responses have been developed, and these help to add objectivity to assessment. These include the Beck Depression Inventory, the Geriatric Depression Scale, and the Centre for Epidemiological Studies Depression Scale.

The following three-tiered approach to detecting depression and assessing its severity has been suggested (Scogin 1997).

▶ First, screen for depression using a self-report instrument such as the Beck Depression Inventory or the Geriatric Depression Scale. The former includes somatic symptoms of depression, and the latter is useful for cognitively impaired people.

▶ Secondly, if the person scores greater than the cut-off score in the screening instrument, a clinical interview should be conducted with a view to seeking evidence of the criteria of DSM-IV (see above).

⦁ Thirdly, severity needs to be assessed using rating scales or the DSM-IV classification, which assesses severity in terms of mild severity, moderate severity, and severe without psychotic features.

The interview

The nurse must talk with the family or the carer of the person, as well talking with the resident. The nurse should attempt to ascertain what the person was like before coming to residential care or before the signs and symptoms developed. The nurse should explore the interplay between precipitating and predisposing factors—an important aspect of which is establishing an understanding of the relationships in the family.

In conducting an interview, the nurse should be patient, and should listen and look for clues. The nurse should resist the urge to talk or put words into the person's mouth. Encouraging words and murmurs on the part of the nurse will encourage responses ('Go on'; 'I see'; 'uh-huh'). It can also be helpful to repeat the person's words to encourage elaboration of what has been said. Nurses should not try to be 'therapeutic' too quickly. Time should be spent talking about other things such as the weather, food, sport, or news. Pressuring depressed people to talk too soon can be counterproductive.

'Pressuring depressed people to talk too soon can be counterproductive.'

The Box on page 180 provides examples of interview techniques that the nurse can use.

Diagnosis made

A depressed elderly person might be relieved to hear that the diagnosis is depression—especially if the person feared a serious physical illness. Once the diagnosis has been made, some of the principles of providing feedback include:
⦁ enlisting the family in the therapeutic process;
⦁ encouraging family to understand the signs and symptoms;
⦁ reducing demands on the person;
⦁ encouraging optimism about therapy;
⦁ monitoring suicidal impulses;
⦁ removing potential weapons and dangerous medications if present;

Examples of interview techniques

Example 1

Person: 'It all seems so useless.'
Nurse: 'It's all useless?'
Person: 'Yes useless, I'm old, tired, no good to anyone.'
Nurse: 'You feel that you are no use to anyone?'
Person: 'Not any more. I used to be.'
Nurse: 'Tell me more about that.'

Comment

In this example the nurse first reflects the term 'useless' in an attempt to clarify what is meant. This communicates that he or she is listening, and it gives the person an opportunity to expand. The last response is on open-ended request for information.

Example 2

Person: 'It all seems so useless.'
Nurse: 'Uh huh . . . OK.'
Person: 'Yes, useless.'
Nurse: 'That's sad.'
Person: 'Yeah all sad. What's the point?'
Nurse: 'The point . . . ?'

Comment

At first the nurse simply acknowledges that he or she is listening, then suggests that feeling useless is sad, and then uses another form of reflection, by repeating the key words 'the point'.

Example 3

Person: 'It all seems so useless.'
Nurse: 'What do you mean by 'useless'?'
Person: 'I mean all those wonderful years and now look . . . '
Nurse: 'Look at . . . ?'
Person: 'You know, my wife's gone, kids don't care . . . our beautiful house . . . '
Nurse: 'Tell me about your house.'
Person: 'My wife loved the garden . . . the roses.'
Nurse: 'The roses?'

Comment

The nurse uses reflection and reminiscence as a technique for giving hope and reminding the person of his worth as an individual. This might also help to resolve grief reactions that are part of the mourning process.

Example 4

Nurse: 'Hello John.'
Person: [no response]

(Continued)

(Continued)

Nurse: 'You're not saying much today.'

Person: [no response]

Nurse: 'Do you mind if I just sit with you for a while. It's nice and relaxing here. I'll read the paper.'

   Some time later . . .

Nurse: 'That was relaxing, thanks for letting me sit here. I'll come back later.'

Comment

Provided that the nurse *does* come back later, the person has not been let down. This might become a foundation for future therapeutic interactions. Some people feel irritable when depressed and the nurse should detect this and not invade personal space.

▶ referring to a family counsellor if it seems that the depression is related to family conflict; and

▶ respecting the confidentiality of the person and seeking his or her consent before making decisions or telling the family.

Family education

The key to educating families is respecting the part they play in the treatment team and involving them by providing clear information and direction. The nurse should explain the meaning of the diagnosis—including a description of what depression is, and how the signs and symptoms exhibited by their elderly family member fit the picture of depression. The nurse should help them understand what they can do to help, and provide them with information in pamphlet or book form, or by referring them to appropriate Internet websites.

> 'The key to educating families is respecting the part they play in the treatment team.'

An opportunity should be provided for family members to become involved with support groups in the community. In general, the nurse should help family members to become involved, and help them make decisions in the best interests of their relative.

If it is considered that there is a risk of suicide, the nurse should talk to the family and explain that it is not unusual for depressed people to feel suicidal. Nevertheless, the family should be aware of dangerous items in the environment—such as knives, and medications.

Treatment of depression

The person should be assessed in terms of physical, psychological, and social factors. Physical illness must be ruled out as a cause, and the medications being taken by the person must be assessed as a possible cause. If no reversible factors (such as physical illnesses, drug effects, or temporary social factors) are apparent, the management of depression involves a combination of drugs and psychotherapy. Electro-convulsive therapy (ECT) is rarely used these days.

Nurses should be aware of the common types of antidepressants, although the question of whether antidepressants should be used to treat people with dementia with coexisting depressive features is a complex one, and research continues (Dening & Bains 2001).

The older antidepressants are the tricyclic antidepressants. These include such drugs as amitriptyline (Tryptanol, Endep) and nortriptyline (Allegron). The newer antidepressants are called selective serotonin uptake inhibitors (SSRIs), and include fluoxetine (Prozac) and sertraline (Zoloft).

The tricyclics have a number of side-effects of which nurses should be aware. The more common and more easily managed side-effects include dry mouth, blurred vision, and drowsiness. More serious side-effects include orthostatic hypotension, memory disturbance, and cardiotoxicity. The person and the family should be educated about the possibility of falls associated with hypotension. They should be briefed about the importance of standing up slowly. Fortunately, the SSRIs have fewer side-effects. With both the tricyclics and the SSRIs, nurses should be aware that compliance in taking these drugs is a problem requiring vigilance.

The common psychotherapies are cognitive-behavioural therapy, inter-personal therapy, psychodynamic therapy, life review therapy, and group and family interventions. Older depressed adults are as likely to benefit from psychotherapeutic intervention as younger adults (Karel & Hinrichsen 2000). Cognitive-behavioural and interpersonal psychotherapies are especially useful, but they are difficult to learn and implement.

Validation therapy is a therapy for communicating with older people who have Alzheimer's disease. A number of techniques and approaches is recommended (Feil 1993), of which the following are the most useful to nurses:

▶ using non-threatening factual words to build trust (such as 'who', 'what', 'where', and 'when'; but *not* 'why');
▶ rephrasing the person's speech to him or her;
▶ encouraging the person to imagine the opposite;
▶ reminiscing;
▶ maintaining genuine, close contact;

- using a clear, low, loving tone of voice;
- observing and matching the person's actions and emotions to create trust;
- touching (although not all people respond well to touch, and this can vary in different stages of depression);
- using music to trigger early memories and thoughts.

A holistic, personalised approach incorporating drug therapy and psycho-dynamic therapy, and involving a team approach that includes the family, is required in the care of depressed people with dementia.

Conclusion

Nurses caring for elderly people are working with people who have vast life experiences, each of whom has experienced a complex of predisposing and precipitating life events.

Nurses must systematically assess and diagnose the problem in association with other team members, and assist in the implementation of relevant strategies. The family is a critical link in the therapeutic process, and community resources such as self-help groups and peer-support groups are increasingly emerging.

'Nurses caring for elderly people are working with people who have vast life experiences.'

Nurses should not merely fulfil vocational requirements, but should keep in mind that extending compassion to another human being is therapeutic in itself, and that being sensitive and sincere is far more helpful than engaging in a premeditated dialogue from a book.

Chapter 16

Aggression

Graham A. Jackson and Colin MacDonald

Introduction
Prevalence and definitions

Aggressive behaviour, in many different forms, often occurs in association with dementia. Many studies have been carried out to establish prevalence, and reported rates vary considerably—from 18% to 65% (Ballard et al. 2000). Moreover, there is no consistent definition of what 'aggression' actually is.

It is important to establish an understanding of what 'aggression' is. Labelling a person as 'aggressive', in any walk of life, alters how others perceive that person. The degree to which others are prepared to accord respect, recognition, willingness to engage, willingness to help, and time to listen are all affected. If a label of 'aggressive' is added to the label of 'dementia', the provision of good-quality care to a person can be seriously compromised.

A label of 'aggressive' also has an effect on whether a person is able to continue to live in any given situation. A 'hierarchy of care' can be described—from living at home, to living with relatives, to residential care, to nursing home care, to specialised care (including hospital care). Behavioural problems, in particular the presence (or even the expectation) of any form of aggression, is the commonest reason for moving up that hierarchy.

The Oxford dictionary defines aggression as: '1. Unprovoked attacking or attack, 2. Hostile or destructive behaviour' (POED 1992). In the context of dementia one widely quoted definition is that aggressive behaviour is: 'an overt act, involving the delivery of noxious stimuli to (but not necessarily aimed at) another organism, object or self, which is clearly not accidental' (Patel & Hope 1992). These and other definitions involve elements of intention and hostility—but these concepts are difficult to establish in the presence of dementia. The belief that such actions are *intentional* makes understanding and tolerating such behaviour difficult.

Documentation

Behaviours that could be described as being 'aggressive' include striking out, shouting in a threatening manner, swearing, throwing items around, biting, scratching, banging doors, and kicking. As well as describing the action it is also important to identify the situation in which such actions occur. For example, it might be occurring because a man finds himself being taken to a strange unrecognisable place by a young woman who is trying to take off his trousers. Perhaps this man does not recognise that he is being taken to the toilet.

The frequency of such behaviours should also be documented. It is possible for a person to be labelled as 'very aggressive' as a result of an isolated incident of limited significance because it involves a 'victim' who happens to take particular offence. Conversely, the label of 'aggression' is less likely to be applied to someone who has otherwise generally likeable traits.

Attitudes, tolerance, and training all play a part in such labelling, and also play a part in how such behaviour is managed. Nurses who work in a home for retired clergy are more likely to be offended by swear words than, say, nurses who work in an area where many of the residents swear frequently (perhaps a working-class area with many ex-miners among the residents).

The extent of the problem therefore needs to be established by asking the following questions:

- ▶ What is the problem behaviour?
- ▶ To whom is it a problem?
- ▶ How often does it occur?
- ▶ How long does an episode last?
- ▶ Who is at risk (the person or others)?
- ▶ How can any such risk be minimised?
- ▶ What are the causes?

Context and management

Most disruptive behaviours exhibited by people with dementia are understandable in the context of the cognitive difficulties experienced by the people involved.

Disorientation in time and place commonly leads to a wish to leave—perhaps to go home, to go to an old address, or to leave for work. A nurse who tries to stop such activity by obstructing it might be perceived to be in the way. In these circumstances, it is no surprise that the person who is obstructed might shout, or try to push, or even hit out.

Disinhibition is another common feature of dementia—particularly if the frontal lobes of the brain are affected. This can lead to inappropriate behaviour—such as a reduced tolerance of others.

Agnosia (failure to recognise) can present particular difficulties. A person who believes that a nursing home is his or her own home might attempt to get others to leave—which can lead to disputes. Similarly, a failure to recognise a spouse or child can cause distress because such relatives might approach a resident in a manner that is perceived by the person as being inappropriate.

Until recent times, dementia care was non-specialist, and was seen as something of a 'Cinderella' speciality. Little interest was shown in it and, consequently, little training was available. Sedating drugs were widely used, particularly neuroleptics, and high doses were often used in spite of there being little evidence of their effectiveness (McGrath & Jackson 1996). This situation is changing, but only slowly. Inappropriate care environments often compound the situation. However, there have been various initiatives in different parts of the world (Burke 1991; SIGN 1999).

Many drugs have been used to manage behavioural problems. The most commonly used drug, until fairly recently, was thioridazine (Melleril)—now no longer in use as greater awareness of its side-effect profile has developed (particularly its anticholinergic side-effects). Other drugs have included haloperidol (Serenace), chlorpromazine (Largactil), trazodone (Desyrel, Trialodine) (and other antidepressants), risperidone (Risperdal), anti-cholinesterase drugs such as donepezil (Aricept), and an assortment of others. In Scotland, SIGN (1999) undertook a literature review and concluded that there was a distinct lack of evidence for the efficacy of these drugs. They therefore recommended that drugs should be used only if there are no alternative ways of managing behaviour.

'Drugs should be used only if there are no alternative ways of managing behaviour.'

A matter that is often ignored is that of consent. Aggressive behaviour, although sometimes due to agitation or distress, usually does not harm the 'aggressor', although it is potentially harmful to others. There is an ethical question as to whether it is right to administer medication to cognitively impaired people, or to use other interventions, simply because of the effect of their actions on others. This ethical question becomes more complex if it involves administering drugs (or using other interventions) with people who are unable to give informed consent.

Medical treatment for aggression also presents a problem because the behaviour is usually of sudden onset, and of short duration. The only way to treat with medication is therefore to try to lower the threshold for reacting to things. In effect, this often means sedation. So, people are sedated because they *might* sometimes annoy or even assault other people. This is not done with other people in the community. For example, football hooligans are not sedated in anticipation of the possibility that they *might* harm others. Is it right to do so in dementia care?

Dementia causes pathological change to the brain. However, two people with the same degree of damage to the same areas of the brain do not necessarily exhibit the same aggressive tendencies. One of

> 'Football hooligans are not sedated in anticipation of the possibility that they *might* harm others. Is it right to do so in dementia care?'

the fundamental principles in working with people with dementia who are aggressive is to remember that aggression is an individual response to a given situation, circumstances, or stimuli. Aggressive behaviour rarely occurs in isolation. No one gets up in the morning and just decides to be aggressive! Every person has his or her own personal 'hot spots', 'hang ups', and irritants. These are often based on individual personalities, beliefs, values, culture, life experiences (good and bad), lifestyles, and vocations. Every person reacts differently to being obstructed or to perceptions of threat. Therefore what works for one person will not necessarily work for another. People with dementia are no different. Management and care strategies should reflect this reality.

Getting to know the person

It is important that nurses make an attempt to understand people who are supposed to be 'aggressive'. Nurses should gather as much information as possible about the person. They should enrol the assistance of family and friends who know the person better than anyone. Information should be gathered about the following aspects of the person in their care.

▶ *Previous personality*—some people might have been 'grumpy' or 'short tempered' all their lives. This has not changed due to the dementia process, and is unlikely to be significantly changed by nurses now.

▶ *Previous lifestyle*—for a man who enjoyed football or rugby matches, shouting and swearing might have been accepted behaviour.

▶ *Previous social role*—someone who has always been in a dominant social role—as a father, a manager, a teacher (or even a nurse!)—might continue to exhibit this behaviour, and this can be interpreted by others as challenging, threatening, or even aggressive.

▶ *Life experiences*—successes, failures, and traumas can be significant, especially if these experiences include physical assault, abuse, imprisonment, or even rape. It is not difficult to understand why the approaches of nurses might be misinterpreted by someone who has had such experiences, and why an aggressive response might result.

▶ *Previous vocations*—in some jobs, aggressive behaviour might have been tolerated or even encouraged (for example, in the armed forces or manual labour).

Assessment and risk reduction
Checking the history
As noted above, nurses should check the history of aggressive incidents—severity, frequency, and circumstances. Who was involved? How many incidents have there been? How were previous incidents managed and resolved?

Following care plans
Nurses should follow any care plan instructions and guidelines. Nurses should be consistent, and should try not to deviate from approaches or strategies that are known to work with any given person.

Not only in people with dementia

My father had an army background—which he never talked about. If startled while sleeping, or woken up too quickly, he would punch out! And yet my father was not an aggressive man! We learnt to avoid this. But what would have happened if he had been admitted to hospital or a nursing home?

Avoiding risk

Nurses should never put themselves in an 'at-risk' situation, especially if the person is known to be, or even potentially, aggressive. In particular, nurses should:

▶ not work alone (or, at the very least, should let someone know where they are);

▶ ensure that extra assistance is readily available, and that someone can be contacted quickly if necessary;

▶ not work in confined areas; and

▶ be aware of possible triggers in their approach, and during personal care tasks with the person.

Facing aggression

If the person is becoming aggressive, nurses should stop and back off. They should ask themselves the following questions.

▶ Does this have to be done right now?

▶ Is there another way of doing this?

▶ Is it safe to leave the person?

▶ Are others safe—especially frail residents? (If not, these people should be removed from the vicinity.)

▶ Is assistance needed and, if so, how many people? (Too many can provoke an aggressive reaction!)

▶ Is someone else better with this person (such as a carer or relative)?

Nurses should never physically intervene or try to restrain a person unless absolutely necessary. To do this will only increases the risk of injury to the nurse and/or the person. Any good work already done in building a relationship of trust will be lost.

Many incidents of aggression occur in situations in which the person's body language and aggressive behaviour make it quite clear that he or she does not like what is happening and that there will be no cooperation. And yet carers often insist on continuing with the task, increasing the risk of injury to themselves or to the person.

Promoting trust and respect

When working with a person who is known to be or is potentially aggressive, the main aim is to avoid provoking the person into an aggressive response. The aim is to help instil feelings of trust, confidence, and respect that will help to promote a better long-term relationship with the person.

Nurses should:

▶ *approach from the front*—they should *never* approach from the back or from the side of a person (because this can frighten or startle the person who might react by hitting out);

▶ *use the person's preferred mode of address*—terms such 'Pop', 'Gran', 'Sweetie', and so on can be perceived as disrespectful or humiliating;

▶ *introduce themselves*—they should tell the person their names, and who they are (a nurse or carer);

▶ *adopt a non-threatening posture*—they should get down to the person's level, but should keep a safe distance (until they know the person well enough); towering over someone can be intimidating;

▶ *use eye contact*—this is a powerful way of communicating trust; but 'staring someone out' can be interpreted as a threatening gesture;

▶ *be calm and unhurried in manner*—they should avoid sudden movements, and avoid showing any signs of tension or anxiety; people with dementia are often astute interpreters of non-verbal communication;

▶ *speak in a clear and gentle voice*—they should avoid shouting, arguing, or any other form of confrontation;

▶ *use touch to reassure the person*—but stop immediately if the person does not like this;

▶ *use empathy*—they should imagine how they would feel if they were in this person's situation now;

▶ *explain what they are going to do for the person rather than to the person*;

▶ *keep any instructions simple*—short sentences, with one question at a time;

▶ *offer alternatives*—based on the person's communication abilities (for example, using short sentences, pictures, or symbols);

▶ *assist and support the person to participate*—for example, with personal care, they should use skills of guiding and coaxing (and perhaps even mild coercion), but should avoid any form of physical restraint, holding, or grabbing;

▶ *respect the person's right to refuse*—nurses can always return later;

▶ *let another nurse try*—sometimes one nurse's face just 'does not fit', or reminds the person of someone else; and

▶ *be consistent*—if an approach/strategy works, it should be documented, and nurses should ensure that everyone does it this way.

Identifying underlying reasons

Certain factors can make aggressive behaviour more likely to occur. In seeking to identify causes of such behaviour, nurses should consider factors in their own attitudes and behaviour, as well as considering factors in the person in their care. The following should be considered:

▶ attitudes of nurses and carers;
▶ care practices and routines;
▶ environmental factors;
▶ physical causes (illnesses, symptoms);
▶ other factors.

Each of these is considered below.

Attitudes of nurses and carers

Negative attitudes of nurses and carers can lead to poor tolerance of aggression. Nurses can have negative attitudes towards their work in general. They might view their work as being difficult, unstimulating, and unrewarding. This, in turn, can make it more likely that they will have negative attitudes towards those in their care.

Nurses might have ageist attitudes in which older people are viewed as dependent, a burden, and worthless to society. Some nurses might perceive older people in terms of certain stereotypes. They might, for example, feel that older people should not swear, talk about sex, or behave aggressively (while tolerating such behaviour in younger people). Such attitudes and stereotypes can lead nurses to have a low tolerance of aggression. They can feel that people should not be allowed to get away with certain behaviour, and feel that something should be done. However, in society in general, standing up for oneself, protecting others, and even being aggressive (for example, in some sports) are often perceived as positive traits.

If nurses do have particular expectations and stereotypes of older people, those who fail to conform to these expectations and views can be viewed negatively. In turn, these people can react in an obstructive manner. When they do, they are labelled as being 'aggressive'.

'If nurses have particular expectations and stereotypes of older people, those who fail to conform to these expectations can be viewed negatively.'

Care practices and routines

Many aggressive incidents occur during direct personal care. Some nurses adopt a 'custodial approach' in which staff always 'know best'. In this approach, the emphasis is on power and control. Nurses have been overheard to say: 'When I'm on, he goes to his bed one way or another'. In such a culture, care is more

---

An early riser

A man who had been a postman all his life was used to getting up between 4 am and 5 am. When he did this in hospital, the night staff felt that this was too early because he might wake other patients.

Nurses were adamant that this man was to go back to bed. A struggle followed, and one of the night staff was punched.

This man's life and care now changed. He was labelled as 'aggressive', and nursing attitudes to him were never the same.

---

likely to be based on punishment, isolation, or restraint. Rather than controlling aggressive behaviours, this approach only increases its severity and prevalence.

Routines in an organisation can lead to nurses adopting a paternalist approach in which all residents are perceived as having the same needs in terms of physical care. These goals of care are pursued irrespective of the views, feelings, and rights of particular individuals. Inflexible routines and the smooth running of the organisation become paramount—for example, with everyone having to be washed and dressed for breakfast at a particular time. If staff resources are limited, this increases the stress on nurses and reduces their tolerance of any behaviour that obstructs the completion of tasks on time. But such routines expect an individual person with dementia to change a lifetime's routines and way of life.

Environmental factors

For a person with dementia, the internal environment of residential accommodation can be perceived in various ways. It might be perceived as a hotel or as a prison. How the person behaves depends on this perception.

Too much noise can be disconcerting. This might come from televisions and radios, from people shouting (including carers), from domestic appliances, or from the clatter of pots and pans.

There might be too much stimulation. Carers, residents, and visitors can 'mill around' and confuse the resident with too much activity and conversation. In many cases, such people are no more than 'strangers' to a person with dementia. Other residents can invade personal space. They can shout and make a noise, thus interfering with and provoking a person with dementia.

People can feel confined. Bedroom doors that are locked, 'no-go areas', and corridors that are shut off can effectively 'pen' people together—thus increasing the risk of conflict. There can be limited access to the outside—thus increasing a sense of frustration. Physical restraints increase feelings of anger and can reinforce ideas of being in a 'prison'.

Physical illnesses and symptoms

Symptoms of illness can be unpleasant and distressing, and can increase confusion. A person with dementia might not be able to communicate his or her symptoms verbally. Rather, such communication might be expressed through the person's behaviour and through his or her reactions to care routines. This might well be interpreted as 'aggressive' behaviour.

A person with painful knees might be unable to communicate his or her distress, but might be expected to walk down a corridor or to some other destination. Conversely, a person who is constipated or desperate to get to the toilet might pace about trying to find the toilet. But this person might be told by carers to sit down quietly.

Increased confusion might be caused by infection, anaemia, low blood sugar, or drugs. Such confusion might lead to 'aggressive' behaviour. Psychiatric disorders can produce hallucinations, delusions, or paranoid ideas. Visual or hearing impairment can cause people to misinterpret conversations, background noises, or other people's actions.

Physical restraint can create anger, frustration, and resentment that becomes directed towards staff. This can increase the level and severity of aggression, which can become worse than the initial behaviour that led to the imposition of restraint.

Failing abilities can produce embarrassment, fear, and anxiety. People might become concerned about being forgetful or incontinent, or become anxious about being in an unfamiliar place surrounded by apparent strangers.

'Physical restraint can create anger, frustration, and resentment that becomes directed towards staff . . . worse than the initial behaviour that led to the imposition of restraint.'

Faced with debilitating symptoms that they cannot understand or communicate, people can use 'aggression' as a form of communication or a defence mechanism. A person hitting out might effectively be saying: 'Leave me alone'.

Other factors

Other 'triggers' could be any act, stimulus, or environmental condition that causes or contributes to aggressive behaviour. By noting common patterns,

ABC of identifying 'triggers'

The 'ABC' of identifying 'triggers' refers to *antecedents*, *behaviour*, and *consequences*. Nurses should ask themselves:

Antecedents

What was happening before the behaviour?
- Who was present?
- What was happening?
- Where did it happen?

Behaviour

What exactly happened?
- What was the person doing?
- Was it of sudden or gradual onset?
- Who or what was it directed at?
- How long did it last?

Consequences

What was the effect of the behaviour on the person or on others?
- What interventions were tried?
- What worked and what failed?
- Did the person calm down in his or her own time?
- Did the person cease the behaviour only after gaining something (food, drink, attention, or other comforts)?
- Was any medication (sedation) or physical restraint used?
- Was anyone hurt or distressed by the behaviour?

themes, and circumstances, nurses can identify such triggers. Ways of removing or preventing triggers can then be considered to reduce episodes of aggression.

By considering antecedents, behaviour, and consequences ('ABC') possible triggers can be identified. The Box above illustrates such an 'ABC' tool.

Use of drugs
Emergency drug use

There are some emergency situations in which drugs are required. Such emergency situations are those which involve a significant risk of violence to others, or a severe degree of distress to the person with dementia. Other ways of managing the situation should already have been tried, and failed. Medication should be used as a last resort. That is, *emergency* treatment should be just that—not something used routinely.

Neuroleptic drugs such as haloperidol, risperidone, or chlorpromazine are often administered in such situations. However, these drugs are relatively non-sedating, and are usually slow to act. Despite this, these drugs are still widely used and repeated doses are given until the recipient eventually becomes virtually non-responsive. The person then takes some considerable time to recover.

Short-acting drugs with more rapid onset of effect are preferable. Low doses should be used. Examples include:

▶ chlormethiazole 192 mg;
▶ lorazepam 0.5–1.0 mg; or
▶ diazepam 2 mg.

The last two drugs can also be used intramuscularly for more rapid effect or if it is difficult to administer an oral preparation.

In all cases, the question of consent must be considered. As in all emergencies in medical and nursing practice, the requirement for consent can be overriden by the needs of the emergency. However, the issue of consent *must* be considered in every case.

Prophylactic drug use

If aggressive episodes occur frequently despite all attempts to avoid or modify such behaviour, prophylactic medication can be considered.

There is a lack of evidence regarding best practice in this regard, but drugs commonly used include trazodone, citalopram, risperidone, carbamazepine, and olanzapine. The potential for side-effects from these drugs is high, and the risk/benefit ratio must be considered. There is little point in eliminating aggression by over-sedating a person if this causes a new set of difficult management issues.

Such drugs are relatively slow to act, and have a cumulative effect. Any drug prescribed should be given time to act. It should be prescribed initially at low dose, and increased only if necessary. At least a few days should have elapsed before changes are made. Drug administration should follow the axiom: 'Start low and go slow'. Such drugs should be used for as short a time as possible, and the need for ongoing administration should be continually reviewed.

Staff education

The cornerstone to successful management of aggression in people with dementia is adequate education of nurses and the provision of sensible strategies and hints. Caring for people with dementia who can be aggressive is no easy task. Education and training can:

▶ help nurses to develop a better general understanding (and tolerance) of aggression in people with dementia; and

▶ develop particular skills and instil confidence in individual nurses that they can safely and effectively manage aggressive situations.

Education and training can prevent problems arising in the first place and/or facilitate a prompt response to any potentially aggressive situation before it develops into something more serious.

General principles

Staff training should emphasise that the keys to success are *observation*, *de-escalation*, and *intervention*.

Observation

Nurses should be aware of *who* needs to be observed, *where*, and *why*. It is obviously impossible to observe every person for every minute of the day. In any event, every person's right to privacy must be respected. Nevertheless, it is prudent to take reasonable steps. For example, the continual presence of a carer in a sitting room can result in more timely responses to potentially aggressive situations and can prevent harm or distress to others (especially to frail or vulnerable residents). Arrangements will vary from establishment to establishment, but prudent observation is the key to prevention.

> 'The keys to success are *observation, de-escalation,* and *intervention.*'

De-escalation

The term 'de-escalation' refers to skills or technique that help to distract the person's attention or defuse a difficult situation. This covers a range of techniques—including verbal distraction, touch, reassurance, empathy, listening, and removing any obvious triggers. Good knowledge of the person is obviously very helpful in this regard.

Intervention

Apart from interventions aimed at de-escalation, nurses might have to intervene physically and quickly in some 'flashpoint' situations to maintain the safety of the person and/or others. This should be limited to immediate safety needs, and should avoid any ongoing physical intervention, restraint, or confrontation—unless absolutely necessary.

Specific hints and strategies

Apart from the general principles of staff education noted above (and discussed elsewhere in this chapter), the following specific hints and strategies might be useful.

Hints for personal interaction

In dealing with people at the interpersonal level, nurses should:

‣ never work alone, or in a situation where assistance cannot be summoned;
‣ never put themselves or others in an 'at risk' situation;
‣ never approach a person from behind;
‣ avoid sudden movements;
‣ avoid confrontations and arguments;
‣ avoid any form of physical restraint;
‣ try to find the reason for the aggressive behaviour, rather than trying to control it; and
‣ de-escalate aggression at an early stage.

Hints for general care

Apart from the above hints dealing with personal interactions, the following hints on general strategies might prove useful in the care of people who demonstrate aggressive behaviour.

‣ *Flexible routines*—these should take account of the previous lifestyles and present needs of individual persons in care.
‣ *Environmental approaches*—these should aim to produce a 'homely environment' (with personal possessions and age-appropriate furnishings), the provision of quiet private areas and a general reduction of noise (with particular attention to television and radio volume), attention to lighting (good natural lighting to maximise visual ability and variable lighting to suit mood), and open-plan areas (where the person can see and be seen).
‣ *Involvement of relatives*—making use of their knowledge of the person, and involving them in a caring role (if appropriate).
‣ *Physical activities*— to burn off physical energy constructively (walking, domestic chores, or gardening).
‣ *Relaxation*—to decrease agitation and enhance calmness (music, hand massage, or simple rest in a chair or bed).
‣ *Distraction*—to divert attention away from any causative factors (invitation to go for a walk or join staff in a cup of tea; encouragement to go to a quieter and more private place).

▶ *Person-centred and consistent approaches*—respecting individual needs and recognising that what works for one person might not work for another.

▶ *Favourite carers*—utilising the fact that many people are more comfortable with a particular, nurse, or relative.

Conclusion

Rather than labelling behaviour (or, indeed, a person) as 'aggressive', nurses must identify particular incidents—including their frequency and their consequences. The use of the term 'aggressive' can, in itself, lead to a change in attitude to that person. This, in turn, can lead to poorer quality of care.

Management of such difficulties usually falls to those carers who have most 'hands-on' care. In a hospital or in a care home these staff members are often the least well trained, and might be the least experienced. It is important that all staff members dealing with people with dementia receive regular training of good quality, and that they are well supported by their managers.

There is no *right* way to deal with problem behaviour. Each person, each carer, and each situation is different. Nurses must persevere, and solutions have to be tailored to particular events. It is not always possible get it right. Nurses should not see a lack of success as being failure. Nurses fail their patients only if they do not try. The key is is to persevere with care that is genuinely person-centred.

> 'Nurses fail their patients only if they do not try. The key is is to persevere with care that is genuinely person-centred.'

Chapter 17

Pressure Sores and Wounds

Geoff Sussman

Introduction

Dementia is a predisposing factor in the development of pressure wounds. Of all of the chronic wounds seen in practice, the most preventable are pressure wounds. In fact, 90% of all pressure wounds can be prevented. The key to prevention is accurate assessment of all people at risk, followed by active intervention.

'90% of all pressure wounds can be prevented.'

A multidisciplinary approach to pressure care and pressure wound management is essential. All hospitals and residential aged-care facilities should put together a team of health professionals to set standards and assist with management.

Pressure wounds can range from simple blisters to extensive pressure ulcers, and are more common in bedridden people suffering from medical conditions such as stroke, spinal injury, multiple sclerosis, and dementia.

Prevalence and costs

Studies of the prevalence of pressure sores in acute hospitals and nursing homes have demonstrated rates of 6.5% to 9.4 %, increasing to 30% in people of more than 65 years of age (Young & Dobrzanski 1992; Rudman et al. 1993; Wright & Tiziani 1996). One study showed that 12% of people developed their pressure ulcers in hospital (McGowan, Hensley & Maddocks 1996).

The annual financial cost to health systems of the management of pressure wounds is huge. This can be illustrated by the fact that the total cost of the management of a single sacral pressure ulcer in an elderly person can be tens of thousands of dollars (Young 1997).

In addition to the financial cost, the social and emotional costs to the people involved must also be considered. The effect of these wounds on the quality of life can be quite severe (Phillips 1994). This is particularly significant in the context of dementia, when the person's quality of life might already be seriously compromised by failing cognition and impaired communication.

What is a pressure sore?

A pressure sore is a localised area of ischaemic cellular damage resulting from direct pressure on the skin or from shearing forces caused by mechanical stress. External pressure that exceeds the mean capillary pressure of 28–38 mm Hg is sufficient to cause tissue damage if it is maintained for long periods—particularly in debilitated patients. Any period exceeding two hours is likely to cause trauma. For cachectic, debilitated, or terminally ill people, tissue damage can occur in less time than this. It is possible for a person to return from an operating theatre with a pressure wound.

Pressure restricts blood supply and this reduces oxygen supply and nutrition to the tissue. In addition, waste products are not removed from the site. The result is hypoxia, tissue acidosis, increased capillary permeability, and the escape of intravascular fluid causing oedema and cell death (Leigh & Bennett 1994).

The most common sites of pressure sores are:

▶ post-sacral (lower back);
▶ post-calcaneal (ankle);
▶ trochanteric (upper femur); and
▶ post-ischeal (buttocks).

Causes

The main causes of pressure wounds are:

▶ pressure;
▶ friction;
▶ shear; and
▶ moisture.

Each of these is discussed below.

Pressure

Direct pressure greater than 30 mm Hg on tissue over a bony prominence causes ischaemia. Pressure of this magnitude can occur as a result of a person being in bed, on a trolley, or sitting in a chair.

The extent of tissue damage depends on the intensity of the pressure, and the length of time that the pressure remains unrelieved. Tissues can tolerate pressure for short periods of time, but even low pressure over a long period of time will have detrimental effects.

Friction

Friction causes a pressure sore when the top layers of skin are worn away by rubbing against an external surface. This can produce a simple blister, tissue oedema, or an open pressure wound. It can be caused by ill-fitting footwear or bed linen.

Shearing forces

Shearing forces cause pressure sores when the skin remains in place, usually unable to move against the surface it is in contact with, while the underlying bone and tissue are forced to move. This force damages deep tissue and obstructs blood vessels in a manner similar to direct pressure.

This type of pressure injury is seen in people who are left sitting up in bed or on a chair. Gravity causes the person to slide down with the skin adhering to the bed linen or the surface of the chair.

Moisture

Continued exposure to moisture causes maceration of the skin, which affects the skin's ability to function normally and makes it prone to damage. Macerated skin is much more likely to stick to bed linen.

Moisture can come form urinary incontinence, faecal incontinence, perspiration, or wound exudate (Allmann et al. 1995; Brandeis et al. 1994).

Risk factors

Why do some people develop pressure wounds whereas others do not? There are many factors, intrinsic and extrinsic, that can contribute to the development of a pressure wound. The major risk factors for the development of pressure wounds are:

▶ lack of mobility;
▶ changes in the skin;
▶ physiological factors;
▶ intensity and duration of pressure; and
▶ tissue tolerance of pressure.

Each of these is discussed below.

Lack of mobility

Lack of mobility might be due to paralysis, sensory defect (such as neuropathy), traction (for example, for management of a fracture), or chronic conditions (such as arthritis, dementia, stroke, or obesity). A person with dementia might not have the awareness to change his or her position frequently, thereby increasing the risk of pressure wounds.

Changes in skin

As previously noted, skin changes can develop from exposure to moisture as a result of incontinence or perspiration. Underweight patients are also at greater risk because they have little fat or muscle to prevent the effects of pressure. A person with dementia might not notice or report skin changes and is therefore dependent on nurses to check all skin surfaces frequently.

Physiological factors

The process of ageing, in itself, predisposes people to pressure damage. The blood supply of the skin dimishes, the skin becomes thinner and skin cells fail to reproduce as quickly, and nerve receptors are less responsive to stimuli (such as touch, pain, temperature change, and so on).

Nutritional deficiencies as a result of a reduced intake of proteins, fluids, electrolytes, and vitamins can cause a breakdown of tissue. A low serum albumin, a lack of amino acids, and low vitamin C can all affect tissue repair. Zinc and iron are essential trace elements.

Systemic disease such as diabetes, anaemia, respiratory disease, carcinoma, and vascular disease can all result in reduced blood supply to the skin causing hypoxia and tissue damage. A person with dementia might have one or more of these diseases, signifying the need for careful assessment of all physiological factors.

Intensity and duration of pressure

Impaired mobility or impaired sensory perception can affect the intensity and duration of pressure. A lack of mobility can mean that a person in discomfort is unable to alter position. A person with sensory impairment might not even experience discomfort, and will not therefore shift position and reduce the potential damage. Those with altered consciousness might have a combination of a lack of sensory input and an inability to move appropriately.

> 'Impaired mobility or impaired sensory perception can affect the intensity and duration of pressure.'

Tissue tolerance

The term 'tissue tolerance' refers to the ability of the skin and its supporting structures to endure the effects of pressure without adverse results. People differ in the ability of their bodies to cushion pressure and to transfer pressure loads from the skin surface to the skeleton.

No matter how appropriate the wound dressing regimen, delayed healing is inevitable if the underlying cause of the pressure-sore is not alleviated.

Risk assessment

People at risk

As a result of the above risk factors, certain people are more susceptible to the development of a pressure wound than others. These include those who have:

- spinal cord damage (especially those with paraplegia);
- cerebral damage (dementia; hemiplegia; unconsciousness);
- nutritional problems (obesity; malnutrition);
- drug-related problems (alcohol; steroids);
- orthopaedic problems (fractured femur; poorly applied traction or cast);
- psychiatric conditions (for example, severe depression);
- vascular disease (peripheral vascular disease; venous congestion);
- surgery (especially major abdominal surgery and neurosurgery); and
- various chronic medical conditions (such as arthritis, diabetes, anaemia, respiratory disease, and carcinoma).

These people should be recognised as being those who are at the greatest risk of pressure sore development, and intervention strategies should be in place to minimise the possibility of damage.

Dementia and pressure wounds

Dementia manifests in many ways, but people with dementia are at increased risk of pressure wounds for several reasons. In general, people with dementia are more likely to:

▶ have potential for self injury;
▶ have long periods of inactivity;
▶ be incontinent; and
▶ have nutritional problems.

For these reasons, research has identified a direct link between dementia and pressure wounds and a greater incidence of pressure wounds among people with dementia in nursing homes (Lyons et al. 1995; Holstein et al. 1994).

'People with dementia are at increased risk of pressure wounds for several reasons.'

Good skin care, good nutrition, general measures to reduce risk, and early intervention to areas of reddened or broken skin are important preventive measures.

Risk-assessment tools

There are several assessment tools that can be used to aid in the identification of people who are at risk of developing a pressure wound. The choice of assessment tool varies, depending on practice setting. The most important issue is that any given risk-assessment tool is used on *all* patients or residents in any one setting. The most commonly used assessment tools are the Norton scale (1989), the Waterlow scale (1985), and the Braden scale (1987).

All of these tools rate the person against a number of criteria including:

▶ mobility;
▶ activity;
▶ mental status;
▶ continence;
▶ general physical condition;
▶ nutritional status;
▶ sensory functioning;
▶ conscious state;
▶ physical and social environment; and
▶ debilitating concurrent illness.

From these various ratings a total score is established so that people who are at risk can be identified. Once a patient has been identified as being at risk, action must be taken to remove or change any risk factors that *can* be changed.

Classification

The classification of pressure sores is based on the level of tissue damage and the depth of the wound as follows (NPUAP 1989).

▶ *Stage 1—non-blanching hyperaemia:* The erythema remains when light finger pressure is applied, indicating that some micro-circulatory disruption is present; superficial damage, including epidermal ulceration might be present; discolouration of the skin, warmth, oedema, induration, or hardness might also be apparent.

▶ *Stage 2—partial thickness:* ulceration with skin loss involving the epidermis and/or the dermis; the ulcer is superficial and presents clinically as an abrasion, blister, or shallow crater.

▶ *Stage 3—full thickness:* skin loss involving damage or necrosis of subcutaneous tissue that extends down to (but not through) underlying fascia. The ulcer presents clinically as a deep crater with or without undermining or adjacent tissue.

▶ *Stage 4—deep full thickness:* skin loss with extensive destruction and tissue necrosis of muscle, bone, or supporting structures (for example, tendon or joint capsule). Undermining and sinus tracts can also be present.

Management

The most important principle in the management of any pressure wound is early intervention. Management involves reducing pressure, turning and positioning the person, reducing friction or shearing forces, and reducing excess moisture by managing incontinence and perspiration. For a person with dementia, prevention involves daily inspection of all skin surfaces and frequent reminders for the person to change position.

> 'The most important principle in the management of any pressure wound is early intervention.'

Any nutritional deficiency should be addressed. It is essential that any person who is at risk is nursed on an appropriate surface to control and reduce pressure.

The presence of necrotic tissue or excessive slough should be treated by surgical debridement of the necrotic tissue, or by the use of amorphous hydrogels to rehydrate the slough, necrotic tissue, and eschar. Enzymatic treatment with proteolytic enzymes can also be used. Slough removal can be assisted by the use of hydrocolloids in the form of hydrocolloid pastes or powders and a hydrocolloid dressing. Failure to remove necrotic tissue or slough will delay or prevent the healing of a pressure wound. The preparation of the wound bed is an essential stage in wound healing.

Infection is always a potential problem for a debilitated patient with a pressure sore. The presence of spreading cellulitis around a pressure sore can be an indication for systemic antibiotics. Infection should be treated with an appropriate antibiotic for any specific organisms identified. If anaerobes are present, the use of metronidazole gels (0.7%–0.8%) is an option.

'Infection is always a potential problem for a debilitated patient with a pressure sore.'

Excessive exudate can delay the healing of a pressure wound. Although it has been common practice to pack a pressure sore with gauze—either on its own or in combination with topical antiseptics—this is inappropriate. The gauze will dry out and stick to the tissue, and this can cause tissue trauma on removal. The use of most topical antiseptics will retard wound healing. If a pressure sore has a lot of exudate, the most appropriate products to use are a foam cavity dressing, an alginate in combination with a surface foam dressing, or a hydroactive polymer dressing.

A decision on the most appropriate dressing products depends on three factors—the stage and colour of the wound, the depth of the wound, and the amount of exudate. Table 17.1 (page 207) provides guidance on dressing choice.

Complications

Complications of pressure wounds include infection, dehydration, and electrolyte imbalance.

The most significant complication is infection. Heavy levels of bacterial colonisation can occur, including methicillin-resistant *staphyloccocus aureus* (MRSA). Infection can progress to cellulitis, generalised sepsis, and osteomyelitis.

Pressure management surfaces

If a patient is assessed as being at high risk, it is essential to use particular devices to prevent the development of a pressure wound, or to prevent it from becoming too severe. These include special air mattresses, water beds, air-fluidised beds, low-pressure air beds, and alternating pressure (ripple-type) mattresses (fixed or driven by air pressure).

These devices fall into two categories.

Table 17.1 Wound types and management

Wound type and aim of treatment	General principles	Superficial	Deep
Black (low exudate)			
Rehydrate; loosen eschar	surgical debridement is most effective method of removal of necrotic material; dressings can enhance autolytic debridement of eschar	amorphous hydrogels; hydrocolloid sheet; proteolytic enzymes	
Yellow (high exudate)			
Remove slough; absorb exudate	surface wounds: hydrocolloids (with or without paste or powder) deeper wounds: hydrogels, alginates, and enzymes aid in removal of slough and absorb exudate	hydrocolloid; alginate; enzymes; hydroactive	hydrocolloid with paste or powder; hydrogel enzymes; alginates; hydroactive cavity; hydrocolloid/ alginate; foam cavity dressing
Yellow (low exudate)			
Remove slough; absorb exudate; maintain moist environment	hydrogels rehydrate the slough; hydrocolloids, films and enzymes aid in autolysis	amorphous hydrogels; sheet hydrogels; hydrocolloid; film dressings	amorphous hydrogels; hydrocolloid with paste; enzymes; foam as a secondary dressing
Red (high exudate)			
Maintain moist environment; absorb exudate; promote granulation and epithelialisation	foam dressings, alginates and hydroactive dressings help control exudate; hydrocolloids with paste or powder for deeper areas	foam; alginates; hydroactive	foam cavity dressing; alginates; hydrocolloid/ alginate; hydrocolloid with paste or powder; hydroactive cavity

(Continued)

Table 17.1 Wound types and management *(Continued)*

Wound type and aim of treatment	General principles	Superficial	Deep
Red (low exudate)			
Maintain moist environment; promote granulation and epithelialisation	hydrocolloid, foams, sheet hydrogels, and film dressings maintain the environment; combination of amorphous hydrogels with a foam cavity dressing in deeper wounds	hydrocolloids; foams; sheet hydrogels; films	hydrocolloids with paste or powder; amorphous hydrogels; foam cavity dressings
Pink (low exudate)			
Maintain moist environment; protect and insulate		foams; thin hydrocolloids; thin hydroactives; film dressings	foams, films, hydrocolloids (thin); hydroactive (thin)
Red (unbroken skin)			
Prevent skin infection		hydrocolloids or film dressings provide best protection	

Author's presentation

- A pressure-relieving mattress moves in a cyclical manner. This subjects areas of the body to low pressures at intervals, and thus allows re-perfusion of tissues.
- A pressure-reducing mattress moulds around the body, thus increasing the area in contact with support. The load is more widely distributed and pressure is reduced over bony prominences.
  The ideal system should have certain features. It should:
- minimise the pressure gradient in the skin and underlying tissues;
- provide good stability for the person;
- allow weight shifts in bed;
- allow easy transfer in and out of bed;
- control moisture accumulation on the skin;

◗ control temperature of the skin;
◗ be lightweight;
◗ be low cost;
◗ be durable; and
◗ be easy to clean

There are many products available on the market including overlay products, mattresses, beds, cushions, and heel protectors. There are also several wool and wool-substitute products used for pressure relief. There is conflicting evidence regarding the value of these products in various circumstances.

Table 17.2 lists some of pressure-management products available, together with their advantages and disadvantages.

Positioning and massage

Pressure can also be relieved by frequently turning bedridden people to reduce friction and shearing forces. People who are bedridden should be turned at least every two hours. This should be achieved by slight shifts of position, rather than by turning the person from side to side. Position changing can be painful for a person with dementia who is unable to articulate feelings of distress and unable to understand the reason for this frequent handling. Resistive responses can occur. In this situation, regular analgesia can be effective.

Chairbound people should be repositioned every hour. If possible, people should be encouraged to shift their weight every 15 minutes. To achieve the

Table 17.2 Pressure management products

Product	Advantages	Disadvantages
Air-filled products	lightweight; inexpensive; easy to clean; effective for many patients	subject to puncture; not easily repaired; inflation needs to be checked frequently
Liquid-filled devices	easy to clean; effective	subject to puncture; heavy
Gel-filled products	adjusts to the body; easy to clean	heavy; expensive
Foam products	widely available; many types; inexpensive; lightweight	wear out quickly; not easily cleaned; properties change with time

Author's presentation

Early appropriate intervention

Mr A was 84 years old and suffered from dementia and cardiac disease. Although not bedridden, he had only limited mobility. He was unable to communicate well, but had good nutritional intake. He spent most of his day lying on the bed.

Mr A had developed a pressure area on his right heel about 15 cm in diameter. The pressure area was partly covered by loose sloughy skin. Although the area was being dressed with a simple product, it was not improving. Indeed, it was enlarging and threatening to become a serious problem.

The dead skin was easily removed, and the wound was irrigated with saline to remove residual exudate. An amorphous hydrogel was applied to the wound and covered with a heel cup of double-layer foam. This was held in place with a lightweight cohesive bandage. A further layer of foam was applied over the dressing and held in place with a lightweight tubular bandage. The dressing was changed every three days.

The aims of this treatement were to remove non-viable tissue, provide a moist environment, absorb exudate, raise the core temperature of the skin, and reduce the pressure.

The wound completely healed within a fortnight. After it had healed, Mr A continued to wear the foam heel cup to protect the new tissue and to maintain pressure reduction.

necessary positioning, a person with dementia might require frequent prompting—perhaps coupled with another pleasurable activity.

Avoid positioning people with their weight directly over the trochanter (the bony prominence at the top of the thigh). It is also useful to use pillows or foam wedges to keep bony prominences from direct contact with one another.

Massage has been long considered helpful in the prevention of pressure sores. It was thought that massage stimulated circulation, aided in comfort and well-being, and prevented pressure sores. However, research has shown that massage decreases skin blood flow, decreases skin temperature, and can damage unhealthy tissue (Ek, Gustavsson & Lewis 1985; Dyson 1978). Other measures of comfort might be suggested by family members. These family members might also be willing to assist a person with dementia in maintaining appropriate skin care.

General management rules

The following rules of management are suggested in the management of pressure areas and pressure wounds:

- clean the skin at the time of soiling or at routine intervals;
- avoid hot water, soap, and any application of force or friction;

- minimise environmental factors (for example, low humidity, or exposure to cold);
- treat dry skin with moisturisers;
- minimise skin exposure to moisture from incontinence, perspiration, or wound drainage;
- use lifting devices to move people (rather than dragging them over mattresses);
- place people who are at risk on pressure-reducing devices;
- treat at the first sign of redness; do not wait until a pressure wound appears;
- provide effective pain relief when necessary;
- communicate clearly and offer reassurance to a person with dementia;
- maintain good nutrition.

The Box on page 210 presents a case study in which these general rules of management, and other suggestions contained in this chapter, were applied with good results.

Conclusion

Pressure wounds are the most preventable chronic wounds in clinical practice and their impact can be significantly reduced by preventive measures. These include the identification of patients who are at risk, and prompt intervention. Appropriate products on the skin or wound and pressure-reducing devices can help to prevent these serious wounds developing or becoming worse. By ensuring that the burden of dementia is not compounded by the preventable occurrence of pressure sores, nurses play a significant role in the care of people with dementia.

'By ensuring that the burden of dementia is not compounded by the preventable occurrence of pressure sores, nurses play a significant role in the care of people with dementia.'

Chapter 18

Palliative Care

Rosalie Hudson

'This is not my mum. This is a different person.'

'I can't face visiting any more. I just can't bear to see him like this.'

'How long will this go on?'

'This is a living death.'

'Shoot me if I ever get like that!'

These are some of the reactions of relatives and staff who are confronted with the relentless progression of dementia. Prompted by a perception of meaninglessness and hopelessness at the end of life, these reactions are typical and understandable. Before exploring some of the practical issues of palliative care in dementia nursing, two quotations help to set this subject in a more hopeful light.

The first is from Kitwood (1997, p. 69):

> Dementia will always have a deeply tragic aspect, both for those who are affected and for those who are close to them. There is, however, a vast difference between a tragedy, in which persons are actively involved and morally committed, and a blind and hopeless submission to fate.

The second is from Killick and Allan (2001 p. 242), who acknowledged the interdependence of nurses and those in their care when facing end-of-life issues for people with dementia.

> . . . we all depend on each other for keeping that precious spark of self alive, and never more so when it is under attack from something like dementia.

Is palliative care appropriate for people dying with dementia in a nursing home, and can palliative care help to reverse some of the negative connotations of such a death? Palliative care can be defined as 'specialised health care of dying people which aims to maximise quality of life and assist families and carers during and after death' (PCA 1999, p. v). The hallmark of palliative care in this context is the active involvement and moral commitment of people depending on each other in a mutuality of relationships. Within this partnership framework, life is sustained and hope is nurtured. Rather than a fatalism born of despair, palliative care focuses on the person who is living until death occurs. Rather than an individual life ending in isolation, palliative care focuses on each person's network of relationships. Thus, healing can occur even when cure is not possible.

This chapter sets out, by means of practical everyday examples, the benefits of offering palliative care to people dying with dementia—benefits that are shared by residents, staff, families, and the whole nursing-home community.

'Healing can occur even when cure is not possible.'

Many questions present themselves. What are the principles of good nursing care in this situation? What practical skills are required? What is the goal of palliative care in this setting? When should it be commenced? What are the options? Is it possible to counter the common perception that being in a nursing home is a 'fate worse than death'? How can nurses challenge the extreme view that suicide or euthanasia are preferable options?

In contrast to the common pessimistic perception of the 'three dreaded Ds'—death, dying, and dementia—this chapter offers a more hopeful view. This does not imply an unrealistic optimism. Nor does it involve reaching for unachievable goals. Rather, the discussion focuses on the personal meaning of this particular experience for this particular resident at this particular time in his or her unique family context. It also explores the meaning of the shared experience of the staff who care.

Commencing palliative care

The story of Mrs Papadopoulos (Box, below) shows how well-established principles of palliative care can be adapted to residential aged care.

Mrs Papadopolous

Mrs Papadopolous, aged 92, had been in a nursing home for six weeks. Her multiple medical problems included osteoarthritis, a past history of breast cancer, two major strokes, and dementia. When she was admitted to the nursing home she had decubitus ulcers over the sacral area, on both shoulders, and on her heels. She was malnourished, and often refused food and fluids. At the time of Mrs Papadopolous' discharge from the acute hospital her family had been told to expect her death 'within a matter of weeks'.

Staff members in the nursing home were anxious about Mrs Papadopolous' increasing debility. They also feared that she was in constant pain, especially when she was moved and her wounds attended. Nurses were also unsure of the family's expectations. Although she was unable to articulate her needs, Mrs Papadopolous' sad eyes seemed to implore: 'Help me please'.

After many weeks, when her death had not occurred as expected, family members became confused, guilty, anxious, and irritable. They said that other family priorities meant that their visiting would now be reduced. An atmosphere of hopelessness prevailed.

In consultation with Mrs Papadopolous' family and local doctor a palliative-care physician was consulted to address the serious issue of pain management. It was agreed that Mrs Papadopolous' osteoarthritis and painful ulcers warranted the administration of oral slow-release morphine, after other analgesia had been tried with no effect. Within days Mrs Papadopolous' appetite improved. She no longer resisted every attempt to change her position. Although she had little independent movement, she readily opened her mouth to be fed.

The family's visits now increased. Family members discussed appropriate food for Mrs Papadopolous with kitchen staff, and provided their own roster to assist her with meals. The despair that they had previously felt was replaced by hope—not hope for a miraculous cure, but hope for improved quality of life. They now felt reassured that her pain was relieved, and had a sense of satisfaction that they were making their own contributions to her care. The palliative-care physician explained that Mrs Papadopolous' death might not occur as soon as had been expected, and that she might 'still have some living to do'.

As her illness took its course, Mrs Papadopolous became unable to swallow oral medication, and a continuous subcutaneous infusion of low-dose morphine was therefore commenced. Because it was agreed by the family that Mrs Papadopoulos would 'hate the indignity and invasion of a tube into her stomach', family members

(Continued)

(Continued)

preferred to offer her small amounts of food and fluid as tolerated. It was now possible to give greater attention to her skin care because the nurses were no longer anxious about causing her pain. Staff members sought expert advice on the most appropriate wound management and discussed various equipment options to prevent further pressure problems. In spite of minimal oral intake Mrs Papadopolous lived for another four months.

During this time, meetings were held with the family to clarify goals and evaluate the outcome of care. All agreed that the goal was not the artificial prolongation of life but the maximising of comfort. Aromatherapy, massage, music, and sunshine were added to the care plan, together with visits from the family's pet dog. The family expressed relief and satisfaction that Mrs Papadopoulos was now so peaceful.

'She even smells nice now', observed her daughter. 'I'm sure she knows who we are and what we're saying to her', said her eldest son. 'It's taken me a long time,' said another son, 'but I've finally resolved some inner conflict I've had about my relationship with mum. Visiting has now become a pleasure rather than a chore. I'm glad we've all had this extra time.'

The story of Mrs Papadopolous is an illustration of the effective early implementation of pain management as an element of palliative care. Although Mrs Papadopolous' diagnoses did not readily fit the criteria for palliative care as it is commonly perceived, early and effective pain management is an essential element of palliative care, and the story of Mrs Papadopolous shows the increasing blurring of the boundaries between death from cancer and death from other causes. What were the options for Mrs Papadopolous and her family? Euthanasia? This had been mentioned by at least one family member as he expressed his frustration at seeing her suffering. Euthanasia can often seem the only option in the face of apparently inadequate care, and family members and staff members had at first expressed concern about the quality of care. But all were at a loss to know how to improve the situation. Because they believed the prognosis provided by the hospital, they had all thought (and perhaps hoped?) that she would die very soon.

The story of Mrs Papadopolous highlights the value of entering the resident's story to build a continuous narrative in which members of the family become key witnesses. In building this continuous narrative, a partnership of care is developed.

'In entering the resident's story to build a continuous narrative . . . a partnership of care is developed.'

The story also highlights the following principles of palliative care within the nursing-home context:

▶ flexibility in adapting to shifting goals and changing family expectations;
▶ increasing family confidence in skilled care;
▶ effective use of narcotics based on comprehensive assessment and review;
▶ understanding dementia in relation to various coexisting diseases;
▶ responding to the present and the living of life now, rather than concentrating on the last hours or days and being weighed down by a pessimistic prognosis;
▶ family and staff in a partnership of care;
▶ frequent review of all care;
▶ ready access to palliative-care physicians and other consultants (for example, for wound care);
▶ maintenance of a pleasant ambience by attention to odour;
▶ creative care planning for holistic care;
▶ options for nutrition and hydration;
▶ understanding the family network and relationships; and
▶ sensitivity to cultural issues.

Interdependent relationships

Palliative care is not provision of care in one direction—from an expert to a patient. Rather, palliative care, especially in the context of dementia, involves care within a mutual relationship. Within such a relationship, the carer is prompted to ask: 'Who is this person I am caring for?', and 'Who am I in relation to this person?'. These deeply philosophical questions form the basis of the person-centred care advocated here. Palliative care in this context is not merely attention to physical tasks; rather, it is a commitment of carers as persons in relation (Kitwood 1997). To sustain life in this situation does not mean the artificial prolongation of life; rather, it means regarding life in all its fullness and potential even in the face of serious debilitating disease. To nurture hope as a person dies with dementia does not mean naïve optimism or anxiously waiting for a miraculous cure. It does not mean desperately clinging to hope for an unexpected reversal of the disease process. In the face of progressive illness, life is sustained

'Life is sustained and hope is nurtured through honest and trusting relationships developed and refined over time.'

and hope is nurtured through honest and trusting relationships developed and refined over time.

Care planning

Care planning is a vitally important aspect of care. Failure to agree on goals and failure to implement a planned course of care are serious obstacles to effective end-of-life care (Travis et al. 2002). Good care planning concentrates on the life to be lived until death occurs, and represents a source of hope for the person and his or her family.

A skilled gerontic nurse should discuss with the person and family every aspect of the physical, emotional, psychological, social, and spiritual care required, and how this particular person's unique needs might be met. If clearly defined goals are established in this way, all those involved experience satisfaction that they are being heard, and reassurance that they will not be abandoned. Within such a climate of trust, hope is nurtured and fears are dispelled. The Box on page 218 illustrates how this can happen.

The story of Mr Fox's family highlights the following questions. Taken together, these questions represent a checklist of desirable features of palliative care in this context.

▶ Do the person and family understand the meaning of palliative care?
▶ Are the person and family reassured that the nursing home is able to provide skilled and appropriate end-of-life care?
▶ Does the nursing home have a documented policy on palliative care, and is it clearly stated in the printed brochure?
▶ Are all visiting doctors and health professionals aware of the palliative-care policy? Have they been involved in the formulation of such a policy?
▶ Does the nursing home provide written material on use of narcotics, facts about dehydration, resuscitation issues, and pastoral care services?
▶ Does the nursing home ensure that the person and family appreciate the importance of their involvement in planning and reviewing the care?
▶ Is the local doctor involved in any discussions about palliative care?
▶ Is there a need to refer to a specialist palliative-care service for medical or nursing advice, or for follow-up bereavement care?

Issues in risk management

The contemporary emphasis on risk management in aged care is founded more on fear of litigation than on a genuine desire to care for the whole person at the

Mr Fox's family

Maria, the unit manager, had made an appointment to meet with Mr Fox's family to discuss the issue of palliative care. During the conversation, she pointed out that the brochure of the nursing home referred to 'end-of-life care', including access to medical and nursing consultants in palliative care. Then she made reference to the major headings in the care plan—covering physical, psycho-emotional, social, and spiritual factors—and asked the family's opinion about the most urgent needs.

Sensitive discussion uncovered the desires of family members for their father's care. They felt that he would never ever want the intrusion of tubes into his stomach and bladder, and they all agreed that they wanted no extraordinary resuscitation measures.

Concerned about their father being in pain, they asked how the nurses would know the extent of his discomfort. Maria showed the family the pain-assessment tool, including the non-cognitive areas of assessment.

'You won't kill him off with morphine, will you?' asked Mr Fox's anxious daughter.

Having come well prepared for this meeting, Maria offered the family a clearly worded pamphlet about the use of slow-release oral morphine. The brochure also covered other issues—such as continence care and skin care, and the role of various allied health professionals.

Mr Fox's eldest son was relieved and hopeful. 'One more thing', he said, 'Dad's never been particularly religious but I think he'd appreciate a visit from the chaplain.' Maria outlined the various options for pastoral care, including procedures for contacting the chaplain.

Asked if they had any further questions or concerns, Mr Fox's son replied: 'I had no idea palliative care covered so much and I didn't think it was an option in nursing homes. The doctor told us there's nothing that can be done for dementia and that's why we had to find a nursing home bed. We were distraught. We didn't want Dad to end up like this. Now you've given us some hope. And what's more, I'll be telling my friends about this!'

end of life. The focus is on physical risk. What if this person falls out of bed and breaks her hip? What if that person with dementia, walking freely, falls and gashes his head?

Such an emphasis on risk focuses on the *deficits* of people while ignoring their *potential*. Why is there no discussion of risk in relation to emotional, psychosocial, and spiritual matters? What if this person dies without her wishes and dreams ever being explored? What if that person dies without his deepest religious longings ever being articulated?

There are real risks when care is less than holistic—for example, when a dying person is not understood in the context of family and social circumstances. There is real suffering if a person is considered unworthy of palliative care simply because he or she is suffering from dementia and has little time to live, or if a resident's spouse of 62 years is left to grieve alone.

Nurses can also suffer if care is less than holistic. Staff members cannot continue to offer quality care if they are never given the chance to talk about the impact of four people dying in their care in one week.

Rather than concentrating on the difficulties of offering palliative care to nursing-home residents the more immediate concern is the cost of *not* providing such care. Nay (2002) has stated the problem in these terms: 'Overzealous risk management may protect a physical body from bruising but it may also damage irreparably the already vulnerable human soul'.

The importance of communication

Insensitive communication can damage a vulnerable person with dementia. Florence Nightingale understood this when she wrote: 'Apprehension, uncertainty, waiting, expectation, fear of surprise, do a patient more harm than any exertion' (Nightingale 1969, p. viii). The way in which carers approach people with dementia has significant implications for fostering hope and trust, and the importance of sensitive, imaginative, and creative communication cannot be overstated.

> 'Apprehension, uncertainty, waiting, expectation, fear of surprise, do a patient more harm than any exertion.'

Palliative care in other contexts (for example, in home care or hospice care) commonly focuses on people who can clearly articulate their wishes and desires. Such people are able to map their pain on a pain scale, are able to describe the effects of particular treatment regimens, can make rational decisions, and can give informed consent about treatment options. In contrast, palliative care in the context of dementia involves thoughtful discussion with those who advocate for a person who is cognitively impaired. It also involves astute observation from skilled nurses who watch closely, intimately know those in their care, and respond intuitively to subtle cues. These cues can be more revealing than the overt signs identified by technology.

Resuscitation

Good palliative care includes a clear articulation of end-of-life wishes, together with appropriate information about issues such as 'resuscitation'. But what can 'resuscitation' mean in the context of a person receiving palliative care as he or she approaches the end of life?

'Resuscitation' means the revival of a person from apparent death. But does this have any meaning in the context of palliative care? Resuscitation is essentially a *physical* perspective on a life that really encompasses so much more than mere physical survival. A holistic view of person-centred care, as advocated in this chapter, does not think in terms of mere 'resuscitation'. Rather than think in terms of *reviving people from apparent death*, nurses should think in terms of *restoring people to the wholeness of life.*

> 'Rather than think in terms of reviving people from apparent death, nurses should think in terms of restoring people to the wholeness of life.'

Can nurses restore life in dying people by the way they accompany them on their journey towards death? Rather than concentrating on the physical beating of a person's heart (as implied by a focus on resuscitation), nurses can reach out to the heart of a person in metaphorical terms: 'She pulls at my heart strings'. Although every arrhythmia can be detected by modern technology, there are other ways of noting a 'broken heart'. In a very real sense, nurses can have their 'fingers on the pulse' of their relationships with those who are dying of dementia. They can detect a change of life's rhythms by observation, intuition, and empathy.

If nurses think in terms of physical 'resuscitation', they think in terms of using a sphygmomanometer to measure vital signs. But if they think in terms of 'restoring life', they think in terms of seeking signs of tension, distress, and spiritual pain. Caring holistically for people dying with dementia encourages nurses to enter into the situation of these people, to explore the meaning inherent in their dying, and to offer a hopeful presence when other forms of treatment are futile. This is the real meaning of 'restoring life', as opposed to mere 'resuscitation'. A trusting relationship, in which a frank discussion of end-of-life issues is encouraged, obviates the need for extraordinary resuscitation measures to be considered, unless in exceptional circumstances. This close personal presence, this entering the 'sacred space' of another person's experience, is the heart of spiritual care.

Spiritual care

Spiritual care in the context of dementia care means any attitude, reflection, or episode that affects an understanding of the whole person in his or her unique family context—thereby sustaining hope, even when death is imminent. An interdependent community provides a safe territory in which stories can be told and in which all people—residents, families, and staff—can freely narrate their fears and concerns, as well as their hopes and wishes.

Spiritual care is an essential part of palliative care, in that it fosters hope and dispels fear. Spiritual care is not dependent on nurses having 'correct' or 'definitive' answers to the mystery of death or to the philosophical questions raised by dementia in all its manifestations. Rather, spiritual care is a willingness to listen, to hear, and to respond. As Carson (1989, p. 163) observed: 'Probably the most effective spiritual intervention is the nurse's offering of self'.

The ordinary human encounter

The individual task at hand understandably attracts a nurse's immediate attention. However, if task-centredness assumes priority over all else, opportunities can be lost for pausing to record a moment in time that might profoundly influence a person's progression towards death. Such a moment in time might be quite ordinary, and not imbued with any apparent importance (Taylor 1994). Sadly, ordinary matters are not always accorded the attention they deserve, and the ongoing enactment of small daily life rituals can often be ignored.

For Gerald and his wife (Box, page 222), the saying of grace before each meal became a symbol of hope—hope that someone was listening to their story and responding. Hope is not merely private wishful thinking. Hope is enhanced or weakened by relationships with others. By their words and actions, family members and health-care professionals can be powerful modulators of hope in people with dementia (Post 1995).

Hope can thus be fostered by the close personal presence of another person in the 'ordinary' moments of being human—as in the story of Jock (Box, page 222).

> 'Hope is not merely private wishful thinking. Hope is enhanced or weakened by relationships with others.'

Caring for people with dementia is not like the transient short-lived affair of the modern hospital. Rather, it is a committed long-term relationship that requires holistic care and faithfulness ('for better or worse') to the end. Palliative care in this context involves a nurse focusing on a person's changing physical signs and symptoms, noting how the person's illness is affecting the family, and entering into the meaning inherent in this last phase of life. Professional nurses and other carers are privileged to share in this hopeful waiting.

Gerald

Gerald was a gentleman of great piety. In a quiet unassuming manner he integrated his faith into his daily life. Following his admission to a nursing home, one of the things he missed was his habit of meticulously saying grace before each meal.

Now aged 92, Gerald had never been away from home before. The relentless progression of dementia had left him severely debilitated both physically and mentally, so his wife acted as his advocate in this matter.

'I'll try to get here at least once a day to share a meal with him', she said. 'It has been our ritual for more than 60 years to say grace before each meal. I have never ever known Gerald to miss. We always say it together. He says the first part and I join in the second part.'

A creative gerontic nurse was confident that some nurses would be comfortable with assisting Gerald in his familiar pattern, but realised that some would need tuition! Gerald's wife printed the brief prayer and response, and it was included in the care plan. It became the responsibility of the nurse delivering Gerald's meal to join with him in his customary giving of thanks before eating. Nurses who felt uncomfortable with this usually found a colleague ready to share in this dimension of Gerald's care.

Jock

Deciding which residents should be given the opportunity to attend a Christmas carol service, or any other activity, is not always an easy matter. Who decides for those unable to discern for themselves?

Some wondered why Jock, who was profoundly affected by Alzheimer's disease, had been brought into the lounge. Some thought that he wouldn't know what was going on, and that he might become more confused.

A nurse chose to sit with him, not expecting anything other than to hold his hands and encourage him to tap along to the music. To her surprise, as the next carol, which was about preparing for Christmas, was announced, the usually inarticulate Jock said in a clear voice: 'We're all living, and we're all waiting'.

Two years later, Jock was still living and still waiting—with trusted carers accompanying him on his slow journey towards death.

Measuring the quality of palliative care

It is difficult to 'measure' the sustaining of life and the nurturing of hope in the challenging role of caring for dying people with dementia. Rewards can be few in the relentless effort to understand a person's needs and to respond appropriately—often without even a 'thank you'. This thanks and praise needs to come from elsewhere if confidence and hope are to be sustained in carers, and if staff 'burnout' is to be prevented. Praise from a colleague and documentation that demonstrates excellent care at the end of life are both indicators of quality (Hudson 1997).

Nurses who use imagination, ingenuity, intuition, and creative responses should be rewarded and supported—for people dying with dementia fit no conventional model (Killick & Allan 2001). This is particularly important in a team that includes non-professional or untrained staff. When the efforts of all staff are acknowledged, the leader of a team engenders self-satisfaction and team pride. Sincere words of praise can make an enormous difference: 'Michael, you've made Jessica look so comfortable this morning. Thank you for taking so much time with her grooming. You seem to have a special way of communicating with her.' Such observations demonstrate an acknowledgment of the integration of all aspects of care. As Rumbold (1986, p. 18) has observed: 'Giving attention to the quality of personal relationships will lead to a corresponding improvement in the effectiveness of the physical care which is offered'.

> 'Nurses who use imagination, ingenuity, intuition, and creative responses should be rewarded and supported.'

Quality can also be identified by personal or group reflection on practice:

- Did I have any idea what life and death meant to this person?
- Did I find out about this person's wishes and dreams as well as his or her identified physical needs?
- Did I provide reassurance that all physical, emotional, psychological, and spiritual issues would be comprehensively assessed and frequently reviewed?
- Did I enter this person's story and gain his or her trust?
- Did I really listen?
- Did I understand the wishes and needs of the family?
- What part did I play in this particular narrative?
- Did I enter as a key witness to this particular drama, or was I merely a bystander?
- Would this be the kind of death that I would welcome for myself or my family in similar circumstances?
- What particular memories am I left with after this death?
- Does our nursing-home community provide an open, welcoming, and trusting environment in which all end-of-life issues can be freely discussed?

Dame Cicely Saunders, founder of the modern hospice movement, famously said: 'How people die remains in the memories of those who live on' (Saunders & Baines 1989). In the midst of this mysterious malady of dementia in which memory disappears, what memories are left with the family? This question should encourage nurses to maintain the highest standards in all aspects of care, and should raise their awareness of the complexities of family visiting.

Cornelius (2001, p. 114), in a superb piece of fiction, described what it is like for a daughter to enter the strange world of a nursing home to visit her mother who is slowly dying of dementia. In the following extract the daughter, who has been trying (with limited success) to break through her mother's strange repetitive speech and actions, visits her mother one morning and finds her in bed. The communication now becomes intensely personal and intensely meaningful in anticipation of 'the final sweet parting':

> I see her in the mornings sometimes when she's still in bed. She moves over and pulls back the covers. I get in. There are some raised eyebrows from the man with the vacuum cleaner. We lay there napping and I wonder whom she thinks she's invited into her bed. My body is enormous around hers . . . I fear I might smother her or push her out of bed onto the hard linoleum floor. I cup her body and we lie quietly. I pick up a lock of her white hair and place it behind her ear. Mum, I whisper. Mum.

'Professional carers will never fully understand the light and shade, the hope and despair, and the frustration and joy of each family member's relationship with a person who has dementia.'

Professional carers will never fully understand the light and shade, the hope and despair, and the frustration and joy of each family member's relationship with a person who has dementia. The best that they can do is to develop, in partnership with families, a mutually agreed plan that includes the very best physical care, thoughtful and sensitive social support, and emotional and spiritual space for each unique parting.

Chapter 19

Intimacy

Malcolm Goldsmith

This day is mine
I've yet to know tomorrow
I'll use it well
For who can tell
If joy will come or sorrow.
What was can be no more
What is can be today
I'll use the day for all it's worth
Before it too will fade away.
            'HELEN' (1994)

Introduction

The little poem that introduces this chapter was written by a 69-year-old woman who was suffering from Alzheimer's disease. She emphasises the significance of the here and now. There is an emphasis upon valuing the small things of the present. This lady's attitude might be called 'the sacrament of the present moment'.

The shift in dementia care that has taken place over the last few years—from a biomedical model to a person-centred approach—is greatly to be welcomed. To focus upon the *person* with dementia rather than upon the person with *dementia* opens up a whole new range of possibilities for care and understanding. But the many important things offered by a biomedical approach should not be dismissed, and a person-centred approach must remain in dialogue with, and be critiqued by, the biomedical perspective. There is always a danger that a person-centred approach can become dogmatic. It can become a 'new orthodoxy' that seeks to negate or ignore any criticisms or suggestions that might be offered.

'To focus upon the *person* with dementia rather than upon the person with *dementia* opens up a whole new range of possibilities for care and understanding.'

What is needed is a shift in the culture—a change in the ways that carers approach and seek to understand both illness and the people affected by illness. This is a point beautifully argued by Waller (2002):

In the last year of my father's life he became a man with Alzheimer's. Although he was called by his name, he was defined by his dementia. He was in the culture of a subset consisting of the oldest-old, the dependent, the infirm, and the senile. Sometimes it seemed that people regarded his dementia as the most important piece of information about him. The condition of Alzheimer's was used as identification, as a reason, and as a predictor. At times, this information was used to hastily decide what he could and couldn't do, understand and feel. It provided reason enough to speak and act in a certain way and not another. It defined the quality of many of his interactions. My father's dementia was at least as much socially and culturally constructed as it was medically defined.

The foundations of person-centred care

The foundations upon which the culture of person-centred care is built, if not directly and consciously, then indirectly and unconsciously, is the work of Martin Buber (1878–1965). Buber was an eminent Jewish scholar and philosopher and, although he wrote a great deal, it is for his little book *I and Thou* (1923, 1958) that he is primarily remembered. In this book Buber discussed the differences between encounter and dialogue, and between an I–It relationship and an I–Thou relationship. An I–It relationship occurs if the 'other' is made an object and if the meeting between the two remains distant and uncreative. But if there is a genuine acceptance of the 'other', the possibility of dialogue and the possibility of change emerge—and an I–Thou relationship develops. These moments need to be seized and valued—because, when they pass, they are inevitably changed into an 'I–It' relationship. They become a commodity of the past. But when they are here, in the present, there are real gifts to be experienced.

> 'If there is a genuine acceptance of the 'other', the possibility of dialogue and the possibility of change emerge—and an I–Thou relationship develops.'

When asked to explain the background to his views Buber explained (Friedman 1995):

> . . . it was an inclination to meet people and, as far as possible to change something in the other, but also to let me be changed by him . . . I felt I have not the right to want to change another if I am not open to be changed by him.

Friedman (1995), who wrote a biography of Buber, has observed:

> I think he never despaired because he was ready to meet the new moment in whatever form it came with all his being. And that, perhaps is the secret, if there is one, of dialogue which can never become a technique or a philosophy, but only a living presence which is present to the present-ness of the situation and calls the other into presence too.

The I–It relationship, against which Buber rebelled, can easily become embodied in the sort of social pathology that Kitwood (1997) has outlined in his analysis of the ways in which people with dementia are often treated as 'it'. Kitwood (1997) referred to the following elements of this social pathology:

- treachery;
- disempowerment;
- infantilisation;
- intimidation;
- labelling;
- stigmatisation;
- outpacing;
- invalidation;
- banishment; and
- objectification.

To this original list, Kitwood later added:

- ignoring;
- imposition;
- withholding;
- accusation;
- disruption;
- mockery; and
- disparagement.

The person-centred approach also contains more than a passing hint of the work of Carl Rogers (1902–87). Rogers spoke of the coming together of congruence, empathy, and unconditional regard. This involves a recognition that I have needs, that you have needs, and that I accept you unconditionally without imposing my own agenda upon you (Rogers 1961; Rogers & Stevens 1968).

At the heart of the person-centred approach there is therefore an emphasis upon *relationship*. This emphasis on relationship is to be contrasted with an approach by which social work practice used to be focused on the 'casework relationship'. This 'casework relationship' described how social workers could be involved with people without this being personally costly. It involved a social worker learning various tools or techniques that gave the impression of intimate involvement without such involvement actually changing the caseworker.

This approach is still around. It can be seen in many professionals—some of whom have not even mastered the technique of *appearing* to be involved. Such an approach hardly passes the test of Buber's I–Thou relationship—a relationship in which there is capacity for each person to discover something new, creative, whole-some, and nurturing in the other. As one of the elderly nuns said to Snowdon (2001, p. 11) in his study *Aging with Grace*: 'They will open up to you, but only if you give of yourself first'.

> 'I–Thou relationship—a relationship in which there is capacity for each person to discover something new, creative, wholesome, and nurturing in the other.'

The vulnerability of carers

Such an invitation to vulnerability should be at the heart of every nurse's approach to caring for, and being with, people with dementia. But it is not easy. Caregivers should not expect to emerge from such encounters triumphant, boastful, or arrogant. Rather, they will come face to face with frustration, failure, anger, incomprehension, tiredness, and near despair. However, if they travel through such foreign and inhospitable terrain, they will almost certainly have discovered new treasures, new depths, new insights, new loves, and new intimacies. Bayley (1999, p. 5) certainly experienced such new discoveries as he cared for his wife, Iris Murdoch:

> A bleak outlook, which left not much room for lightness of heart in the sufferer, or for those who attended the sufferer? Not necessarily. There may be rewards and alleviations on the way, for all parties. As well as anxiety in the patient there may be a kind of merciful indifference, even lightness of heart, a shrugging off of responsibility for the things most of us feel we have to do every day . . . As her condition worsened, and our imprisonment became more complete, the compensations mounted up—they had to. For her as well as for me? I can hope so, at least. We both still have our small pleasures, which have become happily and mutually important: more and more important, not only because they are all we have left but because we can still share them.

Of course, everyone's experience is not the same. People are different—both those with dementia and those who care for them—and there are dangers in drawing universal generalisations from particular cases. Nevertheless, for many people who struggle with the experience of dementia there can be rich rewards. It might not be the pathway that people would choose to tread, but it does not necessarily mean that all is gloom and doom. There are treasures to be discovered en route—small gems to enrich both caregivers and those in their care as they struggle to live creatively within the context of a terrible illness.

'Small gems enrich both caregivers and those in their care as they struggle to live creatively within the context of a terrible illness.'

A kaleidoscope of experience

It is important to recognise that people take their individual personalities with them into their illness. To understand dementia it is necesary to hold together the personality, the biography, the general health, the specific neurological illness, and the network of relationships that make up the person (Kitwood 1997). Each is important, and each has a bearing on how the person will experience and live with his or her illness. The same is true of carers. Each instance of dementia is unique because each person is unique. Dementia care must embrace the kaleidoscopic range of human personality and experience.

The relationship between a person with dementia and a caregiver is not a relationship of equals. But it can still be an 'I–Thou' relationship. Imagine a photograph of a young mother holding, high above her head, her infant child. They are looking into each other's eyes and both are beaming with sheer delight. It is a photograph that encompasses complete tenderness and trust. Although both persons are necessary for the photograph, the scenario could never have taken place without the mother's initiative. It is she who has taken the step to hold her daughter aloft. It is she who is providing the structure and the support, and the small child is totally dependent upon her. Yet both of them are delighting in this moment, and the interaction could not have taken place unless both were participating. They are equal partners in a moment of magic. This is not a relationship of equals, in the usual understanding of the term, but each, from her own perspective, is contributing a vital and essential element. A similar relationship is possible in dementia care. This is not always possible, but it is possible for many people and on more occasions than are often recognised.

People need the moments such as the one described in the Box on page 231. Walking alongside someone with dementia can be a very difficult and lonely journey. In addition to the sadness of witnessing a serious illness there are the times of utter bewilderment, incomprehension, and frustration. No matter how skilled a nurse might be and how saintly he or she might have become, feelings of guilt are never far away.

> 'No matter how skilled a nurse might be and how saintly he or she might have become, feelings of guilt are never far away.'

There is a moving scene near the end of the film 'Schindler's List'. In this scene, Schindler witnesses the virtual salvation of hundreds of Jewish workers. But, as he leaves them, a sense of remorse overwhelms him. He reflects that he might have done more; that he could have saved more. Those who experience the death of someone from dementia often feel the same. While the person is still alive there are times of depression, despair, frustration, and anger. There can be raised voices and times of withdrawal. The person with dementia is also going through a whole range of emotions. How important it is to discover moments of tenderness and intimacy. How important it is to recognise these moments and cherish them. How important it is to establish an environment in which such moments can be recognised, nourished, and enjoyed.

' . . . but you are very, very nice'

A friend of mine told me a little story about his wife who had died a year ago after suffering from Alzheimer's disease.

One day he looked at her and gently asked her if she knew who he was. She looked at him, gave him a wonderful smile, and said: 'No, but you are very, very nice'.

It was a moment of sheer gold for him, and the memory of the exchange has delighted him over the months as he begins to come to terms with her death.

This is an example of what Bayley (1999, p. 18) calls growing 'closer and closer apart'.

Moments of silence

A person with dementia can take much longer than others to receive information, process it, and respond to it. It is therefore important to set aside time, not be rushed, and not be agitated if things seem to be moving along too slowly. Gibran (1926, p. 16) has spoken of letting there be 'spaces in your togetherness'. It is important to value silence, and to recognise that it can be a uniting bond that requires nothing more than a committed presence from the carer. As Ignatieff (1993) has observed in a much-quoted sentence:

> I learned as much from my mother when she couldn't speak to me, when she couldn't communicate, when she simply stared and received our kisses on the cheek, as I learned when she was joking and laughing.

Many people in our busy output-orientated culture find silence difficult. Many feel an overwhelming urge to fill the spaces because they cannot cope with the absence of noise or distraction. There is a tendency to believe that a person must be lonely if he or she is not speaking or listening. It is important to recognise the difference between loneliness and solitude, and to realise that solitude can be a state of peace and serenity. For the carer, silence is not necessarily a shutting-down and a time of nothingness. Rather than being a time to 'switch off' or have a snooze, a period of silence can be a time of being with someone that goes beyond words. It is important to recognise the difference between positive silences and negative silences.

> 'It is important to recognise the difference between loneliness and solitude . . . solitude can be a state of peace and serenity.'

Touch

The experience of touch can be a vehicle for tenderness and intimacy. But it can also be a non-verbal sign of rejection and resentment. Cultures, families, and individuals differ in their attitudes to physical contact. A touch for one person might be a form of endearment. But, for another, this same touch might be an intrusion of privacy and an abuse of personhood.

Nevertheless, most people grow and delight through physical contact, especially from those whom they love. In dementia care there are many opportunities for nurses, consciously and unconsciously, to use touch. Deliberately taking a hand, kissing a cheek, or massaging a part of the body can express the worth and value of the person and his or her body. Touch can also be used unconsciously when a nurse assists a person in personal care, washing, dressing, and toileting.

Touch can be a passing gesture—while the nurse is thinking of something else or talking away (perhaps even to another person). Or touch can be the full focus of a desire to care and to communicate. For some people with dementia, these moments might be the only time that they have physical contact with anyone, and touch can therefore be of enormous significance.

Sexual intimacy

The most intimate form of physical contact is sexual activity, and the fact that a person is growing old or has dementia does not mean that they do not have sexual needs. Indeed, some people with Alzheimer's disease experience increased sexual activity (Derouesne et al. 1996). Recognising these needs, and helping people with dementia to deal with them appropriately, are significant challenges. This is an area that can be problematic for some carers, and sexuality is therefore often ignored in the hope that it will go away. It can disappear, only to reassert itself in other forms of behaviour. Alternatively, it might remain overtly sexual in various forms. Problems in this area can be manifested as: (i) problems with sexual modesty; (ii) problems with specific sexual behaviours; (iii) changes in sexual patterns in marriage; (iv) effects of behaviour changes on family members; and (v) illicit relationships (Sherman 1998). Such changes in sexual activity could be due to damage to the cerebral cortex, the effect of

> 'Physical contact and sexual activity with someone whom they love can provide those moments of intimacy that are of enormous significance and value.'

drugs, or decreasing possibilities of enjoying other pleasurable activities (Sherman 1998).

Although this is an area that is often fraught with difficulties, it must be recognised that, for many people with dementia, physical contact and sexual activity with someone whom they love can provide those moments of intimacy that are of enormous significance and value. Words are not needed and the reality of the distressing illness can, for a time, subside.

Conclusion

Relating to people with dementia as a 'Thou' rather than an 'It' can lead to the discovery of special sparks of humanity that make them precious—no matter who they are, what they have done, or what their present state might be. John Clare (1793–1864) was a poet who spent many years in what were then called 'lunatic asylums'. Clare's poetry (1997, p. 90) conveys something of what, for some people, is the experience of dementia:

> I am—yet what I am, none cares or knows,
> My friends forsake me like a memory lost,
> I am the self-consumer of my woes,
> They rise and vanish in oblivion's host.

It is of the essence of good care to esteem people with dementia—such that they experience something of their worth and delight in moments of intimacy. It is all about a long journey inwards—which is perhaps the most difficult and the most important journey for all to make.

In recent times there has been an increasing willingness to explore the spiritual dimension of dementia, and to give space for a search for ultimate meaning in life. This is not only a cerebral exercise. For many people, it is intuitive. By freeing themselves from the pressures and distractions that can threaten to overwhelm them, people can focus upon the central 'stillness' that many people call 'God', but for which names are not necessary. As de Luca (1996, p. 53) has put it:

> Having lost the past and the future
> it seems that you are pure being;
> that you have made each instant
> your stillest dwelling.

When nurses open themselves up to the world of people with dementia, they are entering into a community of the dispossessed. They need to discover

'Nurses need to discover the resources that enable them to approach this . . . with hope, love, time, grace, gentleness, and faith.'

the resources that enable them to approach this community with hope, love, time, grace, gentleness, and faith. Then they will recognise those moments of intimacy that enliven the days of people with dementia, and also their own. This is a shared experience.

As Waller (2002) has observed:

What do we miss when we don't pay rapt attention to the other—to the arms and eyes, to the rhythm of the body, to the broken chain or words, to the touch, to the spaces of silence, to our own frailty? We miss ourselves; we miss the divine.

Chapter 20

Listening to the Person with Dementia

Julie Goyder

The everyday act of storying

The usual routines that govern the care of people with dementia can mean that even otherwise compassionate nurses can carry out their nursing duties without hearing what has actually been said by those in their care. Nurses concerned with the routines of work can find themselves talking to one another over the head of a bedridden patient who is also talking, and who might even be attempting to engage the nurses in conversation and share a story. In these circumstances, nurses can talk over or *through* the talk of the patient. Sometimes they might bend down to give a cursory response to what seemed like nonsense, but they are more likely to ignore the person, and then move on to the next bed or the next room, perhaps without even saying goodbye. The present author has been as guilty as others in this regard—having failed for many years to recognise the vital importance of listening to stories and engaging in this significant act of 'storying'.

Everyone engages in 'storying'. Indeed, it is something that people do virtually every hour of the day. But when people are diagnosed with dementia it is often immediately assumed that what they have to say is no longer worth listening to—because it does not make sense, or because it is about times long past and now apparently irrelevant. The stories told by people with dementia can seem nonsensical and crazy, and this can be exacerbated by the disorientation and confusion often associated with institutionalisation.

'When people are diagnosed with dementia it is often immediately assumed that what they have to say is no longer worth listening to.'

The everyday act of 'storying' is an essential part of being human. 'Storying' is not just telling a story. It is telling, listening, and responding. It involves exchange and interaction. It entails particular people in a particular context. Although dementia can make the 'storying' disjointed, a person with dementia is still trying to connect with others in attempting to tell a story. If no one listens, if no one engages in the act of 'storying', the isolation, frustration, and suffering of the person is all the more severe.

The story of Joe

In relating the story of Joe (see the beginning of the story in the Box, p. 237), an important aspect of 'storying' becomes apparent. 'Storying' is a malleable activity. It is often full of contradictions, inconsistencies, fantasy, exaggeration, and omission. People with dementia are not alone in relating stories that evolve with time, often in the space of a few seconds or minutes. All people do this when they engage in 'storying', and it is useful to keep this in mind when listening to the stories of people with dementia. Inconsistencies and 'nonsense' in story-telling are not restricted to those with dementia!

The story of Joe also demonstrates that no one should be 'lumped together' with many other people into one alienated mass of what might be called 'them-ness'. Nursing routines can easily lead to nurses treating people as *them*—waking *them*, showering *them*, dressing *them*, feeding *them*, toileting *them*, and putting *them* to bed—in an unchanging, unchangeable routine. This routine usually does not include (except perhaps in the last moments before the end of a nursing shift) listening to *them*. The story of Joe shows how listening to people—as individuals, not as *them*—can produce quite astonishing results.

As a result of this 'breakthrough' in communication, Joe now changed from a miserable old man to an interested communicative fellow. He even became a somewhat amorous suitor! He asked his nurse to 'marry' him, and was delighted when she (wishing not to hurt his feelings) 'accepted' his proposal. The story goes on (Box, p. 238).

'Storying' with Joe (1)

Joe was in his nineties when I met him. I do not know why I became so fascinated by Joe, who was the most cantankerous and difficult resident in the nursing home. He was morose, nasty, and violent, and even the other residents disliked him. For most of the time he was silent, although sometimes he would sob loudly or shout angrily. But he *did* express himself—by yelling, swearing, and singing in a very loud voice (often, it seemed, merely to annoy others). Sometimes he lashed out physically, and the first time that I tried to have a conversation with him that is what he did. I was crouching by his chair when he punched me in the arm, and I nearly fell backwards. I had been asking him if he could remember my name. I had been curious to see if I could 'connect' with him, even though everyone regarded Joe as being impossibly difficult and discourteous.

After he struck me, I went into the panroom and wrote my name in big letters on a paper towel. There was no pen available, so I had to use lipstick. This seemed to be an insignificant detail at the time, but it became important in the story.

I returned to Joe and showed him the paper towel with my name written in large letters in lipstick. He laughed. I had never seen him laugh before. He chuckled some more before taking the paper towel and asking: 'Julie, eh?'.

It was weeks before it finally became unnecessary to show Joe the piece of paper. Each day I wrote another 'name-tag' every time I was on duty, and showed it to Joe. Then suddenly, one day, he knew me! This took me quite by surprise because I had always assumed that it was impossible for people with dementia to remember recent things. When Joe first recognised me, he called out 'Julie!'. Everyone within hearing stopped and stared.

From that day on, my name stuck in his memory. Whenever I came on duty Joe sat up from his slumped position and exclaimed: 'Julie! There's my Julie!'—eliciting chuckles from staff and patients alike.

Learning to listen

The story of Joe, and the way he changed, should encourage nurses to listen to all people in their care who have dementia. The nurses who do listen will feel that they must have been 'deaf' in the past! Every person has such an abundance of interesting detail. There are so many fascinating lives. Although disjointed by time, space, and the effects of disease, these memories still mean so much to the tellers who have retained them, and who now speak of them with such reverence. These stories are like snapshot photographs. And like photographs they can be hazy. But sharing them can be heart-warming. It can also be disturbing. It might even be hilarious.

Nurses who listen and respond as best they can—rather than rushing off, or talking over, or talking *through*—will find that many of those in their care will

'Storying' with Joe (2)

Joe took every opportunity to tell everyone that we were to be 'married'. We were to be married in Fremantle. Sometimes he'd even call me 'Sarah'—his wife of many years ago. Joe even started 'flirting' with other nurses. Sometimes I would come into the lounge room to find him holding the hand of another nurse. But, on seeing me, he would quickly let go of her hand. Later he would reassure me: 'You're the only one I love, Julie'.

Some of nursing workmates teased me about Joe, and some even registered disapproval. For the most part, however, my colleagues were amazed at the transformation in Joe. He even began to sing happily in the loungeroom. His favourite song was 'Goodnight Irene', and he often sang this at night in the shared bedroom—sometimes to a chorus of disapproval from the other residents.

Joe still became grumpy at times, and he still cried occasionally. He became quite jealous of my tending to other male residents, and would often whisper to me that when we were married I was to leave this job immediately. 'I'll look after you,' he would say with a soft smile.

Joe's personality was, I discovered, part-rascal and part-gentleman. Sometimes he would shock me with his naughty amorous comments. And then he would follow these comments with a reassuring: 'Don't you worry, my darling . . . I am a *gentleman*'.

But what amazed me most were his stories—stories about his youth, stories about his wedding, stories about his wife. These stories did not come out in a coherent flow, but fragments were told of the courtship ritual he now seemed to be reliving. I often reflected on what a wonderful wedding and marriage he must have had with Sarah. The fact that he wanted to relive it in such detail showed how much it must have meant to him. He described the Fremantle church, the smell of the air, and the dress Sarah wore.

At this time I became engaged to be married in real life. On the first day that I wore my engagement ring to work, Joe was the first one to notice.

'I hope you like it, Julie. It took me so long to choose.'

begin to talk more often. They begin to 'story' more often. The simple act of having someone actively *listen* can bring great pleasure to story-tellers.

Most nurses do not have enough time to organise a structured 'listening session' in a semi-formal therapeutic setting set aside for the express purpose of listening. But they *can* actively listen while showering, feeding, toileting, and otherwise caring for those with dementia. These informal episodes of active

> 'The simple act of having someone actively *listen* can bring great pleasure to story-tellers.'

Real persons in their own right

At about the same time as I entered into Joe's fantasy story of our 'courtship', I also got to know David. David was a new resident who just wanted to go home, and who told poignant stories about home—not his recent home, but his childhood home on a farm in a house with snakes under the floorboards and rats in the roof.

Then there was Nelly who was haunted by a white man with a black face who was going to come in the window and do something terrible to her. But it can't have been too terrible because she would relate this with a twinkle in her eye and a wicked cackle.

And there were many more stories and story fragments about the distant past and the recent past—but rarely, the present. The stories would often be a collage of distant past and recent past, of mixed locations, and of the fantastic and the credible.

The pleasure I gained from listening was immense and I began to realise how much I had missed during the years when I had not listened. The stories extricated their tellers from that anonymous category of 'the demented' and re- individualised them as real persons in their own right.

listening, no matter how unstructured, can give meaning and purpose to the 'storying' of those in their care. Fragmented stories, even if apparently nonsensical, then take on a therapeutic role for both story-teller and listener. The Box above brings this to life as real persons emerge from the anonymous category of 'the demented'.

People like Joe can have a profound effect on the professional and personal lives of caring nurses. Nurses are confronted with the question: 'Who is this person with dementia?'. And the answer is that this person is everyone of us—

Joe's story ends

The silences gradually became more frequent. Joe was dying.

I would chatter away, holding his hand, sitting on the side of his bed. He would look at me, then look away, then look at me again. His eyes, which had been so blank and uninterested when I first met him, and had then, for such a short time, become so twinkly and mischievous, now alternated again between blankness, bewilderment, and obvious physical pain.

Then Joe stopped speaking altogether.

I cannot presume to know what he was thinking, what he was trying to say when he opened his mouth and tried, and nothing came out.

Goyder (2001, p. 204)

formed, as we are, by a culmination of life's experiences and emotions. This person is someone who has so many stories. This person *is* those stories.

Joe's story, and Joe's story-telling, came to an end. But the re-telling of it here might encourage nursing colleagues to take the time to listen to those in their care, and ask themselves the question: 'Who is this person with dementia'?

> There is the idea of the story-taker, the necessary collaborator in the act of telling, the one who listens, shapes the narrative by assuming that there is something there to be told; who takes the story, not as appropriation, but as part of a deal, so that the outcome—an entity, a story—might be placed there, in the space between the listener and the teller. The presence of the story-taker wards off the question 'So what?'
>
> STEEDMAN (1992, P. 171)

Chapter 21

Leisure

Sally Bowen

Introduction

Although people with dementia have a diminished framework for understanding leisure activities, life skills, and independence, they continue to experience the cognitive, physical, emotional, social, and spiritual dimensions of life. Carers are witnesses to the emotional dimensions of disability and the way in which disabilities affect every aspect of the life of a person with dementia. To respond effectively to people with dementia who experience such disabilities is a challenge and a joy.

Leisure provides opportunities for the pursuit of pleasure and fulfilment, and offers a means of improved self-image through the achievement of goals. Positive leisure experiences provide hope and enthusiasm. The quality of life of those with dementia is significantly improved by the quality of leisure experiences. In turn, the quality of these leisure experiences is influenced by:

> 'Positive leisure experiences provide hope and enthusiasm.'

- the role that the individual person plays in determining his or her level of involvement in the leisure experience;
- the individual person's social relationships and friendships;
- the environment in which the activity takes place; and
- the kind of activity chosen.

Objectives of leisure

The objectives of leisure in the context of dementia care can be summarised as follows:

- *immediate personal objectives*—satisfaction, quality of life, learning new skills, fun and laughter;
- *therapeutic objectives*—improving social, physical, affective, and cognitive skills to foster independence and assist in adjustment to the illness (particularly adjustment to institutional life); and
- *preventive objectives*—nurturing existing skills and competencies, and motivating the person to maintain his or her present level of functioning.

These objectives for leisure care are developed in consultation with the person and/or family. Whenever possible, objectives are based on the person's own stated wishes.

Assessing needs and making plans

Kitwood's person-centred dementia care celebrates the person, rather than focusing on the illness (Kitwood 1997). Learning more about the person's experience of dementia has significant bearing on care practices for the entire health-care team. The implications of such a progressive illness, together with the implications of the ageing process, can demoralise a person. Wilcox (1999) has stated that occupation is a major biological mechanism for health. In being provided with opportunities for leisure, a resident with dementia is assisted to create a new self and to shape a new world, even within the unfamiliar environment of residential care. Carers have a responsibility to facilitate the self-determination of people with dementia by meeting their identified needs, maintaining

'In being provided with opportunities for leisure, a resident with dementia is assisted to create a new self and to shape a new world.'

and enhancing their health, enriching their environment, and influencing their well-being.

In this context, the leisure plan is an important component of the overall care plan. Within that overall care plan, the role of leisure activities is complementary to the role of traditional medical and nursing interventions. The two come together in an holistic overall plan of care that caters for the needs of the whole person.

Social history

The first step in discussing the needs of an older person with dementia is to ask the person what he or she considers those needs to be. This directly informs the program that carers will design for that person. If any one carer does not have the skills to enable the person to fulfil his or her needs, the members of the care staff can form partnerships and create those opportunities.

The recording of the person's social history provides a blueprint for all that the leisure team will try to achieve. Although it is of importance to assess a person's functional capacity, research has shown that age can be a more significant determinant of reduced lifestyle than particular impairments such as visual difficulties (Clark, Bond & Sanchez 1999). That is, it must be recognised that a person with dementia is the sum total of all of his or her life experiences—childhood, working life, family, and all the various personal relationships of life with their attendant joys and difficulties. It is important to identify which life experiences remain important to a person, particularly in the context of that person's present life in residential care. Perhaps a sibling relationship is sustaining the resident's interest in life and providing a valuable link with family and outside interests. Perhaps a man who spent all his working life as a supervisor on a factory floor is still thinking in terms of managing the workers around him and reminding them of 'clock off time' (because that was the time in his life when he felt most useful and valued).

A comprehensive assessment of a person's social background is best conducted with that person and family members together. Responses should be sought to questions about:

◗ past attitudes to risk-taking;
◗ the value of friendships;
◗ significant role changes;
◗ attitudes to leisure;
◗ coping with loss; and
◗ time given to recreation.

Compiling a careful social history is particularly important in caring for those men and women who experienced major social and cultural upheavals during their lives—of a type that younger carers have never experienced. For example, the period of the Great Depression between the two world wars was, for many, a time in which lives were often more about survival and family rather than the pursuit of leisure. Similarly, there are many older women who were primarily 'homemakers', and who often had no circle of friends outside the family. This isolation was seen as being quite normal. For older migrant men and women, the learning of a new language was not required because younger family members took care of contact with the wider community.

Having taken sensitive note of the social history of such people, there is often scope to develop new interests for them. It is the responsibility of carers to provide meaningful individual contact and discussion, together with appropriate activities, particularly in a new environment of care. The need for mastery and control of one's environment is a basic human motivation (Patterson 1998), and is a social determinant of health.

> 'The need for mastery and control of one's environment is a basic human motivation, and is a social determinant of health.'

Following such a comprehensive assessment, a leisure plan is developed in collaboration with the resident, the family, and other members of the care team. This plan should not focus on the person's deficits, but should explore the person's capacities for leisure, maintenance of life skills, and independence. One of the distinguishing features of such a leisure plan is exploring a wide variety of leisure activities and options for new life skills to be developed. Enshrined within this philosophy are the principles of choice, personal growth, and independence. Such a leisure plan, developed with these principles in mind, is a genuine response to the needs and desires of a person with dementia, and is the wellspring from which care for the resident will come.

Different levels of need

The social history thus informs carers about the person's leisure and lifestyle choices. It also informs them about the person's likely reaction to change. Was this person's former lifestyle busy and active with the involvement of many friends, or was it a quiet reflective lifestyle? A person who had previously enjoyed an active lifestyle might readily adapt to the new environment, meeting new people, and becoming involved in the activities provided. A quieter person might need a longer period of adjustment that allows time and space for quiet reflection.

Entering a residential aged-care facility is a significant life transition, and it requires a period of adjustment. This can be facilitated by sensitive support that acknowledges the difficulties of the transition and aims to reduce the negative aspects of the experience. It might be possible to link a person in some way to his or her former working life, or facilitate direct association with others in the community, or incorporate some of the person's former skills within the new environment. Encouraging the development and maintenance of friendships contributes to morale, adjustment, and life satisfaction (Patterson 1998).

Carers who are sensitive to the needs of people with dementia will not make assumptions about the current capacities of those in their care, even if these appear to be very limited. Rather, such carers will assist residents to engage in skills that are of particular interest, even when some of the necessary skills appear to have been lost. Reminiscing about a particular skill can be far more enjoyable than actually doing it, and a resident with dementia might want to try something new, rather than trying to recapture previous skills.

An encouraging, reassuring relationship can facilitate the learning of new skills. It might be a lack of opportunity and encouragement (rather than incapacity) that prevents people with dementia from engaging in meaningful leisure and life experiences.

It is important, however, to offer people alternatives, no matter how small or trivial the matter might seem. Denial of choice can be perceived as infantilising and controlling. These approaches are resented by older people. Even when a person with dementia is manifesting difficult behavioural responses, it is important to offer the person choice. With choice comes hope, dignity, freedom, and empowerment.

Individual needs

Dementia is complex, and every person with dementia is different. Some abilities are lost entirely, whereas others are enhanced, and the progressive nature of dementia means that each person experiences continuous change in functional abilities. Assessment of leisure needs must therefore be ongoing, and a large part of the daily assessment is the development of a one-to-one relationship.

'Assessment of leisure needs must be ongoing, and a large part of the daily assessment is the development of a one-to-one relationship.'

In this relationship, simple questions become important. 'How are you feeling today?' and 'What would you like to do today?' reveal significant information. It is important to observe the person's body language while the question is being asked, and then to sit quietly and wait for a response, rather than quickly interposing an answer. Becoming an informed and patient listener is one of the hallmarks of good dementia care. If a person's ability to answer even a simple question is underestimated, that person's independence is compromised, and this can lead to further erosion of abilities. On the other hand, overestimating a person's abilities can lead to frustration and an increase in that person's feelings of inadequacy.

It is also important to understand a person's tolerance of activity. Being encouraged to increase activity beyond the level of tolerance can lead to distress, whereas a lack of sufficient stimulation can result in withdrawal and a sense of boredom or despair.

Respect for the dignity of each individual leads to an acknowledgment of the varied activities that a person with dementia might choose—from brewing beer to reciting poetry. Fun and leisure take many forms, and to honour this diversity is to honour the individual.

Benefits from engaging in leisure

The benefits of engaging in leisure include the following:

- relief from the stress of disorientation;
- enhanced self-esteem and feelings of well-being through sensory stimulation;
- enhanced feelings of productivity and usefulness;
- reduction in isolation and loneliness;
- relief from dependency;
- distraction from boredom; and
- relief from physical disability, pain, or anxiety.

These benefits are maximised if leisure activities are chosen carefully. This means avoiding actitivies that accentuate disabilities in people, demean or demoralise them, or inhibit their autonomy. As noted above, whenever possible, residents with dementia should be involved in the planning and preparation of their leisure activities.

The role of the carer

Developing relationships

Building a genuine relationship of trust takes time. Communication is not always easy because people with dementia often live in an 'experiential' world made up of their own thoughts, emotions, and perceptions (Dresser & Whitehouse 1994). Carers should:

- be conscious of how they present themselves to the person with dementia;

- avoid discrepancies in voice tone, language, and manner;
- recognise the importance of non-verbal communication such as walking together, dancing, music, art, massage, and food;
- try to tune into the world of the person with dementia;
- search for the meaning behind the person's behaviour;
- develop the art of listening; and
- respect the wisdom of the person with dementia.

Developing an authentic therapeutic relationship produces significant results and should not be underestimated. Carers should be aware that time constraints and routines often drive patterns of care. These patterns of care often go unquestioned, but can be transformed by carers who strive to improve their communication skills.

Reminiscence and generativity

Reminiscence is a therapeutic review of a person's life. It can allow a person to come to terms with his or her life and derive satisfaction from that life. Reminiscence can be an important leisure activity for some residents. It can foster an acknowledgment of situations that might have been unpleasant or regretted. Feeling positive about one's life, or even just being accepting of one's life, can help in the achievement of a good self-image.

> 'Feeling positive about one's life, or even just being accepting of one's life, can help in the achievement of a good self image.'

Generativity refers to the production of new meaning in this particular phase of life and involves redefinition of one's life in order to enter the next phase of life. This can involve the same life skills or the acquisition of new ones. This process can be painful for some people. For others, although the transition might be distressing, it is followed by acceptance.

There are many reasons for poor self-esteem in an older person with dementia. Physical, social, and emotional losses can cause despair, withdrawal, and depression. People with dementia can experience disturbance in their self-concept as a result of altered lifestyle, changes in role, changes in body image, and a diminution of autonomy.

Carers can assist people with dementia to regain pleasure and meaning in life by learning new skills to replace those that are lost. A resident might become a bartender serving drinks, or a keeper of the rose garden, or a person who reads mail to others, or a proofreader of the monthly newsletter.

The importance of humour

Laughter can facilitate social interaction and is an effective communication tool. From a gentle smile to a spontaneous 'belly laugh', humour can build better personal communication. Laughter helps the self to shine through and promotes genuine dialogue. Fun and games are an important component of leisure activities for people with dementia.

People with dementia often display a keen sense of humour. However, humour should be respectful and constructive. It should not demean a person or undermine dignity. There is a distinction between 'laughing with someone and laughing at them' (Killick & Allan 2001, p. 90).

Adaptation of environment

Carers can do a great deal to adapt the environment to individual needs so that life is better for residents and carers alike. Factors such as space, light, colour, noise, temperature, texture, touch, air, and objects should all be carefully assessed. An environment that accentuates people's dependency and debility can be reversed with good planning and imagination.

Meaningful leisure activities

Leisure activities should take account of the specific cognitive impairment and communication difficulties of each individual person. The story of Mr A (Box, below) provides a good example.

This example of 'reading' the newspaper shows the benefit of staff understanding and support in leisure activity. This kind of support:

▶ assists the resident to deal with some past losses;
▶ offers autonomy to the person;

Reading his newspaper

Mr A insisted on 'reading' his newspaper each morning. It was apparent that Mr A was no longer able to read and that he had lost the cognitive ability to associate the purpose of spectacles with the routine of wearing them. However, Mr A's family and the staff who cared for him were aware that this activity of 'reading' the paper was an important link with his former life as a husband and father—a person committed to the daily discussion of current affairs—and it was important for him to continue the habit of having the newspaper delivered daily.

After 'reading' the paper, Mr A would fold and unfold the paper, and then proceed to 're-read' the paper. He repeated this procedure several times until he was ready to put it aside and move to some other activity.

- provides choice to participate in activities that are consistent with personal talents, interests, and values;
- provides opportunity for decision-making and personal control;
- notes verbal and non-verbal cues;
- provides opportunity for discussion of learned memories;
- acknowledges the importance of the routine even when it is not supported by a logical rationale ('He can't read the paper so what's the point of giving it to him!');
- provides an opportunity for the person to sit quietly and engage in a dignified activity (as an alternative to agitated or restless behaviour);
- provides stimulation that minimises withdrawal, inhibition, and depression; and
- maintains privacy and dignity at all times.

Useful resources

Local groups such as gardening clubs, service clubs, museums, repertory companies, dancing schools, and car clubs should be encouraged to visit to build continuity of relationships with the wider community.

Volunteers are a rich resource for assisting in activities that require more than one person, and such relationships often develop into lasting friendships.

Conclusion

The provision of leisure activities for people with dementia in residential care requires a team effort, and all nurses are encouraged to include this aspect of care in the daily routine.

If approached with foresight and imagination, supported by sound education and collegiate support, leisure activities can change the culture of residential care. Laughter and play, together with serious concentration on meaningful activities, permeate the workplace, and provide a positive energy that benefits individual residents, their families, and professional carers.

Chapter 22

Creative Care

Introduction
Sally Bowen and Rosalie Hudson

The term 'creative care' is used here to refer to any of the options presented in the various sections of this chapter. This is not intended to be a comprehensive list. Rather, it is a representative selection of creative options that can be employed in the care of people with dementia in residential aged care. In accordance with the theme of this book, the application of any of these options should be based on an accurate, ongoing, and skilled assessment of the needs of each resident, rather than an idiosyncratic preference of the program facilitator. Creative care is a finely tuned response to each resident's unique abilities and wishes, rather than an indiscriminate use of generic programs.

> 'Creative care is a finely tuned response to each resident's unique abilities and wishes.'

Careful matching of appropriate activities to the abilities of a person with dementia requires flexibility rather than routine programs. The choice of an activity should be based on the maintenance of independence, a sensitivity to cultural needs, and an understanding of the person's previous life style. 'Good dementia care is about creating opportunities for people to respond appropriately and utilise their abilities' (Alzheimer's Australia 2003).

Group programs are not appropriate for all people with dementia. It is important, however, for residents to be asked frequently about their choices, as these might change from day to day. When a group is formed, attention to the needs of each person takes precedence over 'a group response'. One resident might come to a group program with a keen sense of interest, curiosity, and anticipation, ready to join with others in experiencing the benefits and enjoyment of socialising. Another resident might have reduced social skills, leading to a sense of anxiety or fear about interacting with others. Yet another resident might suffer reduced self-esteem from an inability to participate in a particular group activity.

Some residents will respond to certain activities with increased motivation, independence, and confidence whereas others will respond by withdrawing from situations they perceive to be threatening. Some residents with dementia will engage in activities that are closely linked to their previous life experiences, whereas others will enjoy new opportunities for self-expression.

When formulating groups it is also important to know about each person's previous employment and professional experience. For example:

◗ a dentist's tools can become excellent carving equipment when working in talc or sandstone, thus providing enormous creative satisfaction;

◗ a former art director might provide the ideas for a water-colour painting group; and

◗ a former radio announcer might wish to share an original tape-recording of a familiar radio program.

These activities can be very simple and can be carried out by anyone with an interest in holistic care of people with dementia.

Providing a variety of opportunities for people with dementia enables them to express a variety of thoughts and feelings. For example, a person who writes poetry or creates a picture or sculpture might reveal thoughts and feelings not expressed verbally. Such creative expression might help such a person to make sense of the strange world of dementia that cannot be accessed directly by carers. In the context of dementia care, expressive arts such as poetry, art, and craft provide opportunities for self-expression that is without artifice or conceit. Expressive arts offer a means of defining a person with dementia at a far deeper level than that revealed in a medical history. Artistic expression reveals the essence of a person in a way that mere physiological characteristics fail to uncover. As the various sections of this chapter demonstrate, people with dementia have much to offer the world of the arts, and carers have the privilege of offering them something in return.

Dementia nursing is dependent on team-work and the fostering of creative partnerships with families and other carers (such as volunteers). Including other people in the planning of holistic creative care often results in others providing time and energy and equipment to put the plan into effect, particularly when it will benefit their own family member.

To provide the kind of creative care described in this chapter, nurses need to be flexible and be prepared to vary their routines in response to the needs of a particular resident. These needs are often expressed spontaneously and require an immediate response—for a person with dementia might not know what is 'the right time' to seek a particular form of care. In residential care, the 'night shift' allows for a variety of creative responses, particularly for a resident who can no longer distinguish night from day. Furthermore, a person with dementia might not recognise the difference between a nurse and a music therapist, or between a volunteer and an aromatherapist. Although nurses quite properly rely on the expertise of other health-care professionals for guidance and direction in creative care, and for facilitating specific programs, the needs of the resident call for creative responses by nurses at any time of the day or night. For example, a resident who responds well to the comfort and care of a doll should not have to depend on the 'doll therapist' being available to enjoy this experience. Nor should a resident who loves dancing have to depend on the prompting of the 'dance therapist' or the annual nursing home 'ball' to nurture this pleasure.

Pets can also be encouraged on frequent informal occasions, rather than waiting for the planned annual 'pet therapy visit'. Other ways in which nurses can provide creative care at any time during the 24-hour care cycle include:

- sharing in the recitation of a poem known by the nurse and the resident;
- providing a resident with the equipment for drawing or artwork;
- dancing with a resident who clearly prefers this activity to structured exercise;
- provision of aromas of a resident's choice;
- singing along with a resident in the shower;
- reminiscing with a resident during other care routines;
- creating opportunities for 'visiting pets'; and
- inviting a restless resident to sit in a quiet area that has a calm ambience.

Suggestions for creative care are not presented here as ideas to be tried when all else has failed, but as integral to the care of the whole person. They can be initiated not only by qualified therapists but also by any member of the care team interested in making a difference to the lives of people with dementia. It is professionally satisfying for a nurse to see each individual resident's needs being met in such a holistic way.

Carers with experience in exploring these interventions attest to the significant positive impact on individual behaviour—one of the most challenging issues in dementia care. There is no one blueprint that fits all, and patience and imagination are needed to discover the care best suited to each person. Sensory deprivation of sound, sight, smell, and touch, and the emotional effects of these losses, can lead to withdrawal and social isolation. In contrast, staying connected to life on the sensory levels, particularly when language has lost its meaning, creates opportunities for pleasure and enjoyment.

'There is no one blueprint that fits all, and patience and imagination are needed to discover the care best suited to each person.'

The variety of creative care techniques and sensory stimulation described in this chapter might need to be initiated by those qualified and experienced in a particular field of knowledge, and nurses are indebted to such skilled colleagues. Following such instruction, and with appropriate oversight, support, and encouragement, creative care can then be included informally and formally within the working day of any carer.

Creative care is, therefore, not an 'option' for good dementia nursing, and nor is it merely the inclusion of 'alternative therapies'. Creative care of the type described in this chapter is not a luxury that is 'added to' nursing. Rather, it is complementary to good clinical care and should be included in every nurse's repertoire of skills. Creative care for people with dementia is not about providing a variety of activity programs to meet external auditing or funding requirements. It goes to the heart of the 'interpersonal connection' (Taylor 2001) that is essential to human-centred dementia nursing. Creative care focuses on the needs of the *person* with dementia .

Poetry
Sally Bowen

The joy of poetry
Poetry is for reading and sharing. It tells a story, explains a situation, gives vent to feelings and, above all, is a celebration of language. Poetry is also a very personal matter. It is one of the highest forms of self-expression and invites the reader to participate in an intimate, personal, and pleasurable experience. Age is

no barrier to the enjoyment of poetry, and people with dementia can participate, depending on their capacity for concentration and understanding. Participants in a poetry group can be engaged at various levels and they can take on different roles of writing, reading, and reciting—as illustrated by the following examples.

▶ One resident is well read and articulate, but she suffers from emphysma and is short of breath, so her role might be to choose several poems to be read in the next poetry session.

▶ Another resident revels in the sense of performance that recitation provides. However, because of the effects of dementia, he requires much emotional support and prompting from the group.

▶ Another resident was an actor, and she engages the group with a 'professional' recitation.

The only prerequisite for the facilitator is engagement with the group in the mutual enjoyment of poetry. When the poetry celebrates current or recent past events—such as the work of Spike Milligan in memory of his life and death, or the Poet Laureate's poem composed for the funeral of Princess Margaret—the session becomes a dynamic response to the world. This vibrancy of content is directly proportional to the research and preparation by the facilitator.

> 'The only prerequisite for the facilitator is engagement with the group in the mutual enjoyment of poetry.'

Getting started

It is important to choose an appropriate venue for the group. Some residents might have hearing impairments that interfere with their enjoyment and participation level. A small unobtrusive voice amplifier can ensure that all participants enjoy this time together.

Careful preparation for a poetry group begins with a comprehensive knowledge of the social history of all participants, particularly their past interest in poetry. The group will evolve according to the mood of the participants and the engaging style of the facilitator—especially if the ambience is relaxed and not forced. An invitation can be extended to all residents who enjoy poetry, including those who have dementia and those who have other medical problems. After the facilitator has engaged the participants, the facilitator's presence becomes less prominent and the participants become more involved.

Those who are able and willing to recite a poem might need several days' notice before the session to allow them time to prepare for their roles in the group. It is important to allow people choice, and to offer suggestions only when asked. Poems in large print, protected by suitable covering, can be distributed for rehearsal.

The facilitator of a poetry group needs to be flexible and prepared to change according to the needs of the group and the level of cognition of each participant. One way to begin is for the facilitator to recite a poem familiar to most of the group. For example, 'The Village Blacksmith' or 'Daffodils' or 'Little Boy Blue' might be selected from a primary school reader. The facilitator might then invite one of the participants to read a verse, and then alternate between facilitator and residents to ensure balance and variety. Discussion after the poem might include recalling the time at which it was written, the biography of the poet, and the poem itself.

Resources

Local libraries are a useful source of anthologies and biographies, and various libraries have different collections. For many people with dementia, there is a strong link to poetry learnt in childhood or enjoyed through small children or grandchildren. Accessing the children's section of the library can therefore prove to be very fruitful. The familiar works of A.A. Milne, Beatrix Potter, and Robert Louis Stevenson are examples of poetry that can provoke a lively response from members of the group. Modern verse, for example from Roald Dahl, might also be appropriate. Tapping into early memories can evoke significant responses. For example, Mrs T, who is a blind centenarian, can recite whole slabs of verse that were read to her by her mother by the fire before bedtime when she was a little girl.

Many of the old anthology books include a biography with a poem, and such anthologies can readily be found on the shelves of second-hand bookshops. The poems in such books are often organised around themes—for example, animals or friendship—and this facilitates planning. A poetry group for older people, including those with dementia, lends itself well to the introduction of themes— military poetry for Remembrance Day, Irish poetry and limericks for St Patrick's Day, and other poems suited to the seasons of the year.

The poetry should be a mixture of the old and the new, the sad and the humorous, the traditional and the modern, and the familiar and the unfamiliar. The choice of poem should be based on the needs and interests of the group. A sensitive facilitator will be aware of mood, and will choose poems carefully for balance and variety. Another option is to intersperse the poems with a short story.

Concluding the session

It is often best to finish on a light or humorous note. Alternatively, it might be more appropriate to conclude a particular session with a quiet period that allows participants time to reflect on the verse or story enjoyed that day.

Joining a poetry group session, even for a short time, can benefit a person with dementia, particularly if that person has demonstrated an interest in the subject. However, even for someone with dementia who has not shown a particular interest in poetry, it can be a pleasurable experience to recall poems learned at school. This can be a way of simultaneously rekindling memories and pursuing a new interest.

Drama
Sally Bowen

The value of drama

Drama is a dynamic and confronting art form that engages people at various levels. Drama can therefore be an effective way of entering the world of dementia, and it can prompt unique, creative forms of expression. Before a resident with dementia is invited to join a structured drama group, a careful assessment is required. This includes an assessment of physical capacities (for example, fatigue), cognitive abilities (concentration span, comprehension level), and emotional responses (pleasure, frustration, anxiety). For a structured drama production, the degree of difficulty of the script and the portrayal of characters needs to be matched to the group's abilities. Careful assessment of the group will determine whether the drama production is a short informal piece, a longer structured play, or a segment from an opera.

Participants should be chosen for their interest and their commitment to the project. Productions can be audiotaped for appraisal and future enjoyment. Drama offers a unique opportunity for residents to work collaboratively and to enjoy the benefits to be derived from group participation. There is no set, no costume, no lighting, and no audience involved—the performance stands alone. Although nothing replaces the value of good acting, a playreading provides an opportunity to utilise gestures, facial expressions, and modulations of

'Drama offers a unique opportunity for residents to work collaboratively and to enjoy the benefits to be derived from group participation.'

voice. Through the portrayal of various characters, the playreading becomes a theatre of the group's own making and imagination.

Successful outcomes depend on the right choice of material and appropriate allocation of characters. A scene from a well-known play, such as *The Importance of Being Earnest*, can be a successful formula in terms of length, character number, and the physical requirements of the actors. As noted above, the group requires no stage—the language and its expression compensate for the absence of a formal stage setting. The stage is set by the emotions and the atmosphere that spring from the language of the play. At the conclusion of a structured performance, celebratory drinks can be enjoyed by the group, their families, and other residents.

Getting started

Opinions and ideas are sought from each individual in the group. Acknowledging each person's feedback makes the session dynamic and responsive. Once the choice of play has been decided, printed notes are provided for those who are able to engage at this level. Suitable non-reading parts can be chosen for a person with dementia who has difficulty with some of the more structured processes. Rehearsal times and forward planning depend on the participants' ability to work to a schedule, and flexibility allows for the spontaneous engagement of a person taking an 'unrehearsed' role. Other planning might involve lengthy but pleasurable preparation—for example, for the performance of a Christmas production. Capturing the performance on tape is an important element that shapes the performance and allows the work to reach a logical conclusion.

Other options

Guests can be invited to join the drama group from time to time. A reader from a radio station or from a local repertory company can join the group to offer suggestions, to discuss the process, and to offer insightful evaluation.

There are informal ways of engaging people with dementia—either in a group setting or individual setting. Fantasy and imagination play key roles for some people with dementia, allowing them a welcome escape from the realities of predictable institutionalised life, and providing a welcome relief from an otherwise inhospitable environment (Killick & Allan 2001).

In both poetry and drama, people with dementia can be encouraged to revisit familiar territory or to enter a new and friendly world that transcends everyday routines.

Art and drawing
Barbara Davison

The value of art

Many people with dementia have drawn or painted at some time in their lives. A few are skilled artists. Whether they are novices or experienced, they will need assistance to take up these activities in a residential-care setting.

Art can be pursued individually or in a group, and is an absorbing and engaging activity. Drawing (with pencil, charcoal, or pastels) and painting (water-based) are relatively inexpensive activities. They are easily portable and can be quickly set up and put away. The materials are usually non-toxic and are readily available. The drawings and paintings are tangible outcomes that can be exhibited or reproduced. Such tangible outcomes provide satisfaction to the artist and to others.

Who should be involved?

Facilitators need to understand painting and drawing techniques, and require skills in dealing with the common challenges of dementia. A ratio of one helper to two or three residents is desirable. Many participants need one-to-one help.

Residents with mild-to-moderate dementia can participate. Facilitators should start with a few residents and build the number up to about seven. Established artists can be reluctant to paint if they are aware that their skills are diminishing. Sometimes people can be encouraged to participate, but they should never be forced.

Choosing a time and place

Painting and drawing are quiet calming activities, so the facilitator should choose a room that is:

▶ free from noise and visual distraction;
▶ well lit, but not glary;
▶ close to a sink, water, and storage facilities; and
▶ provided with chairs and one or more tables with washable plain surfaces.

Social interaction before the session puts residents and helpers at ease. During this time, the facilitator can set up the tables with materials and equipment for each person.

The facilitator should choose a time of day when activities that are quiet and calming are desired. It is helpful to start with a half-hour session and increase the time as tolerated. Some people eventually sit and concentrate for more than one-and-a-half hours.

Choice of tools and materials

Quality papers, paints, pastels, pencils, and brushes should be used, and the activity should be presented in an adult way. Toxic pigments should be avoided because some people with dementia might ingest them. Finished works can be displayed in coloured mounts so that others can enjoy the work.

What to paint or draw?

Most residents require stimulus materials and assistance to start. Objects for a still life can be arranged, or the artist can be allowed to select an object to paint or draw. Photographs from magazines, books, cards, and calendars can be used. Different themes can be the focus of the activity. For example:

▶ a seasonal theme such as Christmas (trees, bells, candles, holly) or Autumn (tracing around autumn leaves); or

▶ objects with simple shapes and clear bright colours (fruit, vegetables, yachts, butterflies, tropical fish, and single flowers).

Getting started

The facilitator should gain some idea of the person's abilities and limitations through trial and error. It will become apparent if the activity needs to be adapted. The following approaches might help.

▶ The facilitator should be be aware of visual impairment, and make sure correct eyeglasses are worn. Pencils or felt pens can be used to make dark outlines that are clearly visible.

▶ The facilitator should avoid complex subjects with busy figure grounds— such as a vase of flowers or landscapes. Subjects with simple shapes should be chosen initially, and more complex compositions can then be attempted if simple activities have been successful.

▶ Abstract designs or patterns (such as stripes or rainbows) are useful for people who cannot copy objects or initiate the activity. The paper can be made wet for the person and a stripe or mark can be painted in a bright colour. A loaded brush with a different colour can then be handed to the person who is then asked to paint a mark or stripe next to the first. Most people will complete a painting with guidance to their hands and verbal encouragement. Colours laid next to each other will mix and form beautiful effects.

▶ For people who are confused, choices should be kept simple (for example, a choice between two colours at a time). Such people should be handed single colour pots rather than a palette. The facilitator can mix colours if necessary.

◗ If the person draws distorted shapes or perseverates on the same spot, colouring-in activities might be more successful. Prepared outlines can be used.

◗ The facilitator should be positive about the artists' efforts. Enjoyment of the activity is the prime goal, rather than the finished result.

When the artwork is finished to the artist's satisfaction, he or she should be encouraged to sign and date it, and perhaps give it a title (if possible). Keeping a journal entry of residents' participation is a good way to document their progress.

Carving, modelling, and sculpture
Graeme Cameron

Introduction and history

The purpose of this contribution to the chapter is not to describe an elaborate art form that is inaccessible to people with dementia. Rather, it is to introduce nurses and other carers to some simple tools and an appropriate setting to stimulate the residents' creativity through the use of carving, modelling, and sculpture.

The origins of sculpture go back to the earliest of times—from simple carving, decoration, and tools to the monumental Easter Island heads carved from a form of bluestone and the Egyptian sphinxes, religious icons, and idols. The desire to create three-dimensional images from natural materials goes back to the beginnings of human development in a similar way to the earliest rock paintings.

This form of art can provoke significant responses from people with dementia, tapping into forgotten creativity or developing new forms of self-expression.

What separates sculpture from art and drawing? Fundamentally, sculpture is a three-dimensional process whereas the others are two-dimensional. Sculpture and related art forms are probably the most comprehensive of artistic categories, and include work in a variety of materials:

◗ clay;
◗ plasticine/play clay/play dough;
◗ wood;
◗ stone;
◗ plaster;
◗ plastic;
◗ metal;
◗ papier mâché;
◗ concrete;

▶ aerated lightweight concrete (Hebel block);

▶ wax;

▶ glass;

▶ ceramics;

▶ bronze;

▶ soap/talc stone;

▶ soft sculpture (fibre-filled fabric or nylon objects creating dolls or toys); and

▶ almost any product or recycled material.

Each of these materials has its own characteristics of texture, hardness, colour, shape, and workability. Each evokes particular feelings of touch, emotion, and memory. Some are quite soft and easy to work (such as clay, papier mâché, and play clay) whereas others (such as granite, marble, and metal) require skill, special tools, and a lot of energy. However, all have a number of similar comparative properties. These include:

▶ texture (smooth/rough);

▶ colour;

▶ shape;

▶ hardness;

▶ softness;

▶ masculinity or femininity;

▶ angularity;

▶ sharpness;

▶ subtlety; and

▶ impact.

They can all evoke a variety of emotions in people with dementia. Sculpture should not only be looked at, but also touched. Because of its three-dimensional character sculpture can be viewed from any angle, and something different will be seen from each angle—be it realistic or abstract. Two-dimensional painting can be viewed from only one direction.

Although sculpture is, in itself, a separate art it can also include a two-dimensional phase. Most sculptors sketch a design from a number of different angles before beginning the actual work. Others simply start with the material and create a form with their hands and eyes as they go. It is probably a simplistic generalisation to say that sculpture is the art of removal of material to reveal an object whereas painting is the art of adding line and colour to create an image. However, for the present purposes, this generalisation suffices to make a useful contrast between the art forms.

For practical purposes in the residential aged-care setting, any hands-on experience introduced to residents is limited to the safer materials that require very little in the way of tools. These are materials such as clay, papier mâché, plaster, and soft carving materials such as balsa wood, very soft wet limestone, or wet aerated concrete. The wetness eliminates dust and makes the material easier to work. However, having been encouraged to begin with basic materials, some residents graduate to more challenging materials and tools.

Tools can include small axes for chipping, blunt knives for scraping and chiselling, small handsaws and perforated rasps for cutting, and power drills for making holes. The power tools must be used only by the group leader on the resident's behalf—doing what the resident has requested.

It is important to note that the background and capabilities of the residents vary considerably. Therefore, a careful assessment of each resident's needs is necessary.

Carving, modelling, and sculpting might prove to be more attractive to male residents—perhaps because some perceive painting as being a more feminine pursuit. Men identify with the more tactile materials found in their 'sheds'. However, many of the best painters have been men (for example, Arthur Streeton), and many of the best sculptors have been women (for example, Barbara Hepworth). Experience has shown that women find these activities fun, and mixed groups create different dynamics from those of single-sex groups.

Results vary from a few scratches on the surface of the material, to abstract shapes and loaves of bread, and even to the finest of serviette rings and bracelets that really push the limitations of the materials to their extreme.

By far the hardest part of beginning any activity is actually making a start. A design is not necessary. It is sufficient to make a start by simply chipping, scraping, or cutting. Remarkable things evolve. In practice, what seems to work is simply to set each resident up with some material and a few tools. Once they see what each tool can achieve, participants invariably follow in their own time, at their own pace, with their own design.

> 'It is sufficient to make a start by simply chipping, scraping, or cutting. Remarkable things evolve.'

When working as a group for the first time, the participants might respond to being presented with a small variety of examples to play with. A simple wooden carving, small animals made of different materials (such as glazed ceramic or bronze), or an item of smooth or textured pottery each produces a different sensory sensation. The various textures, colours, and shapes have the potential to awaken forgotten or hidden feelings, pleasures, and creativity. Soft materials such as clay, wet plaster, or papier mâché might be likened to the old 'mud pies' of childhood.

As noted above, sculpture is more often than not the removal of material to expose a design. However, this technique can also be used in reverse—by adding material using moulds and filling them, or simply by building up material into a shape or form. Simple items such as a plate or jelly mould can be used. Other simple rubber moulds of animals and objects are also available for filling with plaster or papier mâché, and simple chickenwire mesh can be used to make a rough shape over which these materials can be applied to make a more refined piece or shape. Once these objects have dried, various coloured paints, stones, shells, textiles, beads, string, glitter, and a variety of bits and pieces can be added. Each resident's design influences the use of these items (with some suggestions from the group leader as required).

Practicalities

This type of work/play is potentially dirty and messy. In practice, it is recommended that a large plastic sheet over a group of tables be used. These tables can be pushed together to create a group atmosphere. The provision of aprons (disposable or otherwise) is recommended. Hand-washing facilities are also useful. For some residents, soft cotton or disposable gloves might be needed to protect delicate skin.

Conclusion

If sculpture is reduced to its simplest form—creating three-dimensional objects from simple and cheap materials—a good deal of stimulation, pleasure, pride, and raised self-esteem in residents is achieved. Men and women who thought that they would never again be able to consider working with any kind of practical material (with which they might have been familiar in their earlier years) are amazed and elevated to discover that they still have the power to achieve.

Working with older people in this way is not only satisfying for them but also a joy and privilege for the group leader—who will learn more from them than he or she could possibly teach.

Dance
Heather Hill

A common response to the idea of dance being part of the care of people with dementia is simple disbelief. What kind of dance could they possibly do? Often the idea is simply dismissed as being a fairly trivial activity—an 'entertainment'. However, dance therapy does, in fact, meet people at the deepest and most meaningful levels of their being.

Human beings are *embodied* beings. They live in and through their bodies. What happens to their bodies affects their minds, and vice versa. As Damasio (1994, p. 226) observed:

> 'Dance therapy meets people at the deepest and most meaningful levels of their being.'

> I am not saying that the mind is in the body. I am saying that the body contributes more than life support and modulatory effects to the brain. It contributes a content that is part and parcel of the workings of the normal mind.

By engaging with the body of a person with dementia, a carer is connecting with the thinking and feeling person in his or her entirety.

Although dance in Western culture has often been regarded as a somewhat peripheral activity (perhaps even an élitist activity), dance is actually part of life. People dance to express their joy and their grief, to join others in community, to teach their young the rituals of their society, and so on. Dance is an essentially *human* activity of expression and communication.

As their dementia progresses, people find it more difficult to communicate at a verbal level. In a dance session, they have an opportunity to express themselves through their bodies. The expression of feelings—humour, anger, sadness, nostalgia—is such a great need, and often it does not find an appropriate outlet elsewhere. Staff and relatives can feel uncomfortable when a person with dementia expresses sadness. However, within the environment of a dance session, people can safely express their feelings—knowing those feelings are accepted and acknowledged.

As one of the arts, the aesthetic aspect of dance has much to offer people with dementia. The art of dance is about structure (through rhythm and shape), and about involvement and focus. These are important matters for people with dementia who struggle to make sense of a fragmented world. Contained within a circle and within the steady beat of the music, they can find some coherence—if only for a short time. The experience of making art (whether it be dance, music, or visual art) is life-enhancing and contributes to a feeling of overall well-being and ease. This makes the experience of dance different from that of other forms of exercises (although these have their own benefits). The difference is in the 'how'—the creation of a space, of atmosphere, and quality of movement. It involves a sensitivity to non-verbal cues and being in the moment. It is not enough to put on some music and wave scarves around!

This work fits well with Kitwood's (1997) concept of person-centred care—which involves focusing on the individual and on the maintenance of that person's personhood. In dance therapy, the other person is approached with humility and respect—as another human being who, despite disabilities, still has something to offer and something to 'say'.

Kitwood also talked of 'positive person work'—recognition, negotiation, collaboration, play, 'timalation' (the word used by Kitwood for pleasure received through the senses), celebration, relaxation, validation, holding, and facilitation. Dance therapy is about affirming and valuing a person through play, humour, relaxation, tapping into the senses, reminiscence, and so on. All of these help to maintain and reinforce a person's sense of self. Many people with dementia need to be reminded who they are. They need to be encouraged to unfreeze their bodies (for both physical and psychological well-being), and they need to be helped to feel at ease and completely involved in something positive. At the same time, the dance experience can encourage people to reach out to others and to have positive inter-action with other people.

> 'The dance experience can encourage people to reach out to others and to have positive interaction with other people.'

There are also benefits for the hostel, hospital, or nursing home. Dance therapists can provide another perspective on people with dementia. Nurses who attend sessions have an opportunity to be with those in their care in a different way—that is, to be just another person, rather than a staff person. Some realise for the first time that a person has more abilities than staff recognised. The atmosphere of the dance room often spills over into the nursing home in general, and offers nurturing and pleasure to everyone.

In summary, dance therapy is about:

- creating a space and giving time for people to emerge;
- expression and communication;
- creativity and feeling alive;
- enjoyment and sociability; and
- self-acceptance and acceptance by others.

Above all, dance therapy is about relationship.

As one resident at a nursing home observed about the dance room: 'That little room gave us a whole lot of room to be ourselves'.

Music
Tanya Ryszczak

The sound of melody coming from the bathroom

His eyes suddenly focused on mine and he stopped for a brief moment to locate the source of my singing. He then continued to pace aimlessly around the room, pushing chairs and tables as they got in his way, and mumbling an incoherent but rhythmical 'mummm, mum, mumm, mum'.

I continued to make my presence known by singing, unaccompanied, a tune that his wife had told me he used to love. Again, he looked up and, this time, as the rhythm of my singing intensified, he smiled—no longer pacing, no longer mumbling, but focused.

I took his hand and tapped the back of it in time with the song. Together we sang and walked in a rhythmical unison that appeared to connect him with his memories and bring him out of his isolation.

His nurse then joined us in our song and directed him towards the shower. The normally difficult task of showering this gentleman with advanced stages of dementia was completed with ease.

All that could be heard was the sound of rhythm and melody coming from the bathroom.

The value of music

The vignette described in the Box highlights how music can be used to enhance the lives of people with dementia. It demonstrates how a music therapist and nursing staff in residential settings can collaborate to make the role of the caregiver more fulfilling.

As dementia progresses and people become less functional, they have an increased need for human contact and sensory stimulation. Music provides stimulation in unique ways. It is often the one stimulus that can be used as an attention-focus for a resident's existing cognitive capacities. Through music, residents with dementia can interact with others or simply be aware that other people are around—thereby coming out of their isolation, even for a short period of time (Clair 1991). Most people who work in aged care have seen the pleasure and emotion that music elicits in people with dementia. They often see music elicit laughter in a depressed person, a flicker of movement in an otherwise non-ambulant resident, or the calming relaxation of a person with agitated behaviour.

The evidence

Music as a therapy has existed in various forms in most cultures for centuries. Today, registered music therapists who are trained as both musicians and health-care professionals at tertiary level have carried out extensive research which shows the efficacy of music therapy in enhancing the social, psychological, and physical aspects of the lives of older people who have degenerative cognitive disorders.

Comparisons of music therapy sessions with discussion-based programs have revealed significant improvements in the music therapy groups with respect to orientation, social behaviour, and verbal participation. Significant decreases were found in non-social behaviour (Riegler 1980; Millar & Smith 1989; Pollack & Namazi 1992; Clair 1996). A study by Burke (1995) found that active participation in group music experiences could positively influence self-esteem, depression, and affect in the elderly.

Some residents with dementia are able to learn new songs even when they are unable to recall new verbal material. Research has shown that cerebral areas used for the execution of musical and language skills are relatively independent. This assists in understanding why people with degenerative cognitive disorders often respond to music more than other interventions (Prickett & Moore 1991; O'Callaghan 1999).

In summary, the research shows that group and individual music therapy is a powerful therapeutic medium. It can be used in dementia care to:

- maintain levels of cognitive functioning;
- reduce isolation and maintain social networks;
- increase verbal and vocal participation;
- increase social behaviour;
- decrease non-social behaviour;
- maintain physical activity;
- enhance quality of life;
- reduce depression;
- increase self-esteem;
- increase orientation;
- stimulate senses; and
- express current and past issues (for example, grief).

As improvements in health care have led to an ageing population, it is important that older adults with dementia are provided with more than a mere existence (O'Callaghan 1999). Opportunities for interaction, communication, and a quality of life with positive experiences can be provided by using music in the day-to-day care of people with dementia. Although music therapists are trained to assess people, set goals, implement music-therapy programs, and evaluate the outcomes of the programs, it is important that non-music therapists also utilise the medium of music to assist in their everyday caregiving.

Implementing a music activity
Selection of music

To provide a sense of security and predictability within the activity, it is important to use music that is both familiar to the person and culturally specific. Although music provided on a live instrument tends to elicit more focus and concentration from people, prerecorded music can work effectively, provided that it has been carefully selected for its quality in sound and performance.

Music techniques

Although there is a variety of music techniques that can be used with residents with dementia, certain techniques are more likely to elicit a response and generate more emjoyment.

It has been found that *movement to music activities* is the preferred music activity for people with dementia (Brotons, Koger & Pickett-Cooper 1997; Hanson et al. 1996). Participants with all stages of dementia show significantly greater response during movement activities than they do during singing activities.

Singing brings a point of contact with other individuals, and this contact is meaningful and emotionally intimate for adults (as was illustrated in the Box on page 266). Singing can enhance the quality of life for people with dementia and their caregivers by encouraging physical contact and more positive visiting experiences by the carers. Although singing is a popular activity, it is important to recognise that responses to this intervention do decline as dementia progresses (Clair 2000; Brotons, Koger & Pickett-Cooper 1997).

Providing a strong sense of *rhythm* can provide an overall organising structure for people with dementia (Aldridge & Brandt 1991). Starting a music activity with a song that has clear and precise rhythmic form—such as a march or a waltz—can help residents to become attentive and focus on the activity.

Family involvement

Family members can be a great source of information regarding their loved one's musical likes and dislikes. This information is important to the success of the music activity. Because the music skills of a person with early to moderate stages of dementia appear to be spared, it can be heartening for family members to be involved in a music session and to see a glimpse of the person who otherwise appeared to be 'lost' (Bright 1991). Hearing a piece of music that elicits memories of special family moments can provide a closeness that cannot be shared verbally.

Contraindications
Carers who provide music activities need to observe the responses of people constantly. If participants are becoming distracted, agitated, or disorientated, it is time to discontinue that particular music activity.

Conclusion
There is no doubt that music therapy is an effective means of improving the quality of life of people with dementia, and that it should be used as part of an overall care program in residential settings. Every tap of the foot, tilt of the head, or flicker of a smile in response to music is a reminder of the people they really are.

Dolls
Sue Piccoli

The value of dolls
Dolls have been used in nursing homes and hostels for many years to improve quality of life for people with challenging behaviour. Staff members who have worked in the field of aged care are well aware that older people with behavioural disturbances can take on caring roles with dolls or soft toys and become more settled in their behaviour.

Dolls can be used with success to manage restlessness, anxiety, wandering, absconding, shadowing, intrusiveness, 'sundowning' behaviours, verbal and physical aggression, withdrawal and, occasionally, even hallucinations and delusions.

Who will benefit from the use of a baby doll?
Dolls can be of benefit in the care of both men and women who have moderate to severe dementia and who are demonstrating challenging behaviour. This is especially so with people who have a history of being caring persons—either with their own children or with children in their families or the wider community.

What are the results for a person with dementia?
The use of dolls can assist people with dementia to:
▶ become more relaxed and contented;
▶ be safer and less likely to wander (with reduced risk of falls); and

▶ behave in socially appropriate ways (through being more stimulated and able to interact better with staff and other residents).

What are the advantages for the caregivers?

Doll therapy is a convenient and effective form of care. The doll is available 24 hours a day and its use is not dependent on recreational staff to organise interventions. Because dolls can assist in reducing incidents of aggression, they can be useful in decreasing stress (and possibly injuries) for staff members.

How are the dolls introduced?

Introducing a doll is as simple as approaching someone and saying: 'Look what I've got!'.

Some people will see it as a doll, agree that it is beautiful, and be happy to pass it on.

Others will think that it is a real baby, but that it belongs to a staff member. In this instance the doll can be valuable in diverting or distracting someone

---

'The children are hurt . . . they are lost'

A woman with a moderate dementia who had been a refugee in both World War I (as a small child) and in World War II (as a young adult) was wandering around the nursing home in an agitated manner. She was crying and calling out: 'The children are hurt, they are crying, I can't find them, they are lost'.

She was given a baby doll and her behaviour settled almost immediately. No further interventions were required.

'A doting grandmother'

A doll was obtained for a lady who was agitated and repeatedly getting up from her armchair. She was at significant risk of falling and sometimes became aggressive when staff members tried to return her to her armchair. This lady had been the eldest daughter of a large family, had raised a large family herself, and was a doting grandmother. When she was given the doll she settled well and her risk of falls was significantly decreased.

Some members of staff felt that it was demeaning for this elderly woman to have a doll, and the doll was therefore withdrawn. The lady's agitation immediately resumed—resulting in an aggressive incident in which a staff member was injured.

At the family's insistence the doll was reintroduced. The lady again became relaxed and less agitated.

'A wonderful husband, father, and grandfather'

A man with dementia had been wandering in a rural area. Because he was at risk of becoming lost, he was placed in a nursing home. For the first four days he roamed around the facility without any sleep at all, attempted to climb the fences, was aggressive when approached, refused to eat, and resisted personal care.

It was decided to take some photographs—just in case the man did manage to abscond. He refused to have his photo taken, shook his fist, and yelled: 'Get out of here'.

Because his wife had described him as a caring person, and as a wonderful husband, father, and grandfather, an inspired carer asked the man if we could take his photo with 'the baby' (a doll). To everyone's surprise, he agreed. He then went inside and fell asleep in an armchair nursing the doll in his arms.

For quite some time after this episode, until his aggressive behaviour diminished, the doll was used to help him settle while medications, food, and personal care could be administered.

---

from an issue that is distressing them—such as wanting to go home because the children will be coming home from school. In these circumstances, dolls can be used for reminiscence, validation, and reality orientation for confused older people.

Others believe that it is a real baby and adopt it as their own. The incidence of a doll being fully accepted is relatively rare. However, when the doll is accepted wholeheartedly, it is important that staff respond to it in an appropriate manner and respect the reactions of the person with dementia.

What should the doll look like?
The doll should be:
- as lifelike as possible;
- soft-bodied, safe, and with no detachable or breakable parts (for example, the eyes);
- dressed in baby clothes (not doll clothes) that are culturally and era appropriate; and
- wrapped in a shawl or similar item.

Do men have the same reaction to dolls?
Dolls can be as effective for a man as for a woman—and for the same reasons.

Conclusion

Dolls do not work for everyone. However, they can be a very useful tool for family and professional carers in managing the confusion and distress so often associated with dementia. Dolls should be part of an overall activity program that makes use of other resources such as photographs, rummage boxes, and other suitable sensory stimulation.

Aromatherapy
Kirsten James

Introduction

Aromatherapy is one way of influencing an individual's environment in a subtle and positive way. In his 1996 book in which he attempted to provide a rigorous overview of massage and aromatherapy, Vickers expressed concern at the lack of sound research in both of these fields. He was particularly critical of aromatherapy, and observed that ' . . . most texts contain vast numbers of unsubstantiated claims' (1996, p. 72).

This is not to say that these therapies are invalid or should be ignored. However, health professionals who are interested in incorporating aromatherapy as part of the care they provide are urged to seek more detailed information from specific texts, and to undertake accredited courses (by recognised professional associations such as the International Federation of Aromatherapists). The following information is merely an *overview* of aromatherapy in dementia care.

What is aromatherapy?

Simply defined, aromatherapy is 'a form of treatment using essential oils extracted from plants for therapeutic effect' (Stevensen 1995, p. 51). The proportion of active chemical constituents of each plant extract determines which oil is appropriate for a particular therapeutic intervention (Franchomme & Penoel 1990). These oils, in their pure forms, are highly concentrated and volatile, and can be adulterated with synthetic chemicals to extend and preserve their fragrance, thereby reducing their cost and quality (Stevenson 1995; Vickers 1996). The use of such adulterated oils does *not* constitute true aromatherapy.

How does aromatherapy work?

There are two main ways in which aromatherapy works—by inhalation and by absorption via the skin. When a person inhales the fragrance of an essential oil, the olfactory nerves stimulate the limbic system in the mid brain. This is where the processing of emotions, moods, memories, and motivation is located, as well as control of the autonomic nervous system and some hormones (Van Toller 1996).

This might explain why people can react positively or negatively to certain fragrances—there are very strong memory associations connected to this experience (which, itself, can be conscious or unconscious). It is therefore important to remember that no matter how 'therapeutic' an oil is purported to be, it will not be therapeutic if a person has a negative memory association with that aroma. This raises particular challenges in the setting of dementia because many people experience changes in memory, personality, and cognition. It is therefore very important to consider each person's individual response.

Inhalation

Effective inhalation methods that are appropriate for use in dementia care include:

▶ vaporisation (using an approved electric vaporiser placed out of the person's reach);
▶ drops of oil placed on a tissue or handkerchief and tucked into the person's clothing;
▶ drops placed on a person's pyjamas or pillow at night; and
▶ compresses.

An effective way of using compresses is to use prepared wash cloths before the serving of meals. Mood-stabilising oils are used on the facecloths—which also act as a ritual to stimulate digestion. Residents can also wash their faces and hands with the cloths—thus promoting good hygiene.

Skin absorption

The other main way in which aromatherapy works is via skin absorption. To achieve this, essential oils can be incorporated into:

▶ baths and foot spas; and
▶ creams, gels, or carrier oils for massage.

These are effective and practical methods that can be utilised in dementia care. Advice on the proportion of essential oils should be sought from a qualified practitioner and incorporated into the facility's policies and protocols. However, many practitioners do recommend that half the usual dosage should be used because of the changing metabolism of the liver and kidneys in older people.

Indications

Four oils are recommended as having mood-stabilising qualities that are well suited to people with dementia. These particular oils combine well together, and are also affordable.

The following oils are recommended:

▶ lavender (*Lavandula angustifolia*);
▶ bergamot (*Citrus aurantium ssp. bergamia*);
▶ sweet orange (*Citrus aurantium*); and
▶ marjoram (*Origanum marjorana*).

Indications for the use of these oils include stress, depression, restlessness, anxiety, and insomnia (Tisserand 1994; Stevensen 1995).

Quality, safety, and professional issues

To ensure maximum therapeutic benefit and to minimise the risk of any unwanted side-effects, the best-quality essential oils should be used. Criteria for selecting quality oils include:

▶ dark bottles (usually amber or blue) with dripolators; and
▶ labelling that includes the oil's botanical name, expiry date, and batch number.

Good-quality essential oils vary in price according to availability, source, and the degree of difficulty in processing a given oil. Nursing staff should not be seduced by cheap products that purport to be '100% natural'.

Equipment (such as electric vaporisers) should conform to minimum safety standards. Before use, they should be checked by the nursing home's engineering department (and labelled accordingly).

Essential oils are relatively expensive, and can be toxic if used inappropriately. They should be used carefully and sparingly. The following points are important to note (Meyer 2001):

▶ essential oils are volatile and flammable;
▶ they are for topical use only;
▶ they should be used in a carrier oil or cream; never undiluted on the skin;
▶ eyes and mucous membranes are to be avoided;
▶ discontinue if skin reaction occurs;
▶ note any precautions and contraindications;
▶ use correct dose and proportions; and
▶ avoid long-term use of the same oils in skin preparations.

The reaction of each individual person to aromatherapy should be assessed and documented. Verbal consent should be obtained from the person (or the person's family), and this should be documented in the resident's care plan. The care plan should be evaluated frequently.

It is recommended that vaporisers not be used in communal areas. Many people are sensitive to certain fragrances and might have negative memory associations and adverse reactions. Vaporisers are therefore best used in individual rooms.

Policies and protocols need to be in place, preceded by staff education that ensures minimum competency standards. A qualified aromatherapy consultant should always be available.

Animals
Kirsten James

Introduction

> Animals make such agreeable friends—they ask no questions, they pass no criticisms.
>
> GEORGE ELIOT (SCENES OF CLERICAL LIFE)

Many people with dementia apparently retain very clear long-term memories of how to relate to animals. If these memories are positive, there is a strong chance that contact with animals will be a therapeutic experience. This is, of course, a fundamental point—carers must never assume that a particular intervention will be of benefit to everyone. Negative memory association and issues such as possible allergies must be considered when assessing the suitability of animal experiences for a person with dementia.

Background

The history of human–animal interaction as a specific therapeutic relationship is relatively recent. In the late eighteenth century, the Quakers at York Retreat in England used pets such as chickens and rabbits in the hope that patients with mental illness would learn self-control by having creatures that were weaker than themselves depend upon them (Beck & Katcher 1996). Since that time, several benefits have been identified and are well supported by research (James 2001).

Animals can be used formally or informally as an intervention with people in dementia. Examples of formal interactions are pet visitation programs or visits to zoos or farms. An example of an informal encounter is the presence of a resident cat or an aquarium.

Benefits

The following benefits of human–animal interaction have been identified and are clearly worth considering as a valid experience for people with dementia (James 2001):

◗ reduction in insomnia, stress, and depression;
◗ improved self-esteem and acceptance;
◗ improved socialisation and reduced aggression;
◗ an opportunity for comfort and nurturing;
◗ a source of distraction and promotion of play;
◗ an opportunity for non-threatening touch (which might be difficult with humans);
◗ a memory stimulus;
◗ promotion of balance, mobility, and activity;
◗ reduced muscle tension;
◗ reduced blood glucose levels;
◗ improved blood pressure;
◗ improved serum triglyceride levels;
◗ increased willingness to be involved in group activities;
◗ reduction of pain;
◗ stimulation of the immune system; and
◗ improvement in mood alteration.

Practical examples

Animals can be included in the lives of people with dementia in several ways. These include:

◗ playing of recorded animal sounds—such as birds, crickets, and frogs;
◗ aquariums—real or played as a video recording;
◗ resident pets—for example, cats, dogs, rabbits, birds;
◗ visiting pets—family members or volunteers can bring a favourite pet from home or animals from professional health-care organisations, mobile farms, or zoos;
◗ visits to parks or beaches to feed the birds; and
◗ visits to sanctuaries, zoos, or farms accompanied by staff and volunteers.

Issues to be considered

In organising visits or other animal programs, the following issues need to be considered:

◗ the suitability of the workplace for such a program—space, layout, quality of floor coverings, ease of cleaning, and opportunities for privacy;

▶ consultation with all key stakeholders regarding the advantages and disadvantages of such a program—allergies to dog hair or cat fur, cultural objections, negative memory associations;

▶ consideration of the costs involved—purchase of animal, vaccinations, veterinary costs, food, toys, grooming, bedding, and so on.

Policy considerations

Staff members should devise a policy that includes consideration of such matters as (James 1998; Moody 1998; Delta 1999):

▶ responsibility for the animal—feeding, training, control, exercising, cleaning and grooming needs;

▶ infection control—vaccination, veterinary checks, cleaning, prophylactic medications, cleaning, reporting of pet soiling, exclusion from certain residents (for example, those who are immuno-compromised and those with open wounds);

▶ insurance cover for any unforeseen liabilities arising from accidents with the animals;

▶ qualifications and suitability of any animal handler who might be visiting the institution—personality, grooming, communication skills, willingness to follow policies; willingness to respect confidentiality;

▶ choice of the animal—health-status check, temperament assessment, grooming and cleanliness;

▶ documentation of the interaction and any outcomes;

▶ incident reporting and protocols for accidents (such as dog bites, cat scratches, pet soiling, and so on);

▶ feeding the animals—avoidance of over-feeding or inappropriate feeding by well-intentioned residents; and

▶ a suitably qualified and experienced animal-therapy consultant (should the need arise).

It should be noted that some animal-welfare experts recommend that dogs should not be kept as residential pets in long-term care facilities because they can become attached to the residents and experience a grief reaction when the residents die. For this reason, it might be wise to utilise dogs in a visiting capacity.

Protocols

Protocols for visiting pets can include the following (James 1998).

▶ *Dogs on leads*: Keep dogs on leads at all times and in the control of the person taking responsibility.

The pregnant mare comes to visit

Many of the residents in a rural nursing home had grown up on farms in an era when horses were more involved in daily life than they are today. A member of the nursing staff offered to bring her gentle pregnant mare in to the hospital grounds. However, the director of nursing, who realised the likely impact of such a visit, encouraged the nurse to bring the mare into the foyer of the nursing home. This meant that even those residents confined to wheelchairs and beds could be close enough to pet the horse and see it up close (which was important with so many of the residents having visual impairment).

Nursing staff were delighted to see some residents—who had not responded to human stimulus for some time—smiling, laughing, and moving in an effort to pet the horse. Some residents were able to regale staff with stories from their youth about their involvement with horses.

The visit was considered a great success, and the nurse planned to bring the mare back with its foal once it had been born.

- *Food protocols:* Some handlers encourage the use of food as a treat to help familiarise animals with residents, but guidance might be required to assess the suitability of such a treat. In the dementia setting, some residents have been known to eat the treat before the animal does!
- *Receptiveness of residents:* Assess the receptiveness of the resident by observing reactions and asking their opinions. Rather than persisting with residents who are indifferent, allow the animal to spend 'quality time' with those who react positively.

Conclusion

With careful planning, the inclusion of animals in the care of people with dementia can significantly enhance the quality of life of many people. Consideration of the requirements of individual residents and care of the animals is essential to the success of such programs. Although effort is required on the part of the staff, the rewards for all involved (including the animals!) will make it worthwhile.

Snoezelen
Carole Quinn

Introduction

People can take for granted the many sensory experiences that enrich their lives—such as walking through a rainforest, touching velvet curtains, or smelling dinner cooking. Residents with advanced dementia have reduced opportunities for such pleasures—indeed, reduced opportunities for sensory experiences in general. These residents typically experience the cumulative effects of:

- vision and hearing loss associated with normal ageing;
- reduced opportunity to explore the environment because of impaired mobility;
- touch deprivation—as a result of no longer being able to reach out to touch or be touched;
- reduced ability to attend to and perceive sensory information due to cognitive deficits; and
- living in an institutional environment.

For these reasons, people with advanced dementia are at risk of significant sensory deprivation (Pinkney 1998).

According to Bowlby (1993), inadequate access to sensory stimulation can accelerate:

- loss of arousal, motivation, and interest in life;
- social and emotional withdrawal; and
- decreased responsiveness and general functional deterioration.

In turn, these losses can diminish independence, esteem, and quality of life.

Sensory activities are especially suitable for residents with advanced dementia because such activities:

- promote interaction with the environment;
- provide a medium for meaningful staff–resident interaction;
- involve minimal cognitive demands, and are therefore non-threatening and usually successful;
- bring pleasure; and
- can be tailored to achieve the right balance between relaxation and stimulation.

Carers should therefore endeavour to provide activities that optimise appropriate sensory experiences for people with advanced dementia. Snoezelen is one way of meeting this need for sensory-based programs.

'Carers should endeavour to provide activities that optimise appropriate sensory experiences for people with advanced dementia.'

An overview of Snoezelen

Snoezelen is a Dutch word meaning to 'sniff and doze'. In recent years it has become a recognised form of therapy for people with advanced dementia.

Snoezelen sessions are usually conducted in a small white-painted room with natural light sources blocked out. The room is fitted with a range of special equipment that can be used to stimulate residents' senses of sight, hearing, touch, taste, and smell. One or two comfortable armchairs are usually included in the room, but there is usually minimal other furniture.

During sessions, carers provide residents with pleasurable multi-sensory experiences in an atmosphere of human contact, trust, and relaxation (Kewin 1994). This enables residents to choose from varied sensory stimuli, and, if possible, to focus on and respond to the stimuli. Should residents be unable to express their choices, carers do so on their behalf, and diligently observe for positive and negative responses. Sensory needs are very individual—so trial and error is often required initially, with the task becoming easier as response patterns and preferences emerge.

Potential outcomes

Although empirical evidence for the exact therapeutic benefits of Snoezelen for residents with dementia is limited, recent studies point to the following outcomes:

- positive manipulation of mood (Pinkney 1997);
- increased focus and concentration (Pinkney 1997);
- increased spontaneous communication (Baker et al. 1997);
- recollection of memories (Baker et al. 1997);
- improved therapeutic relationships and shared 'quality' time (Pinkney & Barker 1994);
- relaxation (Hope 1997);
- improved culture of care (Hope 1997);
- decreased occurrence of disturbed behaviour (Baker et al. 1997);
- increased happiness and interest (Moffat, Baker & Pinkney 1993);
- decreased anxious behaviour (Moffat, Baker & Pinkney 1993); and
- increased expression of feelings to which carers can then to respond (Pinkney 1998).

The special atmosphere and closeness created by Snoezelen empowers carers to do something meaningful for residents with advanced dementia. In addition, it allows them to get to know, appreciate, and respect residents more effectively.

To maximise the benefits of Snoezelen, it is important to:
- identify the individual sensory abilities and needs of residents;
- formulate specific aims against which the program can be evaluated;
- select and implement the appropriate balance of sensory experiences;

◗ ensure that residents are wearing their sensory aids; and
◗ ensure that carers have the required knowledge and skills to utilise all the equipment, activities, and techniques available in the Snoezelen room.

Visual stimulation

A Snoezelen room usually includes a large source of moving visual stimulation such as:

◗ *a bubble column*—in which bubbles are pulsed up a two-metre column of water that changes colour via lamps positioned underneath; large mirrors behind this are often used to multiply the effect four-fold;
◗ *a solar projector with panoramic rotator*—which displays moving thematic or abstract images onto the walls and ceiling; and
◗ *a revolving mirror ball, spotlight, and colour wheel*—which projects a pattern of coloured sparkling coloured stars of light, and which can rotate around the room or be held stationary.

Other sources of visual stimulation that are suitable adjuncts include:

◗ bundles of fibre-optic tubes;
◗ books, magazines, and calendars with large coloured images;
◗ posters and photographs;
◗ videotapes with slow-moving and defined images;
◗ brightly coloured balloons or balls;
◗ items from the garden;
◗ bubbles;
◗ and so on.

Auditory stimulation

Soft, gentle music with predictable tone and rhythm (such as nature sounds) are suitable because they do not distract attention from the other sensory experiences and because they promote a sense of tranquillity and well-being. A good quality CD player and a stock of appropriate CDs is essential.

Other possible auditory equipment and activities include:

◗ a large wind chime that residents can reach;
◗ a rain stick;
◗ soothing percussion instruments;
◗ bells and chimes; and
◗ a small electronic keyboard for residents or staff to play;
◗ and so on.

Tactile stimulation

Touch is a very powerful therapeutic tool and is crucial to well-being. Hugging, holding, and stroking are very effective ways to provide validation, reassurance, and pleasure. Through tactile activities residents are also enabled to experience such concepts as temperature, texture, and shape, and can interact and respond to the world around them.

Possible sources of tactile stimulation include:

▶ a vibration cushion;
▶ massage to the hands, face, shoulders, and feet;
▶ a foot spa that can be used with or without water;
▶ a beauty-care tray;
▶ soft toys or dolls;
▶ pets;
▶ a sensory box or bag full of items to touch—such as, feathers, fabrics, familiar objects, artificial flowers, shells, and so on.

Smell and taste

A range of sources can be used to provide pleasurable olfactory experiences and simultaneously rekindle memories. However, care must be taken not to overload stimulation or mix these smells.

Useful sources include:

▶ aromatherapy oils;
▶ scented candles (if safe);
▶ perfumes, lotions, beauty-care and grooming products;
▶ flowers, pot-pourri, and lavender;
▶ common kitchen and household aromas;
▶ and so on.

If using food and drinks to stimulate taste, care must also be taken to allow for any swallowing difficulties or food sensitivities that residents might have.

Movement and vestibular stimulation

Opportunities to experience movement—such as gentle assisted exercises and music and movement—can be incorporated into Snoezelen sessions. These provide additional tactile stimulation as well as proprioceptive and kinaesthetic stimulation—all of which can help maintain body awareness.

A rocking chair can also be incorporated in a Snoezelen room to provide pleasant and relaxing vestibular stimulation.

Suggested session guidelines

The following guidelines are suggested for successful Snoezelen sessions.

▶ Sessions are usually of about 20 minutes duration and are provided on a 1:1 basis. Sessions with 2–3 residents can also be attempted if required.

▶ Put on some quiet background music and the aromatherapy burner, and ensure suitable temperature control before bringing residents to the room.

▶ Start with normal lighting only.

▶ Shut the door—so that there are no interruptions and distractions.

▶ Seat residents appropriately, and promote comfort and security by adding cushions. Bringing residents in their special water-cushion or comfort chairs reduces the need for transfers.

▶ Spend time talking with the residents to help them feel welcome, settled, and secure before starting.

▶ Introduce one light source—for example, bubble tube or solar projector— before turning off the main light.

▶ Observe closely for positive and negative reactions—particularly if a resident cannot verbalise.

▶ When changing to another light source, turn it on before turning off the other so that there is not a period of darkness.

▶ Do not have more than one large piece of equipment on at any time because this can cause sensory overload.

▶ Remember to utilise the smaller sensory activities fully—sensory box, foot spa, massage oils, soft toys, bubbles, windchime, and so on.

▶ Remember that different sensory experiences used simultaneously should enhance each other, and not conflict.

▶ Remember that the carer is the most important therapeutic ingredient in these sessions. Use communication and facilitating skills well. Utilise knowledge of the resident and of the equipment and activities available to ensure that the best outcomes are achieved.

Reminiscence
Sandy Forster

Introduction

All people possess memories and all reminisce as a natural part of everyday life— sometimes privately, and sometimes in the company of others. Although the act of reminiscing takes place in the present, it can be about things that happened years ago, months ago, or two minutes ago. Reminiscing usually involves a

---

In need of love and compassion

A woman was referred as a result of her non-compliant, aggressive, and noisy behaviour.

Through reminiscing, it became apparent that she had spent time as a teenager in a German concentration camp during World War II. In addition, she had been sexually abused before marriage—although her husband refused to believe this, and suggested that she must have been a willing party.

For 45 years she had kept this secret. Without knowledge of her story, carers had misinterpreted her 'troublesome behaviour'. This woman clearly deserved love and compassion in her remaining years.

---

relationship between a storyteller and one or more listeners, and this relationship is of special significance in dementia care.

Effective reminiscing

Effective reminiscing involves always putting the best interests of residents first. Carers must demonstrate through their words and deeds that they genuinely care. They should listen carefully, and hear what is being communicated. Not 'being heard' is a common cause of frustration for many people, but it can be especially distressing for people with dementia.

Older people often have a need to resolve conflict issues before they die. Carers need to face whatever fears they might personally have about dementia and loss of functioning.

Carers need to be alert, and take time to listen. For residents there is urgency, and they are likely to confide in anyone at any time. These moments need to be cherished. Carers should be sympathetic, empathetic, non-judgmental, and compassionate in all their dealings with residents.

Carers should be respectful, courteous, and polite. They should ascertain the appropriate means of address ('Mr', 'Mrs', 'Miss', or by given name). Respect should be shown for all comments and all means of communication—no matter how bizarre they might seem.

Killick (1994), who has sensitively attended to people with dementia, believes that they express themselves in language nearer to poetry than they used before. For example, a woman struggling to recall her past expressed herself in the following words (Killick 1998):

It isn't fair when your heart wants to remember.

And another put her feelings this way (Killick 1998):

> What is the use of having lived so long, travelled so widely, listened and
> looked so hard, if at the end you don't know what you know?

All behaviour should be viewed as a means of communicating a need that is not being met. An attempt should be made to identify the emotions behind the behaviour.

The life that a person has led before the onset of dementia should be recognised, acknowledged, and celebrated. Lives should be affirmed as having meaning and purpose. In this respect, family, friends, and colleagues of residents can share their knowledge, skills, and insights. This information can be used in flexible ways to reach residents with dementia.

Life storyboards, life storybooks, or memory boxes can be produced as a source of pride for owners, as well as providing communication triggers for carers and visitors. Agency staff report that such communication aids are especially helpful in enabling them to establish meaningful interaction with residents. As a carer observed (Forster 1998, p. 71):

> There is no doubt that when you get to know someone a bit better, your
> attitude changes. The resident is no longer just a resident. She has had an
> interesting life that you have just discovered, where you can now think of
> her, and treat her, as a friend.

Time should be taken to find out what gives residents joy and pleasure. Reminiscing should be seen as a means of empowerment that builds on self-

---

No need to go out to work

A very distressed resident aggressively banged daily on the door of his nursing home demanding that he be let out to go to work. Investigation revealed that he had worked for fifty years as a filing clerk.

A filing cabinet was set up and this resident happily spent a couple of hours each day sorting through 'current documents'.

As his need to 'go out' diminished, he assumed a much calmer disposition.

Memories of past skills

A woman who made soft toys in her early life surrounded her bed with examples of her talent. She found this comforting and reassuring.

Similarly, an old horse collar and bridle provided much pleasure for a visually impaired man who had spent many years as a horse trainer.

esteem and feelings of worthiness. Utilising long-term memory keeps residents socially connected to other people, whereas bringing them back to reality is usually a distressing and futile exercise.

People with dementia who no longer possess the ability to reminisce still enjoy listening to the reminiscences of others.

Other means of triggering responses should be explored when words fail. Music, drama, dance, painting, and objects with distinctive aromas and specific tactile surfaces can all be used for this purpose.

Ineffective reminiscing

In contrast to the above suggestions, reminiscing will be ineffective if residents are patronised or treated in a condescending manner. Even if people sometimes behave in a child-like manner, such people should never be labelled as being 'childish'.

Residents should never be ignored, and it should never be assumed that residents with dementia cannot understand what is being said about them.

The reminiscences of residents should never be trivialised; they own their stories.

Reminiscing should never be viewed negatively as 'living in the past'. Reminiscing is therapeutic in the present.

Chapter 23

The Eden Alternative

Dawn MacKenzie

The Eden Alternative™ seeks to challenge the traditional models of aged care and the environment in which these operate. As the generation born in the decade following the end of World War II approaches retirement age, the question of what this generation wants for its aged care becomes more important. Not surprisingly, the 'medical model' practised in many places does not appeal to these people who are demanding a different lifestyle for their senior years. The need to assess the current model against the 'wish list' of the future has become more urgent.

The origin of the Eden Alternative

In the United States of America in 1990, Dr Bill Thomas was working in a large geriatric long-term facility when a resident asked him for help. The lady said that she was lonely. Dr Thomas looked around and wondered how she could possibly be lonely because there was so much hustle and bustle in the place—with care staff, allied professionals, catering and cleaning staff, and visitors in the home. He told the lady that he would get back to her. Dr Thomas pondered this incident and ultimately identified what he termed 'the three plagues' of long-term aged care, concluding that many people were suffering from *loneliness*, *helplessness*, and *boredom*. Rather than treating these problems with medication, he sought to treat the cause. He looked at the needs of the human spirit and searched for a solution.

Loneliness

To treat loneliness in an aged-care facility, it is important to understand the changes that occur in people's lives when they enter a home. Family and friends often perceive that the resident is now with other people and does not need the company of family and friends. Some feel uncomfortable about visiting in what they perceive to be a depressing environment.

The community contacts that the person once enjoyed often diminish because the person is now thought to be unable to make a meaningful contribution. Should the resident have signs of early dementia, people in the community often feel that there is no point in visiting because the person 'will not remember anyway'.

Loneliness for residents can also be due to grief at the loss of their home environments in which their memories and chores kept them occupied. In some instances, a pet might have been left behind, and this might have been 'adopted' by someone else. Grief at the loss of home, lifestyle, and independence is often not fully understood by other people.

> 'Grief at the loss of home, lifestyle, and independence is often not fully understood by other people.'

Helplessness

The terms 'aged care facility' or 'long-term care home' can send the wrong messages to the community and to staff members who work in such an environment.

When people enter a 'home' they believe that they will become the recipients of care. Their families and friends expect total care, and the staff members understand that they have a 'duty of care' to deliver total care. In such a scenario, there is potential for residents to become helpless over time. The responsibility of ensuring ongoing independence lies with the resident and the caregiver. Perhaps the 'carer' should be called something else other than 'carer', and perhaps the residents should be educated about life enhancement, and about giving as well as receiving.

As aged-care professionals, nurses do 'care' about the residents. However, perhaps they should also aim to provide assistance with living.

Boredom

If the human spirit is not valued, a person's self-esteem begins to erode. Little by little, piece by piece, there is a gradual decline in a person's ability to feel positive about his or her personal self and environment. This feeling is often exacerbated in people with dementia.

> 'If the human spirit is not valued, a person's self-esteem begins to erode.'

A lack of purpose leads to reduced initiative, and this can produce a 'nothingness' that can culminate in a serious decline in health. Unfortunately, this appears to occur in many traditional aged-care facilities.

The Eden Alternative solution

Dr Bill Thomas developed solutions to loneliness, helplessness, and boredom by changing the environment from a clinical medical model to a social model with the introduction of animals, plants, and children.

Changing the environment

The environment needs to change from a clinical medical model to an environment that is homely in atmosphere and appearance. The Eden Alternative model offers diversity and spontaneity in all aspects of daily living. This focuses on spiritual and emotional wellness, as well as on physical independence. It promotes growth through close and continuing contact with family, staff, animals, plants, and children.

Residents with dementia cope favourably with 'smaller' living environments that are intimate and provide easy access to the outdoors. Smaller intimate environments remind residents of their childhoods or their previous home environments, thereby creating settled familiar places that can alleviate the stress and anxiety commonly experienced in the traditional model. If nurses create a 'home' environment, they diminish the desire for residents to abscond and decrease the incidence of comments such as: 'I want to go home!'.

The environment needs to create a homelike environment (or what might called a sense of 'homeness'). This includes suitable soft furnishings and a safe, small, personalised space. This is a difficult challenge because most aged-care facilities need to be large to amortise costs and keep staff/resident ratios at acceptable levels. A culture change is necessary whereby the environment is changed from that of a large institutional setting to one of small communities of 'like' residents. In the wider community, people gravitate to other people who have similar abilities and interests to seek stimulation, sociali-sation, and friendship. Aged care should not be any different; rather, it should be an extension of life in the wider community.

> 'Aged care should be an extension of life in the wider community.'

The ten principles of the Eden Alternative

The Eden Alternative is guided by ten principles.

1. The three plagues of loneliness, helplessness, and boredom account for the bulk of suffering in a human community.
2. Life in a truly human community revolves around close and continuing contact with children, plants, and animals. These ancient relationships provide young and old alike with a pathway to a life worth living.
3. Loving companionship is the antidote to loneliness. In a human community, we must provide easy access to human and animal companionship.
4. To give care to another makes us stronger. To receive care gracefully is a pleasure and an art. A healthy human community promotes both of these virtues in its daily life, seeking always to balance one with the other.
5. Trust in each other allows us the pleasure of answering the needs of the moment. When we fill our lives with variety and spontaneity, we honour the world and our place in it.
6. Meaning is the food and water that nourishes the human spirit. It strengthens us. The counterfeits of meaning tempt us with hollow promises. In the end, they always leave us empty and alone.
7. Medical treatment should be the servant of genuine human caring, never its master.
8. In a human community, the wisdom of the elders grows in direct proportion to the honour and respect accorded to them.
9. Human growth must never be separated from human life.
10. Wise leadership is the lifeblood of any struggle against the three plagues. For it there can be no substitute.

The three stages of the Eden Alternative

There are three stages for the introduction of the Eden Alternative:

▶ vision;
▶ education; and
▶ implementation.

Vision

Before any changes can occur in an organisation, passion, knowledge, and vision need to come from the directors or board of management. These people need to:

▶ understand the 'soul' of the business;
▶ research, understand, and accept the Eden Alternative principles and culture change;
▶ plan a budget;
▶ have the ability to develop a strategic plan;
▶ develop a learning culture;
▶ communicate the vision and philosophy; and
▶ actively participate in person-centred planning, learning circles, and other innovative concepts.

Education

The educational process needs to be planned and must be communicated to the residents and their families, as well as to staff, service providers, and volunteers. To be informed and empowered unites all stakeholders on this journey. Everyone needs to understand the vision and understand the benefits and challenges that exist.

Members of the wider community can make a valuable contribution—including veterinarians, animal trainers, gardeners, teachers, and so on.

Implementation

This process involves the introduction of animals, plants, and children, along with the empowerment of residents, staff, and others to develop a human habitat in which all would want to live. There is a need to promote individual growth for everyone on this never-ending journey. It is important at this stage to develop some baseline data so that it is possible to measure the results of 'Edenising'.

Introduction of animals

Animals are introduced into the home after a thorough planning process and the development of a pet-care plan. Good planning will eliminate the potential for problems in the implementation process. An Eden Alternative committee can be established to research and plan for the introduction of animals in consultation with all people involved. Often there will be some objections from staff or residents who do not like certain animals or claim to be allergic to animal hair. These are common concerns. However, with more than 300 homes fully committed to the Eden Alternative, this issue has been successfully addressed and overcome. Staff members and residents who are allergic to animals should have *no contact* with the animals. Although allergy to animals has not been a problem in the experience of aged-care accommodation facilities that have adopted the Eden Alternative, it is wise for nurses to ensure that residents at risk are not exposed to possible allergy or to unwanted contact with animals.

Fresh air and good housekeeping practices are also important in reducing the potential for adverse reactions. Should a resident have a fear of cats, for example, a water pistol works very well. However, animals appear to sense fear, and generally respond to people who like them.

Residents are permitted to bring pets of their own into the facility. However, a trial period is adopted to ensure that the environment remains harmonious for everyone. Any such pet remains with the resident concerned, and is not expected to be shared as an 'Eden pet'.

All pets undergo aggression testing for suitability. Puppies and kittens are not accepted because their personalities need to develop in a smaller, one-owner environment before being involved in a wider environment. Pets of 3–4 years of age are best for all concerned. Lap dogs are generally more appropriate for the elderly.

Criteria to consider with the residents are:

▶ preference of animal;
▶ safety;
▶ expense to purchase and train; and
▶ maintenance issues.

Residents in our care state that they are happier, healthier, and calmer. And they take on the responsibility of caring for the pet with enthusiasm.

> 'Residents take on the responsibility of caring for the pet with enthusiasm.'

Introduction of plants

This is perhaps the easiest and cheapest component of the Eden Alternative to introduce. Residents can be asked about their favourite plants. They can be asked for cuttings that can be propagated, planted, and raised in garden beds. Seedlings are economical and are practical for the residents to tend to. Having indoor plants is very important so that residents can appreciate the aroma, beauty, and growth of the plant on a daily basis. Artificial plants are not acceptable because they do not offer the same benefits and there is no sense of empowerment in caring for them in a meaningful way.

Vegetable gardens are always popular—especially given the current interest in organic home-grown foods. Some plants are not suitable for various reasons, so professional advice should be sought before planting.

> 'Plants lift the human spirit, provide a therapeutic perfume, and visually enhance the environment.'

Plants provide an opportunity for residents to give care. They lift the human spirit, provide a therapeutic perfume, and visually enhance the environment. Residents with dementia appreciate the benefits of a garden, and gain enjoyment from the indoor and outdoor experience

Introduction of children

This component of the Eden Alternative is perhaps the most challenging and time-consuming. However, the effort is very rewarding for staff, residents, and the children.

In the past, schoolchildren have been introduced into aged-care facilities as a 'token' to sing songs at Christmas time or to deliver Easter eggs. These are pleasant experiences while they last. However, they merely reinforce the isolation that exists for these residents once the children have gone. The Eden Alternative involves children in the aged-care facility on a daily basis in a meaningful way. It is recommended that animals and plants be introduced into the home before the children because animals and plants provide an environment for the children that is vibrant, interesting, fun, and comfortable.

Children should initially be introduced in a limited and planned manner such that they are woven into the daily activities of the residents. Children of various ages should be introduced, and the activities in which they are involved should also be varied—such that spontaneity and diversity provide stimulus for all participants.

Organisations and groups that can be contacted to join the program are:
- local primary schools;
- secondary schools;
- Scouts and Guides;
- after-school programs;
- church playgroups;

- childcare and pre-school groups;
- children of staff members; and
- grandchildren.
  The benefits for the children include:
- one-to-one caring;
- sharing of knowledge;
- respect for the elderly;
- ability to teach;
- empathy for people with disabilities;
- friendship;
- sharing of life experiences;
- listening skills; and
- valuing giving and receiving.
  The benefits for the residents include:
- one-to-one caring;
- sharing of knowledge;
- empowerment;
- friendship;
- sharing of life experiences;
- stimulation; and
- the ability to give and receive companionship.

Residents with dementia usually love interaction with children and babies. Doll therapy often works well for some residents, so the 'real thing' must be beneficial on a daily basis. Children often read aloud to residents with dementia, play board games, paint, dance to music, and develop special relationships.

Children learn about respect for the elderly, as well as learning about life and death. One facility was anxious about how young children would cope with the death of a resident. However, the ability of the young to cope should never be underestimated. Grief and loss were acknowledged, and death was accepted as an inevitable part of life.

Intergenerational experiences enrich life and promote personal growth through acceptance of each other.

Eden Alternative data

Research results from Southwest Texas State University's two-year study of homes that adopted the Eden Alternative (Ransom 2000) show:

- a 60% decrease in behavioural incidents;
- a 57% decrease in pressure sores (stage 1 and stage 2);

◗ an 18% decrease in use of restraint;
◗ an 8% increase in chairbound residents;
◗ a 25% decrease in bedfast residents;
◗ a 48% decrease in staff absenteeism; and
◗ an 11% decrease in employee injuries.

Culture change

Many organisations are searching for an alternative to the institutional medical model in residential aged care. With the introduction of the Eden Alternative and Culture Change, we are changing our environments to include the following:

◗ small, personal communities;
◗ plants and flowers;
◗ dogs, cats, birds, fish, and furry friends;
◗ children, family, friends, and neighbours;
◗ music;
◗ fun, laughter, and spontaneity;
◗ familiar caregivers, a person-centred approach, and a model of self-directed work teams and learning circles.

Changing the culture of aged care is about personal conversion at all levels of the organisation. Hierarchy barriers are flattened so that responsibility, recognition, and value are bestowed on the team.

According to Norton (2003), there are six phases of Culture Change.

◗ *Phase I The study circle:* This first step requires high involvement to assess an organisation and to investigate social models that are working inside the profession.

◗ *Phase II The design team:* In this step, the changes that are possible are determined, given the financial resources and unique characteristics of the organisation.

◗ *Phase III Skills assessment and development:* The key to success is to create a learning climate within the organisation in which leaders are inspired to help others to learn and grow.

◗ *Phase IV Team development:* This step is an ongoing process and gives decision-making authority to self-directed work teams that are close to the residents.

◗ *Phase V Implementation:* This step is the final dividing line between the old way and the new. When an organisation crosses this line, it wants everyone stepping over together, hand in hand.

▶ *Phase VI Evaluation:* This is the final stage when established baseline data for continuous quality improvement (CQI) indicators are identified in the study circle and are compared with new data that the organisation have been tracking.

Routines

It is difficult for residents entering an aged-care facility, particularly those suffering with dementia, to adjust to a new environment, new routines, and new carers, and to deal with the grief and loss of their homes, lifestyles, and frequent contact with family.

The daily lives of people in the general community do not revolve around the same routine day in day out, 365 days a year. In aged care, life should be spontaneous and diverse, and should involve minimal routine. Residents with dementia can have poor self-esteem, restricted communication skills, and a lack of opportunity to make decisions. They can feel pressured by routines. It is important to educate staff and families about breaking out of routines, and it is important that they be provided with an explanation of the desirability of an altered lifestyle. Residents do not want to be rushed under the shower at designated times, bustled into the dining area to eat or drink because it is morning tea time, or woken from a 'catnap' because some people believe that they won't sleep at night. If such residents were residing in their own homes, they would 'potter around' enjoying their daily life pleasures.

Daily pleasures are things that are important to people and make them feel good each day. They include playing with the dog, talking to children, the first cup of tea for the day, and reading the paper in bed on weekends.

> 'If residents were residing in their own homes, they would 'potter around' enjoying their daily life pleasures.'

The following are questions that can be asked of a resident with dementia (or his or her representative) in an aged-care facility:

▶ What are some of your daily pleasures?
▶ Thinking about the little things in your day, what do you enjoy the most each day?
▶ What little things would make your life more enjoyable?

Changing the routine allows for the enjoyment of daily pleasures that provide people with their inner well-being. Residents with dementia have the same needs and desires but cannot always express them. Rather, their frustrations are often displayed as behavioural problems.

Staff

For a long time nurses and carers in aged care have been subject to routines in their daily work lives, and to change this culture requires education, constant reinforcement, and support. In the traditional aged-care setting, with many residents requiring assistance with their activities of daily living, it is quicker for carers to perform the daily tasks for residents rather than encouraging independence and empowerment. If a large group is segregated into small communities of 'like' people, empowerment increases and there is more quality time available for the staff members to spend with residents. Permanently assigned staff members have an opportunity to learn the idiosyncrasies of individuals, and residents with dementia have the stability of recognising (and trusting) familiar faces.

Teamwork is about valuing and treating each other as key assets, recognising the opportunity for a learning climate, and acknowledging the emotional needs of staff members. Self-directed work teams have proved to be very successful in changing the culture. Staff are encouraged to self-roster to accommodate their lifestyle. Rather than rotating throughout different communities, staff can nominate the community of preference to work in, thus encouraging the development of valuable relationships with residents and fellow staff members. Because staff members know residents well through such a work environment, there is a significant decrease in time that would otherwise be wasted by having to assess each individual resident's daily needs.

> 'Valuing each team member assists in building a friendly, inspired, unified, and motivated team.'

Valuing each team member daily assists in building a friendly, inspired, unified, and motivated team.

Residents

All decisions in aged care should be based on a person-centred approach whereby choice and decision-making routinely occur through the resident or people closest to the resident.

With the community model, some residents voluntarily assist other residents when appropriate, and their self-esteem and self-worth can improve as a result.

A real sense of belonging and ownership of the community develops. Recently, a group of residents who wanted to be supportive of a friend during palliative care chose to sit with this person, hold hands, read to the person, and pray together. Imagine the peace and reassurance this must have provided for the dying resident—to be among friends and to die with love and companionship. This process also allows for residents to grieve for their loss in an active and supportive manner. The community model and culture change allows for the giving and receiving of the human spirit.

Families

To accept the Eden Alternative and a Change in Culture can be challenging for some family members who already have had to deal with many changes relating to their loved one. Children often grieve for the loss of caring for a parent. If the person is suffering from dementia, children can also grieve for the loss of the parent as an authoritative figure. However, role reversal has to take place, and families need to understand that, although a person with dementia might appear childlike at times, the person should still be valued for his or her personality and lifetime experiences. In this way, his or her self-esteem can be affirmed. Education and active participation of families is encouraged so that useful skills are developed for effective communication and worthwhile interactions.

The most important people in an elderly person's life are his or her family and, although roles have changed, this is a great opportunity for families to make a difference in the life of their loved one. It is a time to learn new skills, enrich their loved one's life, and give of themselves to strengthen the bond at a time of need. To be involved in a special community of special people has its own rewards, and to be empowered as part of the care team is a great privilege for everyone.

In the traditional aged-care facility, the environment, the processes, and the atmosphere are not as friendly as they might be. By introducing animals, plants, children, small communities, and a change in culture, the aged-care model has been revolutionised to focus on a person-centred approach with self-directed work teams.

The organisational hierarchical structure has been levelled out, and recognition has been given to the fact that everyone has a valuable contribution to make in changing the culture in aged care.

Chapter 24

Dementia Care Mapping

Virginia Moore

Introduction

Dementia care mapping (DCM) is a structured observational method for recording what a person with dementia is engaged in, and the quality of his or her response to that engagement. Observations are measurable and can be presented in quantifiable terms.

DCM is a tool that refines the observer's skills to look at events through the eyes of the person with dementia. Data are collected and are used to reflect on the care that is being provided—in particular, whether that care reflects the principles of person-centred care as described by Kitwood (1997a, 1997b).

The value of DCM is that it provides evidence-based data for improvements in both individual care-planning and wider manage-ment decisions. DCM also has a

'The value of DCM is that it provides evidence-based data for improvements in individual care-planning and wider management decisions.'

significant influence on the awareness of individual care workers in their personal approaches to care practices (Barnett 1995).

Underlying philosophy

Kitwood's person-centred theory was based, in part, on psychotherapeutic approaches developed from the 1950s onwards—among them the work of Rogers (1961). Rogers' explorations of a theory of personality led him to the concept of 'client-centred care', in which the therapist took on the role of facilitator or companion, rather than that of an expert with the answers. Rogers' theory fostered the idea that a therapist walked alongside people, accepting the uniqueness of each person and the importance of each person's feelings and experiences. It was essentially a non-judgmental approach to therapy. Morton (1999, p. 12) outlined how these principles, as developed by Rogers, can be applied to a person-centred approach in dementia care.

In developing his approach, Kitwood challenged the concept that the signs and symptoms of dementia are purely a result of neurological damage, and that they should therefore be 'managed' only as the manisfestations of an organic disease. Rather, he suggested that a much broader spectrum of factors was contributing to the signs and symptoms of dementia. The significance of the neuropathological changes was not denied, but Kitwood's approach included psychological and social factors in addition to physical factors (Morton 1999).

When put together this theory forms what is essentially an equation (Kitwood 1993):

$$D = NI + PH + B + P + SE$$

in which:

D = dementia
NI = neurological impairment
PH = physical health
B = biography of the person
P = personality of the person
SE = social environment of the person

These factors are explored in greater detail below. However, before describing these, another factor deserves to be considered for inclusion in the equation. The physical and sensory environment also has an effect on the functional capacity of people with dementia and their resultant behavioural responses (Calkins 1998). Anecdotal evidence supports the contention that pleasant, less-institutionalised physical surroundings promote physical and emotional well-being. For this reason, a sixth contributing factor can be added to Kitwood's equation—that of the physical sensory environment (PSE).

The equation now becomes:

$$D = NI + PH + B + P + SE + PSE$$

All of these factors are now considered in more detail.

Neurological impairment

It is accepted, given the current state of knowledge in this area, that the neuropathological changes of dementia are irreversible. Much research has been done, and several types of medication are now available that improve cognitive function in the initial stages of dementia. However cognitive impairment, from a day-to-day care perspective, is a factor that must be accepted and worked with. Good medical diagnosis and ongoing monitoring are essential. However, in isolation, these are not sufficient for good care.

Physical health

Older people have an increased susceptibility to a number of health problems, including arthritis, cardiovascular disease, and certain infections. Many people with dementia also have longstanding physical problems or have developed problems after the onset of dementia. Difficulty in clearly verbalising their needs puts these people at increased risk of having their physical health needs overlooked or mismanaged. Simple needs can be at risk. For example, inadequate fluid intake can lead to constipation and increased agitation. Similarly, unrelieved pain can cause agitation, perceived non-compliance, and resistance to care. The story of Mr X (Box, page 301) is one such example of pain affecting behaviour.

Insightful management of physical health promotes emotional and physical well-being. However, if the physical problems of people with dementia are mismanaged, or not recognised, these physical factors exacerbate the symptoms of dementia (Kitwood 1997b).

Biography

All lives are shaped by background history and critical incidents in the past. Being aware of some of the losses and stresses experienced by people with dementia over their lifetimes can be of assistance in understanding some of the behavioural responses that otherwise have no meaning (Loveday & Kitwood 1998). Collecting and sharing this knowledge is critical.

A change in behaviour explained

Over the past 4–5 weeks, Mr X had become reluctant to sit down and was walking about incessantly, both day and night. It was difficult to get him to sit for meals and he was constantly getting in the way of other residents.

When time was taken to talk with Mr X, it became clear that he was expressing discomfort about something. His conversation was very jumbled, but he was trying to explain something in his own way. When staff members discussed his problem and checked his health record, it was noted that Mr X had suffered a minor fall, with no apparent injury, just before the onset of the increased walking. Further investigation revealed a fractured coccyx.

Quite simply, Mr X found sitting or lying too painful. His only alternative was to walk. Because he was confused, he often invaded other people's rooms or personal space—thus precipitating reactions that required staff to intervene. When good pain management was provided, Mr X settled very well.

Personality

The personality of a person with dementia has developed over his or her lifetime and is reflected in how that person now reacts to stress. How people cope with stress, and the personal resources and strengths that they have to draw on, affect how people deal with the experience of increasing loss of self and identify. It is critical that nurses learn as much about these matters as possible to help them understand individual responses.

Social environment

People create a certain interactive, social 'atmosphere' by the way in which they respond to, and communicate with, others. The dynamics created by individual interactive styles can make a person feel valued or devalued. What people say and do, and how they say and do it, have direct effects on the emotional well-being of others. The social environment thus created can support or undermine a person's sense of personal value.

Personal and sensory environment

People respond to information from the physical environment by adapting their behaviour. This response is based on prior learning and recognition of the cues around them. This can occur at a subconscious level and allows people to regulate their responses appropriately to a given situation. For example, a classroom setting gives people cues about the function of the room and the likely required response. In contrast, a lounge room gives people a clear indication of a different function, and thus produces a different response. For people with dementia, the physical environment can be enabling or disabling (Calkins 1996).

Similarly, the sensory environment can be a powerful initiator of positive and negative behavioural responses. An environment devoid of sensory experiences can contribute to withdrawal by the person. Conversely, an enriched sensory environment can elicit responses that might have been previously considered lost (Wylie 2000).

> 'The physical and sensory environments can have a powerful effect on the signs and symptoms of dementia.'

Taken together, the physical and sensory environments can have a powerful effect on the signs and symptoms of dementia. If this issue is ignored, a vital part of the equation is missing.

Personhood

Kitwood defined personhood as 'a standing or status that is bestowed upon one human being by others, in the context of relationships and social being. It implies recognition, respect and trust' (Kitwood 1997b, p. 8). For a person with dementia, this sense of self-identity and personal value is under threat. As his or her cognitive capacity declines, there is an increased need for nurses to reinforce the person's sense of identity by reinforcing feelings of acceptance and belonging. The person needs to be engaged in life in a meaningful way and to be reassured that comfort will be provided when required.

> 'There is an increased need for nurses to reinforce the person's sense of identity by reinforcing feelings of acceptance and belonging.'

It is important that nurses understand that a decline in cognitive capacity does not equate to a decline in 'feeling' capacity. A person with dementia continues to relate emotionally to events and people. The difficulty that he or she experiences is connecting this emotion to the wider context of what is happening—that is, interpreting the emotion at a cognitive level. The person is left with a sense or 'memory' of feelings of acceptance, or rejection, and achievement or failure. The person's behaviour in response to these feelings is dependent on these 'feeling memories'.

All behaviour is thus an attempt to communicate these feelings to others. For people who can no longer use meaningful verbal language to communicate, behaviour is a means of communication. Behaviour understood as communication is a two-way interaction that can often be understood and responded to in a way that supports personhood.

Well-being and ill-being

A person's emotional response to engagement (or lack thereof) can be interpreted as an indicator of his or her personhood being sustained or eroded (Morton 1999). These emotional responses to engagement are measurable (Kitwood 1997b, p. 8). A list of emotional responses that are reliable indicators for people with dementia has been drawn up. This list can be divided into two groups as indicators of well-being and ill-being (see Table 24.1, page 305).

These indicators form a core part of the DCM process, and are the basis of tracking whether personhood is being maintained. The concepts of well-being and ill-being have been found to be of value to care staff in several respects:

▶ the terminology and concepts are quickly grasped and meaningful to staff;
▶ having clear indicators can significantly focus the observations of staff members, thus improving sharing of information and feedback;
▶ the development of a common descriptive language used by all staff members improves the consistency of the information shared;
▶ a conscious looking for well-being can heighten awareness of the significance of these often-overlooked responses; and
▶ identifying well-being has a positive effect on staff, and provides a positive feedback system for desirable care practices.

In summary, the identification of a common language for information-gathering and information-sharing provides nurses with a significant tool.

Personal detractors

Various types of interactions (or relationships) have a damaging effect on people with dementia. These can be termed 'personal detractors'. Such interactions undermine personhood—that is, they devalue the person.

Personal detractors are important in the area of dementia care because these people are unable to remove themselves physically from the environment in which they find themselves, and they are also unable to put the total interaction into a broader context and see the whole picture. Rather, they retain a 'feeling' related to these interactions.

Table 24.1 Bradford Dementia Group indicators of well-being and ill-being

Well-being indicators	Ill-being indicators
Assertiveness or being able to express wishes in an acceptable way	Unattended sadness or grief
Bodily relaxation	Sustained anger
Initiating social contact	Despair
Affection	Boredom
Self-respect (such as being concerned about hygiene, tidiness and appearance)	Anxiety
Helpfulness	Physical discomfort/pain
Humour	Apathy and withdrawal
Creative self-expression (such as singing, dancing or painting)	
Taking pleasure in some aspects of daily life	
Sensitivity to the emotional needs of others	
Expressing a full range of emotions (both positive and negative)	
Acceptance of others who have dementia	

Bradford Dementia Group (1997); published with permission

Examples of personal detractors are:

- *labelling*—for example, referring to someone as 'She's a soft diet', 'These are the dementias', 'He's aggressive', and so on;
- *ignoring*—for example, two nurses talking to each other over a person's head while showering him or her;
- *disruption*—for example, pulling a person's chair out from the table (from behind the person) without telling him or her what the nurse is intending to do;
- *intimidation*—using threats to seek compliance: for example, 'There's no breakfast until you've finished dressing';

▶ *accusation*—blaming a person for actions that are due to disability: for example, 'Oh you've spilt your drink again'; and
▶ *outpacing*—giving a person information at a pace that leaves him or her bewildered and excluded.

Personal detractions should not seen as deliberate acts of malice on the part of staff. They often pass completely unnoticed, but they have a negative cumulative effect. For example, if a person is repeatedly 'outpaced' over several weeks, it is likely this person will respond with the following signs of ill-being:

▶ withdrawing and becoming less responsive;
▶ becoming more agitated;
▶ walking constantly;
▶ becoming distressed; and/or
▶ becoming angry and frustrated.

Table 24.2 lists 17 personal detractors that impact negatively on personhood.

Table 24.2 Bradford Dementia Group interactions that undermine personhood

Interaction	Description
Treachery	Using some form of deception in order to distract or manipulate a person, or force them into compliance.
Disempowerment	Not allowing people to use the abilities that they do have: failing to help them to complete actions that they have initiated.
Infantilisation	Treating a person patronisingly (as an insensitive parent might treat a young child).
Intimidation	Inducing fear in a person, through the use of threats or physical power
Labelling	Using a pattern of behaviour (for example, 'wanderer') or a category (such as 'dementias') as the main basis for describing and interacting with a person.
Stigmatisation	Treating a person as if he or she were a diseased object, an alien, or an outcast.
Outpacing	Providing information, presenting choices, and so on at a rate too fast for the person to understand; putting people under pressure to do things more rapidly than they can bear.

(Continued)

Table 24.2 Bradford Dementia Group interactions that undermine personhood (*Continued*)

Interaction	Description
Invalidation	Failing to acknowledge the subjective reality of a person's experience and especially what he or she is feeling.
Banishment	Sending a person away or excluding him or her physically or psychologically.
Objectification	Treating a person as if he or she were a lump of dead matter to be pushed, lifted, or filled—without proper reference to the fact that this person is a sentient being.
Ignoring	Carrying on (in conversation or action) in the presence of a person as if that person were not there.
Imposition	Forcing a person to do something, overriding desire, or denying the possibility of choice.
Accusation	Blaming the person for actions (or failures of action) that arise from the person's lack of ability or misunderstanding of the situation
Disruption	Roughly intruding on a person's action or inaction; crudely breaking that person's 'frame of reference'.
Mockery	Making fun of a person's 'strange' actions or remarks; teasing; humiliating; making jokes at a person's expense.
Disparagement	Telling a person that he or she is incompetent, useless, worthless, and so on; giving messages that are damaging to a person's self esteem.

Adapted from Bradford Dementia Group (1997); published with permission

Methods and results of DCM

DCM is a system for collecting and analysing data to reflect a person's response to engagement—that is, what the person is *doing* and how he or she *feels* about that activity. Observations are recorded every five minutes—based on the behaviour in which the person was predominantly engaged during this timeframe. A list of 24 behaviour codes is available and the choice of code is determined according to a predetermined set of rules. For each timeframe, a behaviour category code (BCC) ('what the person was doing') is assigned. The quality of that interaction from the person's perspective is reflected in his or her emotional well-being or ill-being. This is recorded as a well-being or ill-being (WIB) value. WIB values range from +5 to +1 (for well-being) and from −1 to −5 for ill-being.

Four main pieces of information are obtained.

▶ *An individual WIB score and profile:* This can be shown in table or graph format. This reflects the total amount of time that the person spent in each category of well-being or ill-being (for example, 65% in +1, 25% in +3, and 10% in −1).

▶ *A group WIB score and profile:* This shows the percentage of time that the group as a whole spent in each category of well-being or ill-being. This can also be represented in graph format.

▶ *An individual profile of behavioural categories:* This shows the behavioural categories engaged in during the observation period, and clearly shows what the person was doing during the observation period and the percentage of the total time spent in each behavioural category. It also clearly indicates the gaps in a person's opportunity for a variety of engagement.

▶ *A group profile of behavioural categories:* This shows the behavioural categories engaged in during the observation period and reflects the distribution and percentage of time spent in each type of behaviour or activity by the group as a whole.

The uniqueness of DCM lies in its capacity to quantify what the person was 'doing' and how the person was 'feeling', and to represent these in graphs that are easy to read and understand by staff and management alike. They provide a clear picture of the quality of life for the person with dementia from his or her perspective.

In addition, two other items of information are observed and recorded:

▶ *positive events*—instances of positive work by staff members are recorded with comments on the resident's responses; and

▶ *personal detractions*—instances of interaction that detract from personhood are coded and recorded.

An experienced mapper can observe and record up to six people during an observation session. Mapping is carried out only in communal areas (such as the lounge, kitchen, or garden). It is considered unethical to map during episodes of personal care. It is important that mappers remain inconspicuous and 'become part of the furniture' during the observation period.

It is important to ensure that staff members know what is happening during the pre-mapping and post-mapping periods, and that they are made aware of the immediate outcomes. Staff issues and concerns must be taken into consideration by the mapper. This process helps to keep staff involved in the process and helps them to improve continuously.

Results can be presented in a simple format with recommendations for individual and group changes. Alternatively, a full evaluation report can be prepared which includes individual and group care summaries, full graphical analysis, training gap, recommended careplan changes, and suggestions for management support systems.

Practical uses of DCM

DCM data are of significant value in supporting decisions and outcomes in a number of areas. It is difficult for nurses who are in close and constant contact with residents to detach from the task at hand and to reflect on the effect of the care being provided. DCM data enable staff members to see a resident's pattern of engagement during their shift and to reflect on the effect that this has had on the emotional well-being of those in their care.

'DCM data enable staff members to see a resident's pattern of engagement during their shift and to reflect on the effect that this has had on the emotional well-being of those in their care.'

Practical benefits from DCM can be considered as immediate, short term, or long term.

Immediate benefits

Observations can be given to staff immediately following a mapping period. This feedback can outline the positive events that occurred, as well as any episodes of personal detractions.

Feedback on positive effects of interventions can be a powerful morale booster for staff. Understanding the positive benefits for the resident of interactions that are often described as 'just part of the job' reinforces that action. The likelihood of the staff member repeating the action is significantly increased, thereby further enhancing the well-being of the resident. In this way, staff satisfaction and resident well-being reinforce one another in a reciprocal fashion.

Short-term benefits

Following discussion with other team members, changes to care plans can be agreed and made effective immediately. Observations recorded in DCM help to identify gaps in the existing care or areas in which a different approach would be of benefit. Examples include:

- increasing the number of drinks offered to people who are constantly on the move;
- changing mealtime seating arrangements to improve social interaction opportunities among residents;
- checking pressure points in a person who has been sitting for prolonged periods; and
- increasing staff interaction with seated residents by stopping to converse briefly each time a nurse passes by.

These are simple cost-free changes that can be effected immediately, and changes in resident well-being can then be noted and measured. The results of such simple interventions can be significant in terms of increased interaction, decreased agitation, and reduced 'pacing'. Results can also indicate a need to investigate physical signs and symptoms (such as constipation or pain). Changes in patterns of behaviour can then be monitored and compared.

Longer-term benefits

Learning and development plans

The results of DCM can be used to identify gaps in staff training. Programs directly connected to need can thus be planned and instigated. Pre-training and post-training mapping sessions can be held to provide valuable measurements of training effectiveness.

Justification for budget submissions is a constant issue for management. DCM data provide evidence of need and also provide results of any budgetary changes that have been made. This might not necessarily imply spending more money. It might lead to a wise redistribution of existing financial resources.

Anecdotal evidence suggests that DCM is an awareness-raising tool that can directly reduce the number of staff–resident incidents that result in injury to either party.

Research and development

DCM is an effective tool for use in research in dementia care. Users should be properly trained and accredited in all aspects of the use of the tool.

Criticisms

DCM is avaluable tool, but it is being continually reviewed and improved as more research is developed. Some of the main criticisms of DCM are that it is:

▶ time-consuming;
▶ used only in communal areas;
▶ insufficiently sensitive;
▶ subject to error because the presence of a mapper is likely to affect care workers; and
▶ very subjective;
Each of these is discussed below.

Time-consuming

DCM is time-consuming. Data collection of any sort takes time, and the quality and value of data are directly related to the time and resources available. Within the normal work day, mapping periods of 30 minutes have provided valuable insight into responses to specific events (for example, mealtimes). A longer observation period is required for research purposes. Within the direct-care field, short periods of mapping are certainly achievable, and can produce valuable results.

Used only in communal areas

As previously noted, DCM is used only in communal areas because it is considered invasive and unethical to map during times of personal care. However, observations made in a mapping period (in a communal setting) are probably reasonably indicative of the overall care style and practice.

Insufficiently sensitive

DCM is not sufficiently sensitive to record the subtle interactions that occur in people with severe dementia. This is a fair criticism, and the problem is the subject of further research (Perrin 1997).

Presence of mapper likely to affect care workers

Although it is sometimes argued that the presence of mappers will affect care workers, a mapper quietly sitting in a corner and observing is soon forgotten by care workers. They are usually far too busy to be constantly aware of an observer.

Subjective

It has been said that DCM is very subjective. A reliability test has been developed and it is important to use this to ensure that results from different mappers are consistent. Although it is true that DCM is somewhat subjective, DCM uses a disciplined approach to observation, thus reducing the risk (Bradford Dementia Group 1997).

Conclusion

Implementing the principles of person-centred approach to dementia care is a powerful way to raise staff awareness of the needs of people with dementia. Dementia care mapping provides evidence-based data that can be used in conjunction with relevant information to enable changes to be prioritised in a systematic and achievable manner. Against this baseline, improvements can be measured. The adoption of DCM is an investment in the residents, the staff, and the future viability of the organisation. However, whilst there is clear evidence to support the importance and usefulness of DCM, it is important to recognise that some researchers still feel that there are limitations around its use and that there is a clear need to continue to develop the work and look at alternative approaches to learning how to care more effectively for the person with dementia (Adams 1996).

References

Chapter 1 History and Issues

Ebersole, P. & Hess, P. 1998, *Toward Health Ageing—human needs and nursing response*, 5th edn, C.V. Mosby, St Louis.

Koch, S. & Garratt, S. (eds) 2001, *Assessing Older People: a Practical Guide for Health Professionals*, MacLennan & Petty, Sydney.

Nay, R. & Garratt, S. (eds) 1999, *Nursing Older People: Issues and Innovations*, MacLennan & Petty, Sydney.

Stevens, J.A. 1996, *Working with Older People: Do Nurses Care For It?*, University of New South Wales Press, Kensington.

Schultz, B. 1991, *A Tapestry of Service: The evolution of nursing in Australia*, vol. 1, Churchill Livingstone, Melbourne.

Watson, J. 1985, *Nursing: Human Science and Human Care*, Appleton Century Crofts, Norwalk, USA.

Chapter 3 The Whole Person

Coulter, D.L. 2001, 'Recognition of Spirituality in Health Care: Personal and Universal Implications', *Journal of Religion, Disability and Health*, 5(2/3): 1–11.

Emmons, A. 1999, *The Psychology of Ultimate Concerns: Motivation and Spirituality*, The Guilford Press, New York.

Frankl, V. 1967, *Psychotherapy and Existentialism: Selected Papers on Logotherapy*, Washington Square Press, New York.

Frankl, V. 1984, *Man's Search for Meaning*, Washington Square Press, New York.

Gardner, H. 1993, *Multiple Intelligences: The Theory in Practice*, Basic Books, New York.

Gunderson, G. 1997, *Deeply Woven Roots*, Fortress Press, Minneapolis.

Kitwood, T. 1997, *Dementia Reconsidered: The Person Comes First*, Open University Press, Buckingham.

McFadden, S., Ingram, M. & Baldauf, C. 2000, 'Actions, Feelings, and Values: Foundations of Meaning and Personhood in Dementia', in Kimble, M. (ed.), *Viktor Frankl's Contribution to Spirituality and Aging*, pp 67–86, The Haworth Pastoral Press, Binghamton, NY.

Post, S. 2000, *The Moral Challenge of Alzheimer Disease*, 2nd edn, The Johns Hopkins University Press, Baltimore.

Chapter 4 Enriching the Environment

ACCS, see Aged and Community Care Services.

Ackerman, D. 1990, *A Natural History of the Senses*, Phoenix, London.

Adams, P. & Mylander, M. 1993, *Gesundheit! Bringing good health to you, the medical system, and society, through physician service, complementary therapies, humour and joy*, Healing Arts Press, Vermont.

Aged and Community Care Services (ACCS) 1996, *Care needs of people with dementia and challenging behaviour living in residential facilities*, Development and Evaluation Report No. 24, Australian Government Printing Service, Canberra.

Armstrong-Esther, C.A., Browne, K.D. & McAfee, J.G. 1994, 'Elderly patients: still sitting clean and quietly', *Journal of Advanced Nursing*, 19: 264–71.

Bradford Dementia Group 1997, *Evaluating Dementia Care. The DCM Method*, 7th edn, University of Bradford, Bradford.

Brooker, D.J.R. 1997, 'Improving the quality of care for people with dementia', unpublished PhD thesis, University of Birmingham, Birmingham.

Crisp, J. 1995, 'Making sense of the stories that people with Alzheimer's tell: a journey with my mother', *Nursing Inquiry*, 2: 133–40.

Ellis, J. & Thorn, T. 2000, 'Sensory stimulation: where do we go from here?', *The Journal of Dementia Care*, 8(1): 33–7.

Garratt, S. & Hamilton-Smith, E. 1995, *Re-thinking dementia: an Australian approach*, Ausmed Publications, Melbourne.

Häggström, T. & Norberg, A. 1996, 'Maternal thinking in dementia care', *Journal of Advanced Nursing*, 24: 431–8.

Hallberg, I.R., Norberg, A. & Johnsson, K. 1993, 'Verbal interaction during lunch-meal between caregivers and vocally disruptive demented patients, *The American Journal of Alzheimer's Care and Related Disorders & Research*, May/June, 26–32.

Hanson, A. 1992, 'The power of touch', *Geriaction*, 11(3): 12.

Kitwood, T. 1988, 'The technical, the personal, and the framing of dementia', *Social Behaviour*, 9: 161–80.

Kitwood, T. 1993, 'Discover the person, not the disease', *The Journal of Dementia Care*, 1(1): 16–17.

Kitwood, T. 1997, *Dementia reconsidered. The person comes first*, Open University Press, Buckingham.

Lawler, J. 1997, 'Knowing the body and embodiment: methodologies, discourses and nursing', in Lawler, J. (ed.), *The Body in Nursing*, pp 31–51, Churchill Livingstone, Melbourne.

Light, K.M. 1997, 'Florence Nightingale and holistic philosophy', *Journal of Holistic Nursing*, 15(1): 25–40.

Marshall, M. 1996, *"I can't place this place at all". Working with people with dementia and their carers*, Venture Press, Birmingham.

Nash, M. 2000, 'The new science of Alzheimer's', *Time*, July, 17: 49–55.

Newnham, M. 1998, 'The essential effects of aromatherapy', *Nursing Review*, 3(11): 21.

Nightingale, F. 1970, *Notes on Nursing*, first published 1859, Gerald Duckworth & Company Limited, London.

Nolan M, Keady J and Aveyard B. 2001, 'Relationship-centred care is the next logical step', *British Journal of Nursing*, 10(12): 757.

Storr, A. 1992, *Music and the Mind*, HarperCollins Publishers, London.

Sutton, L.J. & Cheston, R. 1997, 'Rewriting the story of dementia: a narrative approach to psychotherapy with people with dementia', in Marshall, M. (ed.), *State of the Art in Dementia Care*, pp 159–63, Centre of Policy on Ageing, London.

Walton, J.A. & Madjar, I. 1999, 'Phenomenology and nursing', in Madjar, I. & Walton, J.A. (eds), *Nursing and the Experience of Illness*, pp 1–16, Allen & Unwin, St Leonards, New South Wales, Australia.

Willcocks, S. 1994, 'Snoezelen in elderly care', *British Journal of Occupational Therapy*, 57(6): 242.

Wylie, K. 2000, 'Valuing sensation and sentience in dementia care', unpublished PhD thesis, University of Newcastle, New South Wales, Australia.

Zingmark, K., Norberg, A. & Sandman, P. 1993, 'Experience of at-homeness and homesickness in patients with Alzheimer's disease', *The American Journal of Alzheimer's Care and Related Disorders & Research*, 8: 10–16.

Chapter 6 Nutrition

Crombie, L. & Kemp, A. 1999, *Special Care for People with Dementia in Non-Specialist Residential Units: Two examples*, Dementia Services Development Centre, Stirling, Scotland.

Dewing, J. 1996, 'Patients' and nurses' experiences of feeding: a phenomenological study', in Biley, F.C. & Maggs, C., *Contemporary Issues in Nursing*, pp 113–69, Churchill Livingstone, Edinburgh.

Gresham, M. 1999, 'The heart of the home—but how are kitchens used?', *Journal of Dementia Care*, March/April 20–23.

Hiatt, L.G. 1995, 'Understanding the Physical Environment', *Pride Institute Journal of Long-Term Care*, 4 (2) 12–22.

Knocker, S. 2001, 'The right mix of ingredients: working alongside care staff', *Journal of Dementia Care*, 9(4) 20–2.

Newton, L. & Stewart, A. 1997, *Finger foods for independence for people with Alzheimer's disease and others who experience eating difficulties*, Creative State, Adelaide.

VOICES 1998, *Eating well for older people with dementia: a good practice guide for residential and nursing homes and others involved in caring for older people with dementia*, VOICES, Potters Bar, Herts, UK.

Walker, J. & Higginson, C. 2000, *The nutrition of elderly people and nutritional aspects of their care in long-term care settings*, Final Audit Report 1997–2000, CRAG, Glenrothes.

Chapter 7 Wandering

Algase, D.L. 1999, 'Wandering: A dementia-compromised behavior', *Journal of Gerontological Nursing*, 25(9): 10–16.

Algase, D.L., Beck, C. & Kolanowski, A. 1996, 'Need-driven dementia-compromised behavior: an alternative view of disruptive behavior', *American Journal of Alzheimer's Disease*, 11(6): 10–19.

Algase, D.L., Kupferschmid, B., Beel-Bates, C. & Beattie, E.R.A. 1997, 'Estimates of stability of daily wandering behavior among cognitively impaired long-term care residents', *Nursing Research*, 46(3): 172–8.

Allan, K. 1994, 'Dementia in acute units: wandering', *Nursing Standard*, 9(8): 32–4.

Arno, S. & Frank, D.I. 1994, 'A group for "wandering" institutionalized clients with primary degenerative dementia', *Perspectives in Psychiatry Care*, 30(3): 13–16.

Cantes, S. & Rigby, P. 1997, 'Freedom to wander safely', *Elderly Care*, 9(4): 8–10.

Cohen-Mansfield, J., Werner, P., Marx, M.S. & Freedman, L. 1991, 'Two studies of pacing in the nursing home', *Journal of Gerontology*, 46(3): M77–M83.

Cohen-Mansfield, J. & Werner, P. 1998, 'The effects of an enhanced environment on nursing home residents who pace', *The Gerontologist*, 38(2): 199–208.

Coltharp, W. (Jr), Richie, M.F. & Kaas, M.J. 1996, 'Wandering', *Journal of Gerontological Nursing*, 22(11): 5–10.

Dickinson, J.I. & McLain-Kark, J. 1998, 'Wandering behavior and attempted exits among residents diagnosed with dementia-related illnesses: a qualitative approach', *Journal of Women & Aging*, 10(2): 23–34

Donat, D.C. 1984, 'Modifying wandering behavior: a case study', *Clinical Gerontologist*, 3: 41–3.

Frolik, L.A. 2000, 'Nursing home liability because of resident wandering and elopement', *Health Care Law Monthly*, 15–18.

Heard, K. & Watson, T.S. 1999, 'Reducing wandering by persons with dementia using differential reinforcement', *Journal of Applied Behavior Analysis*, 32(3): 381–4.

Heim, K.M. 1986, 'Wandering behavior', *Journal of Gerontological Nursing*, 12(11): 4–7.

Henderson, V.W., Mack, W. & Williams, B.W. 1989, 'Spatial disorientation in Alzheimer's disease', *Archives of Neurology*, 46: 391–4.

Hewawasam, L.C. 1996, 'The use of two-dimensional grid patterns to limit hazardous ambulation in elderly patients with Alzheimer's disease', *NT Research*, 1 (3): 217–27.

Hiatt, L.G. 1985, 'Interventions and people who wander—contradictions in practice', *Gerontologist*, 25: 253.

Hoffman, S.B., Platt, C.A. & Barry, K.E. 1987, 'Managing the difficult dementia patient: the impact on untrained nursing home staff', *American Journal of Alzheimer's Care and Related Disorders Research*, 2(4): 26–31.

Holmberg, S.K. 1997, 'A walking program for wanderers: volunteer training and development of an evening walker's group, *Geriatric Nursing*, 18(4): 160–5.

Hope, T., Tilling, K.M., Gedling, K., Keene, J.M., Cooper, S.D. & Fairburn, C.G. 1994, 'The structure of wandering in dementia', *International Journal of Geriatric Psychiatry*, 9: 149–55.

Hope, T., Keene, J., McShane, R.H., Fairburn, C.G., Gedling, K. & Jacoby, R. 2001, 'Wandering in dementia: a longitudinal study', *International Psychogeriatrics*, 13(2): 137–47.

Hussian, R.A. 1982, 'Stimulus control in the modification of problematic behavior in elderly institutionalized patients', *International Journal of Behavioral Geriatrics*, 1(1): 33–46.

Hussian, R.A. 1985, 'Severe Behavioral Problems, in Teri, L. and Lewinsohn P (eds), *Geropsychological Assessment and Treatment*, pp 121–43, Springer, New York.

Hussian, R.A. & Brown, D.C. 1987, 'Use of two-dimensional grid patterns to limit hazardous ambulation in demented patients', *Journal of Gerontology*, 42(5): 558–60.

Kiely, D.K., Morris, J.N. & Algase, D.L. 2000, 'Resident characteristics associated with wandering in nursing homes', *International Journal of Geriatric Psychiatry*, 15: 1013–20.

Martino-Saltzman, D., Blasch, B.B., Morris, R.D. & McNeal, L.W. 1991, 'Travel behavior of nursing home residents perceived as wanderers and nonwanderers', *The Gerontologist*, 31(5): 666–72.

Mayer, R. & Darby, S.T. 1991, 'Does a mirror deter wandering in demented older people?', *International Journal of Geriatric Psychiatry*, 6: 607–9.

McEvoy, C.L. & Patterson, R.L. 1986, 'Behavioral treatment of deficit skills in dementia patients', *Gerontologist*, 26(5): 475–8.

McGrowder-Lin, R. & Bhatt A. 1988, 'A wanderer's lounge program for nursing home residents with Alzheimer's disease', *The Gerontologist*, 28(5): 607–9.

McShane, R., Hope, T. & Wilkinson, J. 1994, 'Tracking patients who wander: ethics and technology', *The Lancet*, 343 (8908): 1274.

McShane, R., Gedling, K., Keene, J., Fairburn, C., Jacoby, R. & Hope, T. 1998, 'Getting lost in dementia: a longitudinal study of a behavioral symptom', *International Psychogeriatrics*, 10(3): 253–60.

McShane, R., Gedling, K., Kenward, B., Kenward, R., Hope, T. & Jacoby, R. 1998, 'The feasibility of electronic tracking devices in dementia: A telephone survey and case series', *International Journal of Geriatric Psychiatry*, 13: 556–3.

Meguro, K., Yamaguchi, S., Yamazaki, H., Itoh, M., Yamaguchi, T., Matsui, H. & Sasaki, H. 1996, 'Cortical glucose metabolism in psychiatric wandering patients with vascular dementia', *Psychiatry Research: Neuroimaging*, 67: 71–80.

Namazi, K.H., Rosner, T.T., Calkins, M.P. 1989, 'Visual barriers to prevent ambulatory Alzheimer's patients from exiting through an emergency door', *The Gerontologist*, 29(5): 699–702.

Negley, E.N., Molla, P.M. & Obenchain, J. 1990, 'No exit: the effects of an electronic security system on confused patients', *Journal of Gerontological Nursing*, 16(8): 21–5.

Nissen, M.J., Corkin, S., Buonanno, F.S., Growdon, J.H., Wray, S.H. & Bauer, J. 1985, 'Spatial vision in Alzheimer's disease. General findings and a case report', *Archives of Neurology*, 42(7): 667–71.

Price, J.D., Hermans, D.G. & Grimley Evan, J. 2001, 'Subjective barriers to prevent wandering of cognitively impaired people' (Cochrane Review), in *The Cochrane Library*, Issue 4, 2001, Update Software, Oxford.

Rader, J., Doan, J. & Schwab, M. 1985, 'How to decrease problem wandering, a form of agenda behavior', *Geriatric Nursing*, 6(4): 196–9.

Robb, S. 1985, 'Exercise treatment for wandering behavior' (Abstract), *Gerontologist*, 25: 136.

Schiff, M.R. 1990, 'Designing environments for individuals with Alzheimer's disease: some general principles', *The American Journal of Alzheimer's Care and Related Disorders & Research*, 5(3): 4–8.

Schlotterer, G., Moscovitch, M. & Crapper-McLachlan, D. 1983, 'Visual processing deficits as assessed by spatial frequency contrast sensitivity and backward masking in normal ageing and Alzheimer's disease,' *Brain*, 107: 309–25.

Snyder, L.H., Rupprecht, P., Pyrek, J., Brekhus, S. & Moss, T. 1978, 'Wandering', *The Gerontologist*, 18(3): 272–80.

Szwabo, P., Woodward, V., Grossberg, G.T. & Shen, W.W. 1991, 'The use of alprazolam for decreasing problem wandering in geriatric patients', *The American Journal of Alzheimer's Care and Related Disorders & Research*, 6: 33–6.

Taft, L.B., Delaney, K., Seman, D. & Stansell, J. 1993, 'Dementia care: creating a therapeutic milieu', *Journal of Gerontological Nursing*, 19(10): 30–9.

Teri, L., Larson, E.B. & Reifler, B.V. 1988, 'Behavioral disturbance in dementia of the Alzheimer's type, *Journal of the American Geriatrics Society*, 36: 1–6.

Chapter 8 Sensory Loss

Erber, N.P. & Osborn, R. 1994, 'Perception of facial cues by adults with low vision', *Journal of Vision Impairment and Blindness*, 88, pp 171–5.

Hickson, L., Lind, C., Worral, L., Yiu, E., Barnett, H. & Lovie-Kitchin, J. 1999, 'Hearing and Vision in Healthy Older Australians: Objective and Self-Report Measures', *Advances in Speech-Language Pathology*, 1: 2, pp 95–105.

Horowitz, A. 1994, 'Vision Impairment and functional disability among nursing home residents', *The Gerontologist*, 34, pp 316–23.

Horowitz, A., Teresi, J. & Cassels, L. 1991, 'Development of a vision screening questionnaire for older people', *Journal of Vision Impairment and Blindness*, 74, pp 42–4.

Klein, R., Klein, B. & Lee, K. 1996, 'The changes in visual acuity in a population: The Beaver Dam Eye Study', *Ophthalmology*, 103 pp. 1169–78.

Lindeman, H.E. & Platenburg-Gits, F.A. 1991, 'Communicative skills of the very old in old peoples homes', *Acta Otolaryngologica Suppl.*, 476, pp 232–8.

Osborn, R.R., Erber, N.P., Rapson, W-M., Galetti, A. & Bennett, J. 2000, 'Effects of background noise on the perception of speech by sighted older adults and older adults with severe low vision', *Journal of Vision Impairment and Blindness*, 94, pp 648–53.

Roper, T.A. 1995, 'The Use of Deaf-aid Communicators in a Salford Hospital: A Failure of Communication?', *Age and Ageing*, 24, pp 160–2.

Tesch-Romer, C. 1997, 'Psychological effects of hearing aid use in older adults', *Journal of Gerontology: Psychological Sciences*, 52B, pp 127–38.

Voeks, S.K., Gallagher, C.M., Lanter, E.H. & Drinka, P.J. 1993, 'Self-reported hearing difficulty and audiometric thresholds in nursing home residents', *The Journal of Family Practice*, vol. 36, pp 54–8. .

Chapter 9 Communication

Crisp, J. 2000, *Keeping in Touch with Someone Who has Alzheimer's*, Ausmed Publications, Melbourne.

Gibb, H. 1990, 'This is what we have to do—are you OK?', Deakin University Institute of Nursing Research, Geelong.

Kitwood, T. 1997, *Dementia Reconsidered*, Open University Press, Buckingham.

Schwartz, M., Marin, O.W.S.M, & Saffran, E.M. 1979, 'Dissociation of language function in dementia; a case study', *Brain and Language*, 7: 277–306.

Touchebeuf, A. 1987, 'La communication verbale entrenue par les personnes âgées démentes': introduction à une approche linguistique pragmatique, *Revue Française de Psychiatrie*, 4: 40–4.

Chapter 10 Restraint

Clarke, A. & Bright, L. 2002, *Showing Restraint*, Counsel and Care, London.

Douglas, M. 1992, *Risk and Blame: Essays in Cultural Theory*, Routledge, London.

Etzioni, A. 1992, 'Normative-affective factors: Toward a new decision making model', in *Decision Making Alternatives to Rational Choice Models*, Zey, M. (ed.), pp 89–111, Park Sage Publications, Newbury.

Furniss, L., Burns, A. & Craig, S.K.L., Scobie, S., Cooke, J. & Faragher, B. 2000, 'Effects of a pharmacist's medication review in nursing homes', *British Journal of Psychiatry*, 176: 563–67.

Gallinagh, R., Nevin, R., McIllroy, D., Mitchell, F., Campbell, L., Ludwick, R. & McKenna, H. 2002, 'The use of physical restraints as a safety measure in the care of older people in four rehabilitation wards: findings from an exploratory study', *International Journal of Nursing Studies*, 39(2): 147–56.

Gallinagh, R., Slevin, E. & McCormack, B. 2001, 'Side rails as physical restraints: the need for appropriate assessment', *Nursing Older People*, 13(7): 22–8.

Hantikainen, V. & Silvia, R. 2000, 'Using restraint with nursing home residents: a qualitative study of nursing staff perceptions and decision-making', *Journal of Advanced Nursing* 32(5): 1196–205.

Kemshall, H. 2002, *Risk, social policy and welfare*, Open University Press, Buckingham.

Killick, J. 1994, *Please give me back my personality!*, DSDC, University of Stirling.

Marangos-Frost, S. & Wells, D. 2000, 'Psychiatric nurses' thoughts and feelings about restraint use; a decision dilemma', *Journal of Advanced Nursing*, 31(2): 362–9.

Molassiotis, A. 1995, 'Use of physical restraints: consequences', *British Journal of Nursing*, 4(3): 155–7.

Opie, J., Doyle, C. & O'Connor, D.W. 2002, 'Challenging behaviours in nursing home residents with dementia: a randomised controlled trial of multidisciplinary interventions,' *International Journal of Geriatric Psychiatry*, 17: 6–13.

RCN, *see* Royal College of Nursing.

Retsas, A. 1997, 'The use of physical restraint in Western Australian nursing homes', *Australian Journal of Advanced Nursing*, 14(3): 33–9.

Retsas, A. & Crabbe, H. 1997, 'Breaking loose: use of physical restraints in nursing homes in Queensland,' *Australia Collegian*, 4(4): 14–21.

Retsas, A. & Crabbe, H. 1998, 'Use of physical restraints in nursing homes in New South Wales', *Australia International Journal of Nursing Studies*, 35(3): 177–83.

Royal College of Nursing (RCN) 1999, *Restraint Revisited—Rights, Risk and Responsibility*, RCN, London.

Chapter 11 Quality Use of Medicines

APAC, *see* Australian Pharmaceutical Advisory Council.

Australian Pharmaceutical Advisory Council (APAC) 2000, *Integrated best practice model for medication management in residential aged care facilities*, 2nd edn, Commonwealth Department of Health and Aged Care, Canberra.

Beattie, J. 2003, 'Addressing inappropriate polypharmacy in residential aged care: An action research study', unpublished doctoral thesis, La Trobe University, Bundoora, Victoria, Australia.

Commonwealth Department of Health and Ageing (DH&A) 2002, *The national strategy for the quality use of medicines*, Canberra.

DH&A, *see* Commonwealth Department of Health and Ageing.

WHO, *see* World Health Organization.

World Health Organization (WHO) 2001, *National drug policies*, <www.who.int/m/topics/national_drug_policies/en/index.html>.

Chapter 12 Incontinence

Fonda, D., Knowlden, S., Kurczycki, L., Millard,R. & Tsokos, N. 1994, 'Incontinence and the older person', NHMRC, Australian Government Publishing.

Fonda, D., Benvenuti, F., Cottenden, A., Dubeau, C., Kirshner-Hermanns, R., Miller, K., Palmer, M. & Resnick, N. 2002, 'Urinary Incontinence and Bladder Dysfunction in Older Persons', in Abrams, P., Cardozo, L., Khoury, S. & Wein, A. (eds), *Incontinence*, 2nd edn, pp 625–95, Health Publications Ltd, Plymouth.

Resnick, B. & Fleishell, A. 2002, 'Developing a restorative care program: a five-step approach that involves the resident', *American Journal of Nursing*, July, vol. 102, no. 7, pp 91–5.

Chapter 13 Falls Prevention

Ackerman, R., Kemle, K., Vogel, R. & Griffin, R. 1998, 'Emergency department use by nursing home residents', *Annals of Emergency Medicine*, 31(6): 749–57.

Buchner, D. & Larson, E. 1987, 'Falls and American fractures in patients with Alzheimer-type dementia', *Journal of the Medical Association*, 257(11): 1492–5.

Campbell, A., Robertson, M., Gardner, M., Norton, R. & Buchner, D. 1999, 'Psychotropic medication withdrawal and a home-based exercise program to prevent falls: a randomized, controlled trial', *Journal of the American Geriatrics Society*, 47(7): 850–3.

Capezuti, E., Strumpf, N., Evans, L., Grisso, J. & Maislin, G. 1998, 'The relationship between physical restraint removal and falls and injuries among nursing home residents', *Journal of Gerontology*, 53A(1): M47–52.

Chapuy, M., Arlot, M., Duboeuf, D., Brun, J., Crouzet, B., Arnaud, S., Delmas, P. & Meunier, P. 1992, 'Vitamin D3 and calcium to prevent hip fractures in elderly women', *New England Journal of Medicine*, 327: 1637–42.

DoH. 2001, *National Service Framework for Older People*, Department of Health, London.

Foy, A. 1993, 'Withdrawing benzodiazepines', *Australian Practitioner*, 16: 12–14.

Friedman, S., Denman, M. & Williamson, J. 1995, 'Increased fall rates in nursing home residents following relocation to a new facility', *Journal of the American Geriatrics Society*, 43(11): SA16.

Hill, K., Smith, R., Murray, K., Sims, J., Gough, J., Darzins, P., Vrantsidis, F. & Clark, R 2000, *An analysis of research on preventing falls and falls injury in older people: community, residential and hospital settings*, Report to the Commonwealth Department of Health and Aged Care, Canberra.

Kellogg International Working Group (KIWG) on Prevention of Falls by the Elderly 1987, 'The prevention of falls in later life', *Danish Medical Bulletin*, 34(Supp 4): 1–24.

KIWG, *see* Kellogg International Working Group.

Koroknay, V., Werner, P., Cohen-Mansfield, J. & Braun, J. 1995, 'Maintaining ambulation in the frail nursing home resident: A nursing administered walking program', *Journal of Gerontological Nursing*, 21(11): 18–24.

Lauritzen, J., Petersen, M. & Lund, B. 1993, 'Effect of external hip protectors on hip fractures', *Lancet*, 341: 11–13.

Lindeman M, Smith R, Vrantsidis F and Gough J. 2002. 'Action research in aged care. A model for practice change and development.' *Geriaction* 20(1): 10–14.

Lindeman, M., Smith, R., Vrantsidis, F. & Gough, J. 2002, 'Action research in aged care. A model for practice change and development', *Geriaction*, 20(1), 10–14.

Menz, H. & Lord, S. 1999, 'Foot problems, functional impairment, and falls in older people', *Journal of the American Podiatric Medical Association*, 89(9): 458–67.

Neufeld, R., Libow, L., Foley, W., Dunbar, J., Cohen, C. & Breuer, B. 1999, 'Restraint reduction reduces serious injuries among nursing home residents', *Journal of the American Geriatrics Society*, 47: 1202–7.

Oleske, D., Wilson, R., Bernard, B., Evans, D. & Terman, E. 1995, 'Epidemiology of injury in people with Alzheimer's disease', *Journal of the American Geriatrics Society*, 43(7): 741–6.

Parker, M., Gillespie, L., Gillespie, W. 2001, 'Hip protectors for preventing hip fractures in the elderly', Cochrane review.

Peninsula Health Care Network (Falls Prevention Service) 1999, *The FRAT Pack*, Peninsula Health Care Network, Mt Eliza, Victoria, Australia..

Ray, W., Taylor, J., Meador, K., Thapa, P., Brown, A., Kalihara, H., Davis, C., Gideon, P. & Griffin, M. 1997, 'A randomised trial of a consultation service to reduce falls in nursing homes', *Journal of the American Medical Association*, 278(7): 557–62.

Rolland, Y., Rival, L., Pillard, F., Lafont, C., Rivere, D., Albarede, J. & Vellas, B. 2000, 'Feasibily of regular physical exercise for patients with moderate to severe Alzheimer disease', *Journal of Nutrition Health & Aging*, 4(2): 109–13.

Rubenstein L, Robbins A, Josephson K, Schulman B and Osterweil D (1990). "The value of assessing falls in an elderly population: A randomized clinical trial." *Annals of Internal Medicine*, 113: 308–316.

Shanley, C. 1998, *Putting your best foot forward*, Centre for Education and Research on Ageing, Concord Hospital, Concord, NSW, Report for the Commonwealth Department of Health and Aged Care.

Schnelle, J., Macrae, P., Ouslander, J., Simmons, S. & Nitta, M. 1995, 'Functional Incidental Training, mobility performance, and incontinence care with nursing home residents, *Journal of the American Geriatrics Society*, 43: 1356–62.

Stein, M., Wark, J., Scherer, S., Walton, S., Chick, P., Di Carlantonio, M., Zajac, J. & Flicker, L. 1999, 'Falls relate to vitamin D and parathyroid hormone in an Australian nursing home and hostel', *Journal of the American Geriatrics Society*, 47: 1195–201.

Tinetti, M. 1987, 'Factors associated with serious injury during falls by ambulatory nursing home residents', *Journal of the American Geriatrics Society*, 35: 644–8.

van Dijk, P., Meulenberg, O., van de Sande, H. & Habbema, J. 1993, 'Falls in dementia patients', *The Gerontologist*, 33: 200–4.

Chapter 14 Pain Management

Castonguay, D. 2000, 'Pain Management 2001', *Nursing News*, 24(4): 6–7 (based on the JCAHO Pain Standards).

Chibnall, J.T. & Tait, R.C. 2001, 'Pain assessment in cognitively impaired and unimpaired older adults: a comparison of four scales', *Pain*, vol. 92, issue 1–2, pp 173–86.

Ebersole, P. & Hess, P. (eds) 1998, *Toward healthy aging: human needs and nursing response*, 5th edn, Mosby. St Louis.

Ferrell, B.A. 1995, 'Pain evaluation and management in the nursing home', *Annals of Internal Medicine*, vol. 123, issue 9. pp 681–7.

Ferrell, B.A., Ferrell, B. & Rivera, L. 1995, 'Pain in Cognitively Impaired Nursing Home Patients, *Journal of Pain and Symptom Management*, vol. 10, no. 8, November.

Gibson, M.C. & Schroder, C. 2001, 'The many faces of pain for older, dying adults', *American Journal of Hospice & Palliative Care*, vol. 18, issue 1, pp 19–25.

Helme, R.D. 2001, 'Chronic pain management in older people', *European Journal on Pain*, vol. 5, supplement A, pp 31–6.

Herr, K.A., Mobily, P.R., Wagenaar, D. & Kohout, F.J. 1998, 'Evaluation of the Faces Scale for use with the Elderly', *The Clinical Journal of Pain*, vol. 14, number 1, March.

Hicks, C.L., von Baeyer, C.L., Spafford, P., van Korlaar, I., Goodenough, B. 2001, 'The Faces Pain Scale—Revised: Towards a common metric in pediatric pain measurement', *Pain*, 93: 173–83.

Landi, F., Onder, G., Cesari, M., Gambassi, G., Steel, K., Russo, A., Lattanzio, F. & Bernabei, R. 2001, 'Pain management in frail, community living elderly patients', *Archives of Internal Medicine*, vol. 161, issue 22, pp 2721–4.

Luggen, A.S. & Gladden, J. 2001, 'Pain management in older adults', *Pain Management Nurse*, vol 2, issue 1, pp 2–3.

Madjar, I. & Higgins, I. 1996, 'The adequacy of pain relief measures in elderly nursing home residents', proceedings of the 8th World Congress on Pain, Vancouver, Canada, Elsevier.

McCaffery, M. 1968, *Nursing Practice Theories Related to Cognition, Bodily Pain, and Man-environment Interactions*, p. 95, UCLA Student's Store, Los Angeles.

Oliver, M. 1996, *The politics of disablement*, Macmillan, London.

Scherder, E.J. & Bouma, A. 2000, 'Visual analogue scales for pain assessment in Alzheimer's Disease', *Gerontology*, vol 46, issue 1, pp 47–53.

Turk, Dennis C. 1993, 'Assess the Person, Not Just the Pain', *Pain Clinical Updates IASP*, vol 1, issue 3, September.

Victor, K. 2001, 'Properly assessing pain in the elderly', *RN Journal*, May.

Zalon, M.L. 1997, 'Pain in frail elderly women after surgery', *Image*, vol. 29, issue 1, pp 21–6.

Chapter 15 Depression

American Psychiatric Association (APA) 1994, *Diagnostic and Statistical Manual of Mental Disorders* (DSM-IV), 4th edn, Washington, D.C.

American Psychiatric Association (APA) 2000, *Diagnostic and Statistical Manual of Mental Disorders* (DSM-IV-TR), 4th edn, text revision, Washington, D.C.

APA, *see* American Psychiatric Association.

Cooper, J. 1994, 'Of dementia, depression and drugs', *Nursing Homes*, 43(2): 44–6.

Dening, T. & Bains, J. 2001, 'Antidepressant drugs for depression in people with dementia (protocol for a Cochrane Review), in *The Cochrane Library*, Issue 4. Update Software, Oxford.

Draper, B. 1999, 'The diagnosis and treatment of depression in dementia', *Psychiatric Services*, 50(9): 1151–3.

Feil, N. 1993, *The validation breakthrough: simple techniques for communicating with people with 'Alzheimer's type dementia'*, Health Promotion Press, Baltimore.

Johnson, J., Sims, R. & Gottlieb, G. 1994, 'Differential diagnosis of dementia, delirium and depression. Implications for drug therapy', *Drugs & Aging*, 5(6): 432–45.

Karel, M. & Hinrichsen, G. 2000, 'Treatment of depression in late life: psychotherapeutic interventions', *Clinical Psychology Review*, 20(6): 707–29.

Kaszniak, A. & Christensen, G. 1997, 'Differential diagnosis of dementia and depression', in Storandt, M. & Van den Bos, G. 1997, op. cit.

LaBarge, E. 1993, 'A preliminary scale to measure the degree of worry among mildly demented Alzheimer's disease patients', *Physical and Occupational Therapy in Geriatrics*, 11(3): 43–57.

Ruggles, D. 1998, 'Depression in the elderly: a review', *Journal of the American Academy of Nurse Practitioners*, 10(11): 503–7.

Scogin, F. 1997, 'Assessment of depression in older adults: a guide for practitioners'. in Storandt & Van den Bos 1997, op. cit.

Steffens, D.C, Skoog, I., Norton, M.C., Hart, A.D., Tschanz, J.T., Plassman, B.L., Wyse, B. W., Welsh-Bohmenr, K.A., & Breitiner, J.C. 2000, 'Prevalence of Depression and its treatment in an elderly population: The Cache County study', *Archives of General Psychiatry*, 57(6): 601–7.

Storandt, M. & Van den Bos, G. (eds) 1997, *Neurophysiological assessment of dementia and depression in older adults: A clinician's guide*, APA, Washington D.C.

Stuart, G. & Laraia, M. 2001, *Principles and practice of psychiatric nursing*, Mosby, St Louis.

Verhey, F., Rozendaal, N., Ponds, R. & Jolles, J. 1993, 'Dementia, awareness and depression', *International Journal of Geriatric Psychiatry*, 8: 851–6.

Chapter 16 Aggression

Ballard, G.B., O'Brien, J., James, I. & Swann, A. 2000, in *Dementia: management of behavioural and psychological symptoms*, p. 63, Oxford University Press, UK.

Burke, W.J. 1991, 'Neuroleptic drug use in the nursing home—the impact of OBRA', *American Family Physician*, 43: 6, pp 2125–30.

Patel, V. & Hope, R.A. 1992, 'A rating scale for aggressive behaviour in the elderly—the RAGE', *Psychological Medicine*, 22, 211–21.

Pocket Oxford English Dictionary (POED) 1992, Oxford University Press, UK.

POED, *see Pocket Oxford English Dictionary.*

McGrath, A. & Jackson. G.A. 1996, 'Survey of neuroleptic prescribing in residents of nursing homes in Glasgow', *British Medical Journal*, 312, 611–12.

Scottish Intercollegiate Guidelines Network (SIGN) 1999, *Interventions in the management of behavioural and psychological aspects of dementia: a national guideline for use in Scotland*, Scottish Intercollegiate Guidelines Network, Edinburgh UK.

SIGN, *see Scottish Intercollegiate Guidelines Network (SIGN).*

Chapter 17 Pressure Sores and Wounds

Allman, R.M., Goode, P.S., Patrick, M.M., Burst, N., Barlolucci, A.A, 1995, 'Pressure ulcer risk factors amongst hospitalised patients with activity limitation', *Journal of the American Medical Association*, 273(11): 865–70.

Braden, B. & Bergstrom, N. 1987, 'A conceptual scheme for the study of the etiology of pressure sores, *Rehabilitation Nursing*,12(1): 8–16.

Brandeis, G.H., Ooi, W.L,, Hossain, M., Morris, J.N, & Lipsitz, L.A. 1994, 'A longitudinal study of risk factors associated with the formation of pressure ulcers in nursing homes', *Journal of the American Geriatric Society*, 42(4): 388–92.

Dyson, R. 1978, 'Bed sores—the injuries hospital staff inflict on patients', *Nursing Mirror*, 146(24): 30–2.

Ek, A.C., Gustavsson, G. & Lewis, D.H. 1985, 'The local skin blood flow in areas at risk for pressure sore treatment with massage', *Scandinavian Journal of Rehabilitation Medicine*, 17(2): 81–6.

Holstein, J., Chatellier, G., Pette, F. & Moulias, R. 1994, 'Prevalence of associated diseases in different types of dementia among elderly institutionalised patients—analysis of 3447 records', *Journal of the American Geriatric Society*, 42(9): 972–7.

Leigh, H.L. & Bennett, G. 1994, 'Pressure ulcers: prevalence, etiology and treatment modalities', *American Journal of Surgery*, 167(1A), 25s–29s.

Lyons, D., Cohen, M., Henderson, T. & Walker, N. 1995, 'Partnership nursing home care for dementia: The Glasgow experience', *International Journal of Geriatric Psychiatry*, 10(7): 5, pp 557–60.

McGowan, S., Hensley, L. & Maddocks, J. 1996, 'Monitoring the occurrence of pressure ulcers in a teaching hospital', *Primary Intention*, 4(1): 9–16.

National Pressure Ulcer Advisory Panel (NPUAP) 1989, 'Pressure ulcers, incidence, economics, risk assessment', Consensus Development Conference Statement, *Decubitus*, 2(2): 24–8.

Norton, D. 1989, 'Calculation the risk: reflections on the Norton Scale', *Decubitus*, 2(3): 24–31.

NPUAP, *see* National Pressure Ulcer Advisory Panel.

Phillips, T., Stanton, B., Provan, A. & Lew, R. 1994, 'A study of the impact of leg ulcers on quality of life: financial, social and psychological implications', *Journal of American Academy of Dermatology*, 31(1): 49–53.

Rudman, D., Mattson, D.E., Alverno, L. & Richarson, I.W. 1993, 'Comparison of clinical indicators in two nursing homes', *Journal of American.Geriatrics Society*, 41(12): 1317–25.

Waterlow, J, 1985, 'A risk assessment card', *Nursing Times*, 81(48): 24–7.

Wright, R. & Tiziani, A. 1996, 'Pressure ulcer prevalence study', *Primary* Intention, 4(1): 18–23.

Young, C. 1997, 'What cost a pressure ulcer', *Primary Intention*, 5(4): 24–31.

Young, J.B. & Dobrzanski, S. 1992, 'Pressure sores. Epidemiology and current management concepts', *Drugs and Ageing*, 2(1): 42–57.

Chapter 18 Palliative Care

Cornelius, P. 2001, 'Sweet parting', in Craven, P. (ed.), *The best Australian stories 2001*, pp 110–14, Black Inc., Melbourne.

Hudson, R. 1997, 'Documented life and death in a nursing home', in Richmond, J, (ed.), *Nursing documentation: writing what we do*, pp 29–38, Ausmed Publications, Melbourne.

Killick, J. & Allan, K. 2001, *Communication and the care of people with dementia*, Open University Press, Buckingham.

Kitwood, T. 1997, *Dementia reconsidered: the person comes first*, Open University Press, Buckingham Philadelphia.

Nay, R. 2002, 'The dignity of risk'. *Australian Nursing Journal*, 9(9), 33.

Nightingale, F. 1969, *Notes on nursing: what it is, and what it is not*, Dover Publications, Inc., New York.

Palliative Care Australia (PCA) 1999, *Standards for palliative care provision*, 3rd edn, Palliative Care Australia.

PCA, *see* Palliative Care Australia.

Post, S.G. 1995, *The moral challenge of Alzheimer disease*, The Johns Hopkins University Press, Baltimore.

Rumbold, B. 1986, *Helplessness and hope: pastoral care in terminal illness*, SCM Press Ltd, London.

Saunders, Cicely & Baines, M 1989, *Living with dying: the management of terminal disease*, 2nd edn. OUP, Oxford.

Taylor, B.J. 1994, *Being human: ordinariness in nursing*, Churchill Livingstone, Melbourne.

Travis, S., Bernard, M., Dixon, S., McAuley, W., Loving, G. & McClanahan, L. 2002, 'Obstacles to palliation and end-of-life care in a long-term care facility', *The Gerontologist*, 42(3), 343–9.

Chapter 19 Intimacy

Bayley, J.1999, *Iris and the Friends*, Abacus London.

Buber, Martin 1958, *I and Thou*, translated by Ronald Gregor Smith, Charles Scribner's Sons, New York.

Clare, J. 1997, *John Clare*, Everyman's Poetry, R.K.R. Thornton (ed.), J.M. Dent, London.

de Luca C. 1996, in *Hearing the Voice of People with Dementia*, Goldsmith, M., Jessica Kingsley, London.

Derouesne, C., Guigot, J., Chermat V., Winchester, N. & Lacomblez, L. 1996, 'Sexual behavioural changes in Alzheimer's disease', *Alzheimer Disease & Associated Disorders*, 10(2).

Friedman, M.S. 1960, *Martin Buber: The Life of Dialogue*, Harper & Row, New York.

Gibran, K. 1926, *The Prophet*, Heinemann Ltd, London.

'Helen' 1994, published in the July issue of *Magazine of the Alzheimer's Association* (USA), Cleveland Area Chapter.

Ignatieff, M. 1993, *Scar Tissue*, Vintage, London.

Kitwood, T. 1997, *Dementia Reconsidered*, Open University Press, Buckingham.

Rogers, C.R. 1961, *On Becoming a Person*, Houghton Mifflin, Boston.

Rogers, C.R. & Stevens, B. 1968, *Person to Person: The problem of being human*, Real People Press, Lafayette (USA).

Sherman, B. 1998, *Sex, Intimacy and Aged Care*, Jessica Kingsley, London.

Snowdon, D. 2001, *Aging with Grace*, Fourth Estate, London.

Waller, S. 2002, 'Dementia as Culture', unpublished paper, quoted with permission.

Chapter 20 Listening to the Person with Dementia

Crisp, Jane 1992, 'Empty Ramblings or Empowering Narratives? The Discourse of the Alzheimer's Sufferer', *Meridian*, 2.2.

Crisp, Jane 1995, 'Making Sense of the Stories that People with Alzheimer's Tell: A Journey with my Mother'. *Nursing Inquiry*, 2.3.

Feil, Naomi 1993, *The Validation Breakthrough*, MacLennan & Petty, Sydney.

Goyder, Julie 2001, *We'll Be Married in Fremantle*, Fremantle Arts Centre Press, Fremantle.

Jolley, Elizabeth 1983, *Mr Scobie's Riddle*, Penguin, Ringwood, Victoria.
Steedman, Carolyn 1992, *Past Tenses*, Rivers Oram Press, London.

Chapter 21 Leisure

Clark, M., Bond, M.J. & Sanchez, L. 1999, 'The effect of sensory impairment on the lifestyle activities of older people', *Australasian Journal on Ageing*, 18(3): 124–9.
Dresser, R. & Whitehouse, P. 1994, 'The Incompetent Patient on the Slippery Slope', *Hastings Centre Report*, July–August: 6–12.
Killick, J., & Allan, K. 2001, *Communication and the care of people with dementia*. Open University Press, Buckingham.
Kitwood, T. 1997, *Dementia Reconsidered*, Open University Press, Buckingham.
Patterson. I. 1998, 'Leisure programs and older people in care', *Geriaction*, 16(3): 24–7.
Wilcox, A.A. 1999, 'Creating self and shaping the world', *Australian Occupational Therapy Journal*, 46: 77–88.

Chapter 22 Creative Care

Aldridge, D. & Brandt, G. 1991, 'Music Therapy and Alzheimer's Disease', *Journal of British Music Therapy*, 5(2): 28–36.
Alzheimer's Australia 2003, *Quality Demntia care: Position Paper 2*, Alzheimer's Australia, Canberra.
Baker, R., Dowling, Z., Wareing, L.A., Dawson, J. & Assey, J. 1997, 'Snoezelen: Its Long-term and Short-term Effects on Older People with Dementia', *British Journal of Occupational Therapy*, 60(5): 213–18.
Beck, A. & Katcher, A. 1996, *Between Pets and People—the importance of animal companionship* (revised edn), Purdue University Press, Indiana.
Bowlby, C. 1993, *Therapeutic Activities with Persons Disabled by Alzheimer's Disease and Related Disorders*, Aspen Publications, Maryland.
Bright, R. 1991, *Music in Geriatric Care: A Second Look*, Music Therapy Enterprises, Australia.
Brotons, M., Koger, S. & Pickett-Cooper, P. 1997, 'Music and dementias: A review of literature', *Journal of Music Therapy*, 34(4): 204–45.
Burke, M.A. 1995, 'Music Therapy Programme Development: Highlights of a Music Therapy Programme for Older Adults', in '1995 Conference Collection of 21st AMTA Inc. National Conference: 28–9.
Clair, A. 1991, 'Music Therapy for a Severely Regressed Person with a Probable Diagnosis of Alzheimer's Disease', in K. Bruscia (ed.), *Case Studies in Music Therapy*, pp 571–80, Barcelona Publishers, USA.
Clair, A. 1996, 'The effect of singing on alert responses in persons with late-stage dementia', *Journal of Music Therapy*, 33(4): 234–47.
Clair, A. 2000, 'The importance of singing with elderly patients', in D. Aldridge (ed.), *Music therapy in dementia care*, pp 91–101, Jessica Kingsley Publishers, London.
Damasio, A.R. 1996, *Descartes' Error: Emotion, reason and the human brain*, Papermac, London.
Delta Society 1999, 'About Animal-Assisted Activities and Animal-Assisted Therapy', <info@deltasociety.org>.
Forster, S. 1998, 'Kingston Centre Reminiscence Programme for Older People', in Schweitzer, P. (ed.), *Reminiscence in Dementia Care*, pp 63–72, Age Exchange, London.
Franchomme, P. & Penoel, D. 1990, *L'aromatherapie exactement*, Jallois, Limoges.
Hanson, N., Gfeller, K., Woodworth, G., Swanson, E, & Garand, L. 1996, 'A comparison of the effectiveness of differing types and difficulty of music activities in programming for older adults with Alzheimer's disease and related disorders', *Journal of Music Therapy*, 33(2): 93–123.
Hope, K. 1997, 'Using multi-sensory environments with older people with dementia', *Journal of Advanced Nursing*, 25: 780–5.
James, K. 1998, in Snyder, M. & Lindquist, R., *Complementary/Alternative Therapies in Nursing*, 3rd edn, Springer Publishing Co., New York.
James, K. 2001, in McCabe, P. (ed.), *Complementary Therapies in Nursing and Midwifery*, pp 215–17, Ausmed Publications, Melbourne.
Kewin, J. 1994, 'Snoezelen—the reasons and the method' in R. Hutchinson & J. Kewin (eds), *Sensations and Disability: Sensory Environmemts for Leisure—Snoezelen, Education & Therapy*, Rompa, Chesterfield.
Killick, J. 1994, 'There's so much to hear when you stop and listen to individual voices', *Journal of Dementia Care*, 2(5): 16–17.
Killick, J. 1998, 'It isn't fair when your heart wants to remember', in Schweitzer, P (ed.), *Reminiscence in Dementia Care*, pp 91–102, Age Exchange, London.
Killick, J. & Allan, K. 2001, *Communication and the Care of People with Dementia*, Open University Press, Buckingham.
Kitwood, T. 1997, *Dementia reconsidered*, Open University Press, Buckingham.

Meyer, M. 2001, 'Aromatherapy', in McCabe, P. (ed.) *Complementary Therapies in Nursing and Midwifery*, Ausmed Publications, Melbourne.

Moffat, N., Baker, P. & Pinkney, L. 1993, *Snoezelen, an experience for people with dementia*, Rompa, Chesterfield.

Moody, W. 1998, 'Animal-assisted Therapy within Hospitals. Suggested Infection Control—a Summary', Therapeutic Solutions Pty Ltd, <redsoil@one.net.au>.

Millar, K. & Smith, J. 1989, 'The Influence of Group Singing Therapy on the Behaviour of Alzheimer's Disease Patients', *Journal of Music Therapy*, 26(2): 58–70.

Neumann, T. 1994, 'Keynote speaker's address at the Inaugural Complementary Therapies in Nursing Conference, Royal College of Nursing, Australia, Canberra.

O'Callaghan, C. 1999, 'Recent Findings about Neural Correlates of Music Pertinent to Music Therapy Across the Lifespan', *Music Therapy Perspectives*, 17(1): 32–6.

Pinkney, L. 1997, 'A comparison of the Snoezelen Environment and a Music Relaxation Group on the Mood and Behaviour of Patients with Senile Dementia', *British Journal of Occupational Therapy*, 60(5): 209–12.

Pinkney, L. 1998, 'Exploring the myths of multi-sensory environments', *British Journal of Occupational Therapy*, 61(80): 365–7.

Pinkney, L. & Barker, P. 1994, 'Snoezelen—an evaluation of an environment used by people who are elderly and confused', in R. Hutchinson & J. Kewin, *Sensations and Disability: Sensory Environmemts for Leisure   Snoezelen, Education & Therapy*, Rompa, Chesterfield.

Pollack, N. & Namazi, K. 1992, 'The Effect of Music Participation on the Social Behaviour of Alzheimer's Disease Patients', *Journal of Music Therapy*, 24(1): 54–67.

Prickett, C.A. & Moore, R.A. 1991, 'The use of music to aid memory of Alzheimer's patients', *Journal of Music Therapy*, 28(2): 101–10.

Riegler, J. 1980, 'Comparison of a Reality Orientation Program for Geriatric Patients with or without Music'. *Journal of Music Therapy*, 17(1): 26–33.

Stevensen, C. 1995, 'Aromatherapy', in Rankin-Box, D. (ed.), *The Nurses' Handbook of Complementary Therapies*, Churchill Livingstone, Edinburgh.

Taylor, B. 2001, 'Research issues in complementary therapies and holistic care', in McCabe, P. (ed.), *Complementary Therapies in Nursing and Midwifery: from Vision to Practice*, pp 81–93, Ausmed Publications, Melbourne.

Tisserand, R. 1994, *The Art of Aromatherapy*, C.J. Daniel Company Ltd, Great Britain.

Van Toller, S. 1996, 'Introduction to the sense of smell', in Vickers 1996, op. cit.

Vickers, A. 1996, *Massage and Aromatherapy, A guide for health professionals*, Chapman & Hall, London.

Chapter 23 The Eden Alternative

Ransom, Sandy 2000, 'Eden Alternative; The Texas Project', Southwest Texas State University, May.

Norton, Lavren 2003, <www.culturechangenow.com>.

Chapter 24 Dementia Care Mapping

Adams T. 1996, 'Kitwood's approach to dementia and dementia care: a critical but appreciative review', *Journal of Advanced Nursing*, 23(5): 948–53.

Barnett, E. 1995, 'A window of insight into quality care', *Journal of Dementia Care*, 3(4): 23–6.

Bradford Dementia Group, University of Bradford 1997, *Evaluating Dementia Care: The DCM Method*, 7th edn, University of Bradford.

Calkins, M. 1988, *Design for Dementia: Planning Environments for the Elderly and Confused*, National Health Publishing, Maryland.

Kitwood, T. 1993, 'Discover the Person not the Disease', *Journal of Dementia Care*, 1(1), pp 16–17.

Kitwood, T. 1997a, 'Cultures of Care: Tradition and Change', in Kitwood, T. & Benson, S. (eds), *The New Culture of Dementia Care*, pp 7–11, Hawker Publications Ltd, London.

Kitwood, T. 1997b, *Dementia Reconsidered*, Open University Press, Buckingham.

Loveday, B. & Kitwood, T. 1998, *Improving Dementia Care*, Hawker Publications, London.

Morton, I. 1999, *Person Centred Approaches to Dementia Care*, Winslow Press Ltd, Bicester.

Perrin, T. 1997, 'The positive response schedule for severe dementia', *Aging and Mental Health*, 1(2): 184–91.

Perrin, T. & May, H. 2000, *Wellbeing in Dementia*, Churchill Livingstone, London.

Rogers, C. 1961, *On Becoming a Person*, Houghton Mifflin, Boston.

Wylie, K. 2000, 'Valuing sensation and sentience in dementia care', unpublished PhD thesis, University of Newcastle.

Index